# MEDICAL RADIOLOGY
## Diagnostic Imaging

Editors:
A. L. Baert, Leuven
M. Knauth, Göttingen
K. Sartor, Heidelberg

G. Maconi · G. Bianchi Porro (Eds.)

# Ultrasound of the Gastrointestinal Tract

With Contributions by

G. Bianchi Porro · E. Danse · S. Daum · C. Del Vecchio Blanco · I. de Sio · M. Fraquelli
D. Geukens · O. H. Gilja · S. Greco · N. Gritzmann · K. Haruma · J. Hata · T. Hausken
J. Hoffmann · T. Kamada · H. Kusunoki · D. H. Lee · J. H. Lim · G. Maconi · N. Manabe
E. Radice · M. Sato · D. Schacherer · J. Schölmerich · T. Tanaka · L. Tarantino · L. Tibullo
S. B. Vijayaraghavan · M. Zeitz

Foreword by

A. L. Baert

With 179 Figures in 347 Separate Illustrations, 57 in Color and 24 Tables

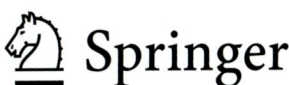

Giovanni Maconi, MD
Gabriele Bianchi Porro, MD, PhD
Chair of Gastroenterology
Department of Clinical Sciences
'L. Sacco' University Hospital
Via G. B. Grassi 74
20157 Milano
Italy

---

Medical Radiology · Diagnostic Imaging and Radiation Oncology
Series Editors: A. L. Baert · L. W. Brady · H.-P. Heilmann · M. Molls · K. Sartor

Continuation of Handbuch der medizinischen Radiologie
Encyclopedia of Medical Radiology

---

Library of Congress Control Number: 2006924827

ISBN 3-540-25826-4  Springer Berlin Heidelberg New York
ISBN 978-3-540-25826-1  Springer Berlin Heidelberg New York

This work is subject to copyright. All rights are reserved, whether the whole or part of the material is concerned, specifically the rights of translation, reprinting, reuse of illustrations, recitations, broadcasting, reproduction on microfilm or in any other way, and storage in data banks. Duplication of this publication or parts thereof is permitted only under the provisions of the German Copyright Law of September 9, 1965, in its current version, and permission for use must always be obtained from Springer-Verlag. Violations are liable for prosecution under the German Copyright Law.

Springer is part of Springer Science+Business Media

http//www.springer.com
© Springer-Verlag Berlin Heidelberg 2007
Printed in Germany

The use of general descriptive names, trademarks, etc. in this publication does not imply, even in the absence of a specific statement, that such names are exempt from the relevant protective laws and regulations and therefore free for general use.

Product liability: The publishers cannot guarantee the accuracy of any information about dosage and application contained in this book. In every case the user must check such information by consulting the relevant literature.

Medical Editor: Dr. Ute Heilmann, Heidelberg
Desk Editor: Ursula N. Davis, Heidelberg
Production Editor: Kurt Teichmann, Mauer
Cover-Design and Typesetting: Verlagsservice Teichmann, Mauer

Printed on acid-free paper – 21/3151xq – 5 4 3 2 1 0

# Foreword

Two to three decades ago only very few radiologists, such as F. Weill and other pioneers in the field, believed in the diagnostic potential of ultrasound for the study of the gastrointestinal tract. The main applications of ultrasound were confined to the study of solid visceral organs, the female pelvis and obstetrics. Rapid progress in computer technology and in transducer design has opened totally new horizons for ultrasound, for instance in musculoskeletal pathology, as well as in the gastrointestinal tract in children and adults.

Today ultrasound plays a major role as the primary imaging procedure in acute abdominal conditions involving the gastrointestinal tract. The indications for surgery in patients suspected of acute appendicitis have dramatically improved due to the widespread application of ultrasound.

I am very much indebted to the editors of this book, Prof. G. Maconi and Prof. G. Bianchi Porro, both internationally recognized experts in abdominal ultrasound. They developed the concept of this volume and have been very successful in involving several other distinguished ultrasound experts from both Europe and the Far East.

I would like to congratulate the editors and the authors most sincerely on this outstanding volume which provides a comprehensive overview of the use of ultrasound in acute and chronic diseases of the gastrointestinal tract.

This book will be of great value, not only for radiologists, but also for gastroenterologists, abdominal surgeons, pediatricians and oncologists. They will find it a very helpful guide in their daily clinical practice.

I am confident that it will meet with the same success among readers as previous volumes published in this series.

Leuven                                                                                    ALBERT L. BAERT

# Preface

In recent decades technological advances, scientific innovations and improved skills of operators have made sonography of the gastrointestinal tract increasingly important in diagnostic work-up and medical decision-making for gastrointestinal disorders, both in acute and non-acute conditions. Thanks to its non-invasiveness, ready availability, repeatability and accuracy, ultrasonographic examination of the gastrointestinal tract is currently employed in many suspected acute and chronic inflammatory conditions, not only for purely diagnostic purposes, but also for management of well-known gastrointestinal diseases. Furthermore, given that ultrasound is usually performed as the first diagnostic imaging procedure for abdominal complaints, its role in detecting or suspecting neoplastic, infectious and inflammatory diseases of the gastrointestinal tract may become even more important in the future as an aid to selecting and driving more expensive and invasive examinations.

Despite the vast mass of scientific literature showing the importance and accuracy of ultrasound in assessing various pathologic conditions of the gastrointestinal tract, it has not yet entered into routine use in clinical practice, and indeed seems to be considered (incorrectly) as a highly specialised application of ultrasound for super-specialist sonographers. The belief that more widespread knowledge of the various applications and usefulness of ultrasound in the assessment of gastrointestinal disorders would be of value in our clinical practice prompted us in to propose this topic for Medical Radiology, Springer-Verlag's prestigious radiological series.

In this context, this book is intended as a high-level volume prepared by authors who are specialist intestinal sonographers, regarded as authorities in their specific fields, with the intention of spreading their experience on the gastrointestinal tract to a much wider audience of sonologists. To this end, a comprehensive overview of ultrasonographic imaging of acute and chronic inflammatory gastrointestinal tract disorders, as well as specific neoplastic and infectious diseases, is provided, and the potential, usefulness and limits of gastrointestinal tract sonography are elucidated.

The topics of the volume cover not only the major gastrointestinal diseases, but also rare conditions, the aim being to help the abdominal sonographer to also interpret incidental findings related to the gastrointestinal tract and to deal with the more common problems encountered during routine abdominal investigations in patients with abdominal complaints and well-known chronic disorders. Specific technical developments and applications of ultrasound devoted to studies of the gastrointestinal tract which promise to be of increasing importance in the future, such as functional and 3D ultrasound, contrast agents and operative US, are also discussed.

The editors of this issue would like to thank the Editor-in-Chief, Prof. Albert Baert, for his valuable suggestions and assistance. A most sincere word of gratitude goes to Ursula N. Davis and Kurt Teichmann of Springer-Verlag and to Marian Shields for their constant, patient and untiring efforts in helping us to collect, edit and revise the manuscripts; their devotion deserves special recognition. We are also extremely grateful to all the authors who have contributed so remarkably in preparing their contributions. Last, but not least, special thanks go to our families for all their encouragement and support.

We hope that readers will share our enthusiasm for this interesting and rapidly developing area of ultrasound.

Milan                                                    GIOVANNI MACONI
                                                         GABRIELE BIANCHI PORRO

# Contents

## Acute Abdomen .................... 1

1 Acute Appendicitis and Appendiceal Mucocele
　NORBERT GRITZMANN .................... 3

2 Mesenteric Lymphadenopathy
　GIOVANNI MACONI, ELISA RADICE, and GABRIELE BIANCHI PORRO .......... 11

3 Acute Colonic Diverticulitis and Diverticulosis
　NORBERT GRITZMANN .................... 19

4 Intestinal Obstruction
　JAE HOON LIM .................... 27

5 Abdominal Hernias, Volvulus and Intussusception
　S. BOOPATHY VIJAYARAGHAVAN .................... 35

6 Ischemic Colitis
　ETIENNE DANSE .................... 55

## Chronic Inflammatory Bowel Diseases .................... 59

7 Crohn's Disease
　GIOVANNI MACONI, ELISA RADICE, and GABRIELE BIANCHI PORRO .......... 61

8 Ulcerative Colitis
　GIOVANNI MACONI, SALVATORE GRECO, and GABRIELE BIANCHI PORRO ....... 73

## Malabsorption .................... 83

9 Coeliac Disease
　MIRELLA FRAQUELLI .................... 85

10 Lymphangiectasia, Whipple's Disease and Eosinophilic Enteritis
　MIRELLA FRAQUELLI .................... 93

## Infections .................... 99

11 Infectious Enteritis
　GIOVANNI MACONI, LUCIANO TARANTINO, and GABRIELE BIANCHI PORRO ...... 101

12 Intestinal Tuberculosis
   Dong Ho Lee and Jae Hoon Lim . . . . . . . . . . . . . . . . . . . . . . . . . . 109

13 Pseudomembranous Colitis
   Etienne Danse and Daphne Geukens . . . . . . . . . . . . . . . . . . . . . . 115

14 Amoebic, Ascariasis and Other Parasitic and Infectious Enteritis
   S. Boopathy Vijayaraghavan . . . . . . . . . . . . . . . . . . . . . . . . . . . 121

**Neoplasm** . . . . . . . . . . . . . . . . . . . . . . . . . . . . . . . . . . . . . . . . . . 127

15 Colorectal Cancer
   Jae Hoon Lim . . . . . . . . . . . . . . . . . . . . . . . . . . . . . . . . . . . 129

16 Gastric Cancer
   Jiro Hata, Ken Haruma, Noriaki Manabe, Tomoari Kamada,
   Hiroaki Kusunoki, Toshiaki Tanaka, and Motonori Sato . . . . . . . . . . . 135

17 Gastrointestinal Lymphomas
   Severin Daum, Jörg G. Hoffmann, and Martin Zeitz . . . . . . . . . . . . . 143

18 Peritoneal Metastasis
   Ilario de Sio, Loredana Tibullo and Camillo Del Vecchio Blanco . . . . . . 151

19 Carcinoid and Submucosal Tumors
   Jiro Hata, Ken Haruma, Noriaki Manabe, Tomoari Kamada,
   Hiroaki Kusunoki, Toshiaki Tanaka, and Motonori Sato . . . . . . . . . . . 159

**Procedures and Technical Developments** . . . . . . . . . . . . . . . . . . . . 167

20 Intravenous Contrast-Enhanced Bowel Ultrasound
   Doris Schacherer and Jourgen Schölmerich . . . . . . . . . . . . . . . . . . 169

21 Oral Contrast-Enhanced Bowel Ultrasound
   Giovanni Maconi, Salvatore Greco, and Gabriele Bianchi Porro . . . . . . . 181

22 Functional Ultrasound of the Gastrointestinal Tract
   Trygve Hausken and Odd Helge Gilja . . . . . . . . . . . . . . . . . . . . . 189

23 Three-Dimensional Ultrasound of the Gastrointestinal Tract
   Odd Helge Gilja . . . . . . . . . . . . . . . . . . . . . . . . . . . . . . . . . 199

24 Percutaneous Gastrointestinal Biopsy
   I. de Sio, Loredana Tibullo, and Camillo Del Vecchio-Blanco . . . . . . . . 213

Subject Index . . . . . . . . . . . . . . . . . . . . . . . . . . . . . . . . . . . . . . 221

List of Contributors . . . . . . . . . . . . . . . . . . . . . . . . . . . . . . . . . . 225

# Acute Abdomen

# Acute Appendicitis and Appendiceal Mucocele

Norbert Gritzmann

CONTENTS

1.1 Introduction 3
1.2 Clinical Evaluation of Acute Appendicitis 3
1.3 Diagnostic Methods 3
1.3.1 Sonography 3
1.3.2 Computed Tomography 6
1.3.3 Magnetic Resonance 7
1.4 Differential Diagnosis 7
1.4.1 Intestinal Differential Diagnosis 7
1.4.2 Gynaecological Differential Diagnosis 8
1.4.3 Urological Differential Diagnosis 8
1.4.4 Diseases of Other Compartments 8
1.5 Mucocele of the Appendix 9
1.6 Conclusions 9
References 9

## 1.1 Introduction

Appendicitis is a common disease in each period of life. Most frequently, appendicitis occurs in children and adolescents. Histologically serous, phlegmoneous, ulcerous and perforated forms are differentiated. These forms usually reveal thickening and enlargement of the tubular organ, whereas chronic or neurogenic forms do not alter the size of the appendix; therefore, neither can usually be diagnosed by imaging.

## 1.2 Clinical Evaluation of Acute Appendicitis

The clinical assessment of the painful right lower quadrant is still the cornerstone in the diagnosis of acute appendicitis. Important signs for acute appendicitis are pain at the Mc Burney's point, axillary–rectal difference of the temperature. In laboratory testing, signs of acute inflammation are present. The C-reactive protein (CRP) is usually elevated, and leucocytosis is often present. Clinical evaluation usually gives significant hints for pathology in the right lower quadrant; however, specificity in diagnosing acute appendicitis is limited. Of all surgically treated appendices, 30–50% do not reveal acute appendicitis at histology. The accuracy in clinical evaluation of acute appendicitis is especially low in young women and older patients (Ueberrueck et al. 2004).

## 1.3 Diagnostic Methods

The main goal of imaging methods is to diagnose appendicitis quickly with high accuracy, non-invasive, cost-effective methods and to provide differential diagnosis without laparotomy (Puylaert 1986a).

### 1.3.1 Sonography

In 1986, Puylaert published a groundbreaking study on the diagnosis of acute appendicitis using sonography with the graded compression technique.

Sonography is used mainly on account of widespread availability and the fact that no radiation is used. First of all, diagnosing appendicitis needs sufficient skill and expertise in the performance of gastrointestinal ultrasound. Various compression techniques are used to visualize the appendix (Lee et al. 2005).

Usually, the abdomen and the retroperitoneum are examined with the 3.5-MHz transducer. Then the caecum, which usually contains gas, is localised. Most

---

N. Gritzmann, MD
Dept. of Radiology and Nuclear Medicine, KH Barmherzige Brüder Salzburg, Kajetanerplatz 1, 5020 Salzburg, Austria

often the appendix originates caudal to Bauhin's valve. The position of the appendix is highly variable. Artrocaecal position or a position within the small pelvis may be found.

The appendix is a blind-ending tubular structure (Fig. 1.1). Normally the appendix is compressible with an ovoid configuration in the transverse section. The antero-posterior diameter is normally <6 mm. Compared with the terminal ileum, no peristalsis is visualised in the normal appendix. In a study by RETTENBACHER et al. (1997), it was shown that the normal appendix is localised sonographically in 50–70% of cases.

Frequently, a high-resolution transducer is used to visualize the appendix during graded compression. In many cases, the appendiceal region can be seen with transabdominal 7.5-MHz transducers. The use of colour- or power Doppler may be useful; however, use of the Doppler methods is not mandatory.

Ultrasound contrast media have been used for the detection of hypervascularisation (INCESU et al. 2004). Harmonic imaging is presently the standard technique in the abdomen. The main advantage is the higher signal-to-noise ratio, but the depth of penetration is lower with this technique (Table 1.1).

Table 1.1. Sonographic signs of acute appendicitis

| |
|---|
| Antero-posterior (a.p.) diameter of 6 mm or more (see Fig. 1.2). In some cases with lymphatic hyperplasia the a.p. diameter is >6 mm (RETTENBACHER et al. 2001) |
| Round configuration in the transverse section (see Fig. 1.2; RETTENBACHER et al. 2003) |
| Missing compressibility (PUYLEART et al. 1986a) |
| Alteration of the periappendiceal fat (Fig. 1.3; NOGUCHI et al. 2005) |
| Missing gas in the appendix (RETTENBACHER et al. 2000) |
| Hypervascularisation of the appendix in colour Doppler (see Fig. 1.4) |
| Moderately enlarged lymph nodes |
| Pain directly above the appendix (PUYLEART et al. 1986a) |
| Faecolith in the appendix, with obstruction (see Fig. 1.5) |
| Localised effusion |

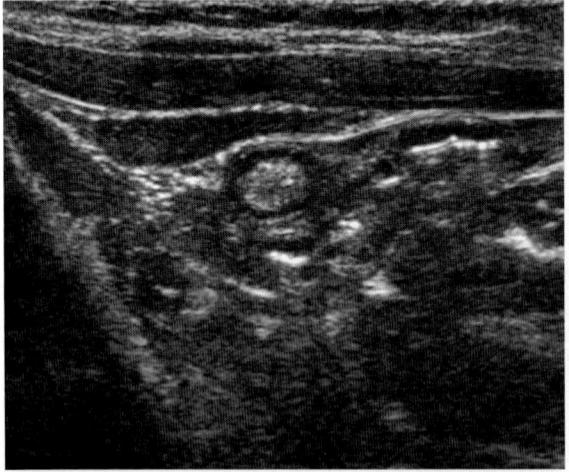
a

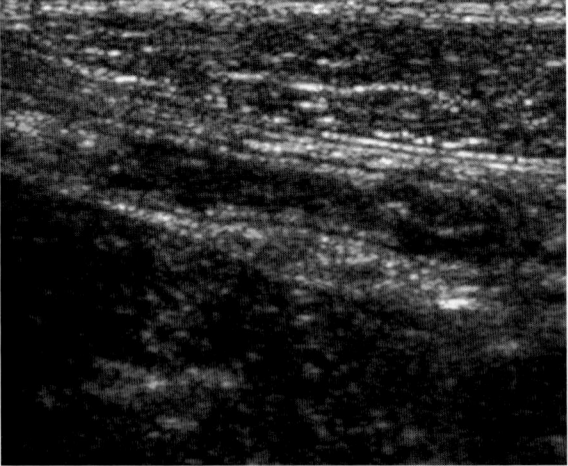
b

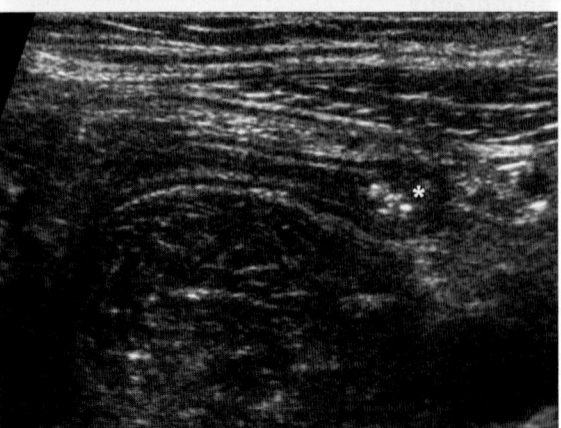
c

Fig. 1.1a–c. Normal appendix. a Transverse section. b Longitudinal section. c Longitudinal section with a variable amount of air within the tip (*asterisk*)

In difficult patients and in women, also a transrectal or transvaginal approach may visualise appendiceal region and appendicitis (Figs. 1.2–1.6).

If severe complications, such as significant perforation (Fig. 1.7) or abscess formation (Fig. 1.8), are present, the appendix often cannot be visualized as the origin of the inflammation. In these cases, computed tomogrphy (CT) should be performed in order to completely delineate the inflammation and to visualise a safe path for a transabdominal drainage; however, the drainage can be performed under US guidance.

The accuracy of sonography in diagnosing appendicitis varies between 70 and 95% depending on the study (CHAN et al. 2005; KESSLER et al. 2004; LEE et al. 2005; PUYLAERT et al. 1986a; RETTENBACHER et al. 2002; VAN BREDA VRIESMAN et al. 2003). In the present author's opinion, accuracies over 90% can be achieved if sonography is performed by an experienced team (GRITZMANN et al. 2002).

It is generally accepted that sonography should be performed in clinically, questionable cases, in order to reduce the high rate of false-negative appendectomies; however, in clinically, highly suspicious cases the incidence of acute appendicitis was only about

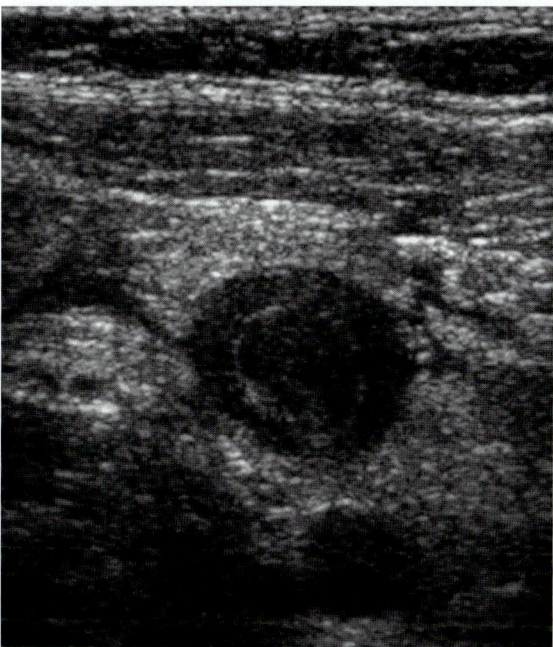

Fig. 1.3. Transverse section in appendicitis. The appendix is enlarged and reveals echogenic alteration of the surrounding fat

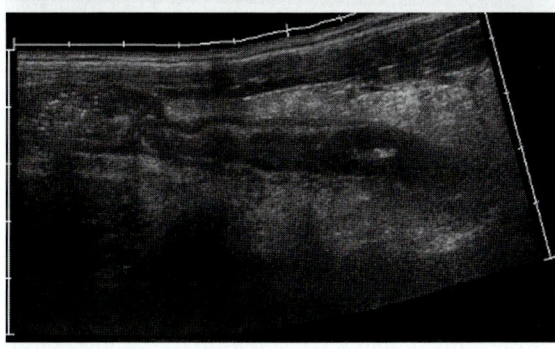

Fig. 1.2a,b. Acute appendicitis. a In transverse section, the appendix is round and measures 12 mm in diameter. b Longitudinal panoramic section

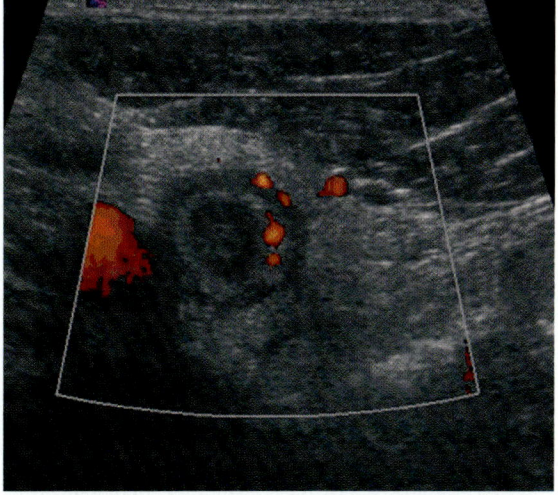

Fig. 1.4. Transverse section in appendicitis with hyperaemia and thickened wall surrounded by echogenic, hyperaemic fat

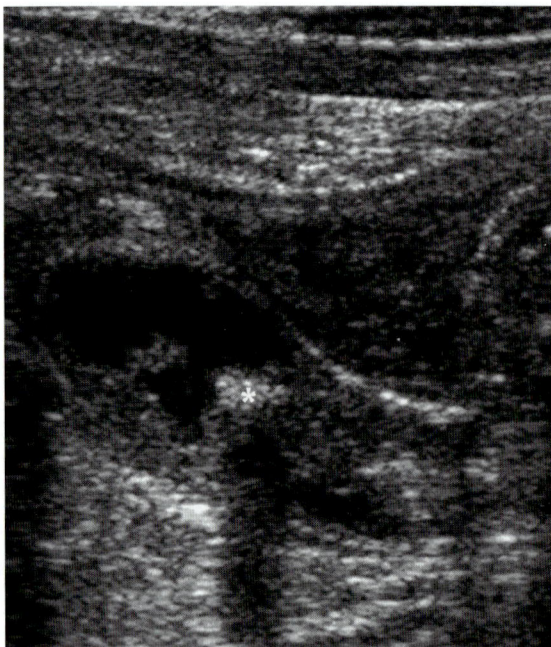

**Fig. 1.5.** Obstructed appendix with faecoliths (*asterisk*) and inflammatory content

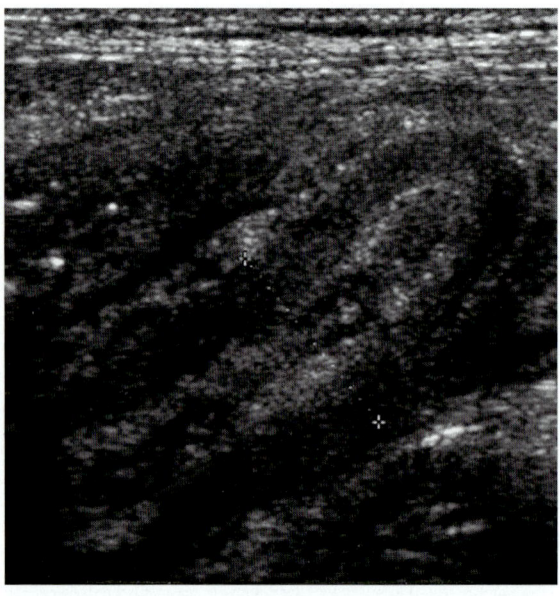

**Fig. 1.7.** Longitudinal section of an acute perforated appendicitis

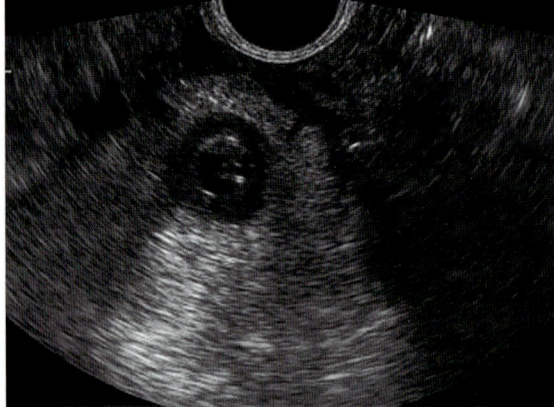

**Fig. 1.6.** Transrectal sonography displays acute appendicitis with echogenic fat reaction

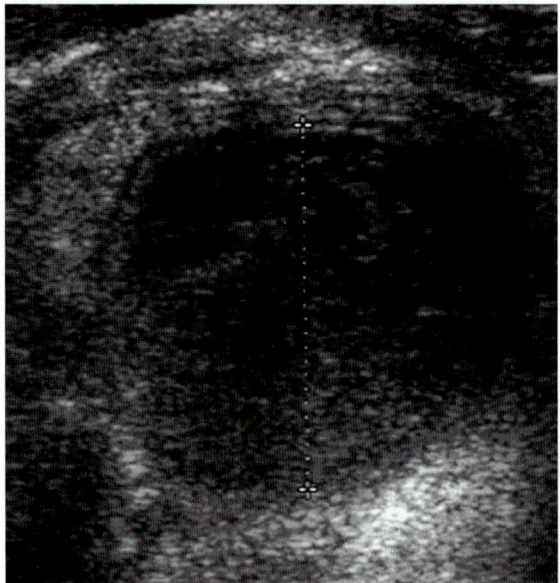

**Fig. 1.8.** Perithyplitic abscess. The appendix can no longer be displayed

70%; therefore, it was advocated that sonography be performed in all cases with pain in the right lower quadrant (RETTENBACHER et al. 2002).

An acute appendicitis can be excluded if the normal appendix can be completely displayed and/or a differential diagnosis that explains the clinical findings can be found.

## 1.3.2
## Computed Tomography

In the United States, CT is the preferred method in the evaluation of acute appendicitis (RAO et al. 1997); however, CT involves significant radiation doses to the patients.

Computed tomography can be performed only in the region of the painful right lower quadrant if it is preceded by sonography. This is a way to reduce radiation, particularly in young patients. Modern multidetector scanners can visualise the abdomen at low doses using modes with a high spatial resolution. The main advantage of CT is that operator dependency is lower than with sonography. Furthermore, the normal appendix can be seen in a higher percentage than with sonography. In European institutions, CT is often used as a problem-solving investigation if sonography fails to give a clear diagnosis (van Breda Vriesman et al. 2003). After oral application of water-soluble contrast media, perityphlitic abscesses or bowel loop abscesses are usually better revealed by CT (see Fig. 1.6).

Table 1.2. Intestinal differential diagnoses of appendicitis

| |
|---|
| Infectious ileocolitis |
| Lymphadenitis mesenterica |
| Invagination |
| Volvulus |
| Right-sided diverticulitis, sigmoid diverticulitis |
| Appendix diverticulitis, perforation, or inflammation of diverticula of the small bowel |
| Meckel's diverticulum (complications) |
| Crohn's disease and ulcerative colitis |
| Tumour (perforated) |
| Ileocaecal tuberculosis |
| Ischaemia of the small bowel |
| Appendagitis |

## 1.3.3
### Magnetic Resonance

Magnetic resonance imaging (MRI) is also used to diagnose acute appendicitis (Hörmann et al. 1998; Birchard et al. 2005). With fast sequences the lower abdomen can be imaged within seconds (i.e., HASTE sequence). The prompt availability is a prerequisite for diagnosing acute appendicitis. Accuracy is reported to be comparable to that of CT (Hörmann et al. 1998); however, its relatively high cost enables only MRI as a problem-solving investigation. In the future, this may change; however, up to now, MRI is not a primary standard imaging modality in the diagnosis of acute appendicitis.

## 1.4
### Differential Diagnosis

The differential diagnosis can be divided into intestinal (Table 1.2), gynaecological, urological and diseases of other compartments (mainly abdominal wall, psoas muscle, gallbladder, pancreas) (Abu-Yousef 2001).

## 1.4.1
### Intestinal Differential Diagnosis

Most often, infectious ileocaecitis is found (Puylaert 1986b; Tarantino et al. 2003). Sonographically, the caecum and/or the terminal ileum are moderately thickened. The caecum shows hyperhaustration. Often, enlarged painful regional lymph nodes are found. The most frequent microbes are *Yersinia*, *Campylobacter* or *Salmonella* (Puylaert et al. 1988). The appendix can be reactively enlarged by these diseases.

When examining children, in the event of a painful lower quadrant, invagination of the small bowel has to be considered. The sonographic picture is typical. A double-layer intussusception can be visualised. With adults, tumours causing invagination have to be excluded. Furthermore, complications of a Meckel's diverticulum (inflammation, bleeding) have to be taken into account (Baldisserotto et al. 2003). Another differential diagnosis when examining children is a volvulus (Patino and Munden 2004). In this condition, the mesenteric vessels show a whirlpool sign.

In adults, diverticulitis of the ascending colon or caecum is an important conservatively managed disease (Macheiner et al. 1999, Wada et al. 1990). Also diverticulitis of the sigmoid colon can be right sided or project on the right side (Hollerweger et al. 2001). Diverticula on the right side are usually true diverticula, which are often large.

Furthermore, a (perforated) tumour of the colon should be considered.

Crohn's disease is a frequent transmural chronic inflammation of the bowel. Usually, segmental thickening of the small bowel is seen. Also other parts of the bowel, appendix included (Fig. 1.9), can be involved. Due to the transmural inflammation, the surrounding fat is frequently affected. Fistulas are often found. In chronic forms, fibrous stenosis is frequently present with dilation of the oral segments

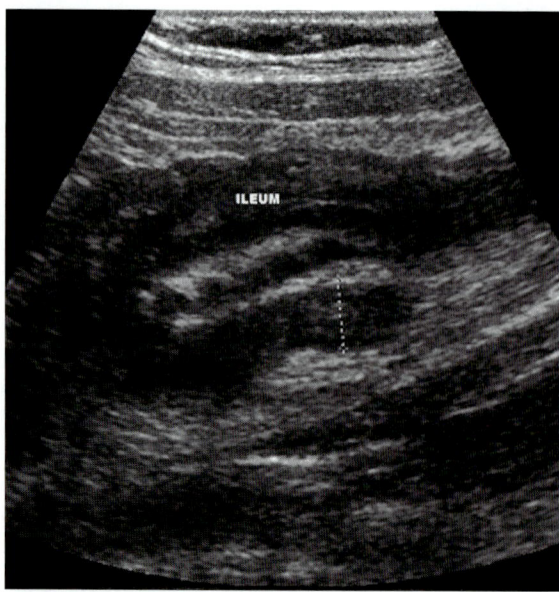

**Fig. 1.9.** Thickening of the appendix in Crohn's disease. The terminal ileum is thickened also

showing fluid-filled bowel loops. Ulcerative colitis is a rare differential diagnoses for appendicitis, since the disease is predominantly left sided.

Another rare disease in the right lower quadrant is tuberculosis of the ileo-caecal region (Portielje et al. 1995).

Appendagitis and omental infarction are further differential diagnoses to acute appendicitis. In appendagitis, an inflammation, torsion or necrosis of the epiploic appendices is present. Sonographically, an ovoid alteration of the pericolonic fat is seen. Usually, the echogenic altered fat is fixed to the ventral peritoneum, whereas the other bowel loops show normal breathing motility with regard to the peritoneum (Hollerweger et al. 2002; van Breda Vriesman et al. 2001).

In colour Doppler, the altered epiploic appendix reveals no vascularisation, whereas the surrounding fat may be hypervascularized (Grattan-Smith et al. 2002). Usually, CT is also performed to verify this relatively rare diagnosis. Appendagitis is treated conservatively. Surgery can be avoided in this self-limiting disease.

### 1.4.2
### Gynaecological Differential Diagnosis

Inflammation of the ovaries is a common differential diagnosis. This diagnosis is made when witnessing a combination of clinical and transvaginal sonographic signs. The most important sign is the pain above the ovary during examination. In a tubo-ovarial abscess, cystoid-hypoechogenic tubular structures can be found in transvaginal sonography. Further differential diagnoses are ruptured adnexal cysts, torque cysts, or cysts with bleeding. All these pathologies may clinically mimic acute appendicitis.

The most important gynaecological differential diagnosis is ectopic pregnancy. In ruptured tubal gestation a haematoma is seen in the adnexal region together with free intraperitoneal fluid. In the uterus a small pseudogestational sac can be depicted.

Transvaginal sonography is used mainly to diagnose gynaecological pathologies. When the appendix is deeply situated in the small pelvis, transvaginal sonography may also reveal appendicitis (Molander et al. 2002).

### 1.4.3
### Urological Differential Diagnosis

Inflammation of the urinary tract may mimic appendicitis. A stone in the right ureter may be a cause of right lower abdominal pain. In acute renal colic, the collecting system may not be dilated. Doppler sonography can be used to diagnose the acute obstruction. Furthermore, a careful search for perirenal fluid at the poles of the kidney should be performed.

Ureter stones are typically located at the three physiological narrowings. Usually, the stone is localised in the intramural part of the ureter, just proximal to the ostium. These stones can be diagnosed with transabdominal and transrectal or transvaginal sonography.

### 1.4.4
### Diseases of Other Compartments

Haematomas of the abdominal wall may mimic acute appendicitis. These cystoid lesions may be easily assessed with high-resolution transducers. They reveal no breathing mobility. Typically these lesions are ovoid or spindle shaped.

Haematomas or abscesses may also be present in the psoas muscle. In these diseases, the psoas muscle is enlarged and reveals tenderness upon pressure.

Either CT and/or MRI should be performed in order to rule out acute spondylodiscitis.

Acute cholecystitis may be caudally situated and may mimic appendicitis clinically. In rare cases, necrotic pancreatitis may be misinterpreted.

In rare cases, dissecting or rupturing aneurysms of the retroperitoneal vessels may cause right lower quadrant pain.

## 1.5 Mucocele of the Appendix

Mucoceles of the appendix are relatively rare lesions. They vary considerably in size. Giant lesions up to 25 cm can be present. The large lesions are most often caused by mucus-producing tumours such as cystadenoma or cystadenocarcinoma. Later, they can rupture and produce a *Pseudomyxoma peritoneii*. Small non-neoplastic lesions are found incidentally during imaging.

Sonographically, mucoceles are cystoid or hypoechogenic lesions. An onion-skin appearance has been described (Fig. 1.10; DGANI et al. 2002; CASPI et al. 2004). This echogenicity is thought to be caused by viscosity differences of the mucus. Colour Doppler is used to exclude vascularisation in the lesion. In *Pseudomyxoma peritoneii* encapsulated cystoid lesions are found in the peritoneum.

## 1.6 Conclusion

Sonography is the first-line imaging method for diagnosing acute appendicitis. Experienced investigators have an accuracy of more than 90%.

Sonography can diagnose many conservatively managed diseases. Sonography can reduce the high rate of false-positive clinical examinations concerning acute appendicitis. It has to be stated that exclusion of appendicitis can only be made sonographically if the normal appendix can be seen in its full length and/or other differential diagnoses can be depicted which explain the clinical symptoms. Mucoceles are rare cystoid lesions of the appendix. They exhibit a typical onion-skin-sign structure caused by mucus. In large mucoceles a tumour causes this lesion.

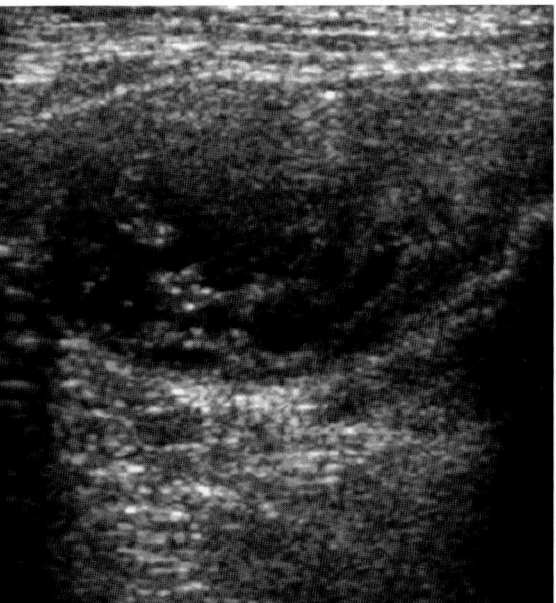
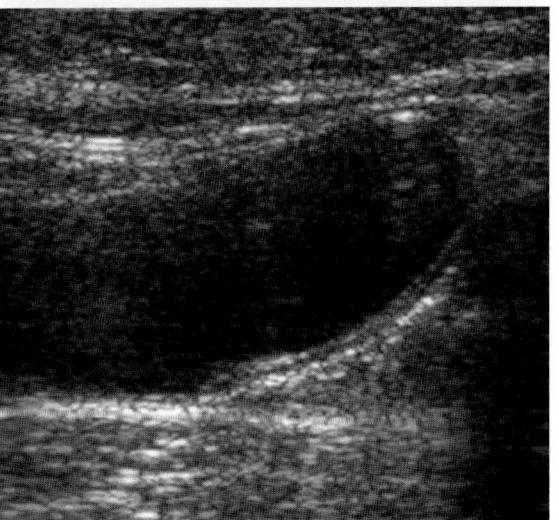

**Fig. 1.10a,b.** Mucocele of the appendix. **a** Cystoid lesion in the region of the appendix with an onion-skin structure. **b** The appendiceal mucocele appears as a cystoid enlargement of the appendix

### References

Abu-Yousef MM (2001) Ultrasonography of the right lower quadrant. Ultrasound Q 17:211–225

Baldisserotto M, Maffazzoni DR, Dora MD (2003) Sonographic findings of Meckel's diverticulitis in children. Am J Roentgenol 180:425–428

Birchard KR, Brown MA, Hyslop WB et al. (2005) MRI of acute abdominal and pelvic pain in pregnant patients. Am J Roentgenol 184:452–458

Caspi B, Cassif E, Auslender R et al (2004) The onion skin sign: a specific sonographic marker of appendiceal mucocele. J Ultrasound Med 23:117–121

Chan I, Bicknell SG, Graham M (2005) Utility and diagnostic accuracy of sonography in detecting appendicitis in a community hospital. Am J Roentgenol 184:1809–1812

Dgani S, Shapiro I, Leibovitz Z, Ohel G (2002) Songraphic appearance of appendiceal mucocele. Ultrasound Obstet Gynecol 19:99–101

Grattan-Smith JD, Blews DE, Brand T (2002) Omental infarction in pediatric patients: sonographic and CT findings. Am J Roentgenol 178:1537–1539

Gritzmann N, Hollerweger A, Macheiner P, Rettenbacher T (2002) Transabdominal sonography of the gastrointestinal tract. Eur Radiol 12:1748–1761

Hollerweger A, Macheiner P, Rettenbacher T et al. (2001) Colonic diverticulitis: diagnostic value and appearance of inflamed diverticula-sonographic evaluation. Eur Radiol 11:1956–1963

Hollerweger A, Macheiner P, Rettenbacher T, Gritzmann N (2002) Primary epiploic appendagitis: sonographic findings with CT correlation. J Clin Ultrasound 30:481–495

Hörmann M, Paya K, Eibenberger K et al. (1998) MR imaging in children with nonperforated acute appendicitis: value of unenhanced MR imaging in sonographically selected cases. Am J Roentgenol 171:467–470

Incesu L, Yazicioglu AK, Selcuk MB, Ozen N (2004) Contrast-enhanced power Doppler US in the diagnosis of acute appendicitis. Eur J Radiol 50:201–209

Kessler N, Cyteval C, Gallix B et al (2004) Appendicitis: evaluation of sensitivity, specificity, and predictive values of US, Doppler US, and laboratory findings. Radiology 230:472–478

Lee JH, Jeong YK, Park KB et al. (2005) Operator-dependent techniques for graded compression sonography to detect the appendix and diagnose acute appendicitis. Am J Roentgenol 184:91–97

Macheiner P, Rettenbacher T, Hollerweger A, Gritzmann N (1999) Diverticulitis of the appendix vermiformis: ultrasonographic appearance. Ultraschall Med 20:115–117

Molander P, Paavonen J, Sjoberg J et al. (2002) Transvaginal sonography in the diagnosis of acute appendicitis. Ultrasound Obstet Gynecol 20:496–501

Noguchi T, Yoshimitsu K, Yoshida M (2005) Periappendiceal hyperechoic structure on sonography: a sign of severe appendicitis. J Ultrasound Med 24:323–327

Patino MO, Munden MM (2004) Utility of the sonographic whirlpool sign in diagnosing midgut volvulus in patients with atypical clinical presentations. J Ultrasound Med 23:397–401

Portielje JE, Lohle PN, van der Werf SD, Puylaert JB (1995) Ultrasound and abdominal tuberculosis. Lancet 346:379–380

Puylaert JB (1986a) Acute appendicitis: US evaluation using graded compression. Radiology 158:355–360

Puylaert JB (1986b) Mesenteric adenitis and acute terminal ileitis: US evaluation using graded compression. Radiology 161:691–695

Puylaert JB, Lalisang RI, van der Werf SD, Doornbos L (1988) *Campylobacter* ileocolitis mimicking acute appendicitis: differentiation with graded-compression US. Radiology 166:737–740

Rao PM, Rhea JT, Novelline RA (1997) Sensitivity and specificity of the individual CT signs of appendicitis: experience with 200 appendiceal CT examinations. J Comput Assist Tomogr 21:686–692

Rettenbacher T, Hollerweger A, Macheiner P, Gritzmann N (1997) Ultrasonography of the normal vermiform appendix. Ultraschall Med 18:139–142

Rettenbacher T, Hollerweger A, Macheiner P et al. (2000) Presence or absence of gas in the appendix: additional criteria to rule out or confirm acute appendicitis: evaluation with US. Radiology 214:183–187

Rettenbacher T, Hollerweger A, Macheiner P et al. (2001) Outer diameter of the vermiform appendix as a sign of acute appendicitis: evaluation at US. Radiology. 218:757–762

Rettenbacher T, Hollerweger A, Gritzmann N et al. (2002) Appendicitis: Should diagnostic imaging be performed if the clinical presentation is highly suggestive of the disease? Gastroenterology 123:992–998

Rettenbacher T, Hollerweger A, Macheiner P et al. (2003) Ovoid shape of the vermiform appendix: a criterion to exclude acute appendicitis: evaluation with US. Radiology 226:95–100

Tarantino L, Giorgio A, Stefano G de et al. (2003) Acute appendicitis mimicking infectious enteritis: diagnostic value of sonography. J Ultrasound Med 22:945–950

Üeberrüeck T, Koch A, Meyer L et al. (2004) Ninety-four appendectomies for suspected acute appendicitis during pregnancy. World J Surg 28:508–511

van Breda Vriesman AC, de Mol van Otterloo AJ, Puylaert JB (2001) Epiploic appendagitis and omental infarction. Eur J Surg 167:723–727

van Breda Vriesman AC, Kole BJ, Puylaert JB (2003) Effect of ultrasonography and optional computed tomography on the outcome of appendectomy. Eur Radiol 13:2278–2282

Wada M, Kikuchi Y, Doy M (1990) Uncomplicated acute diverticulitis of the cecum and ascending colon. Sonographic findings in 18 patients. Am J Roentgenol 155:283–287

# Mesenteric Lymphadenopathy

Giovanni Maconi, Elisa Radice, and Gabriele Bianchi Porro

CONTENTS

2.1 Introduction 11
2.2 Normal Mesenteric Lymph Nodes 11
2.3 Neoplastic Conditions 12
2.4 Inflammatory Conditions 14
2.5 Infectious Conditions 16
2.6 Primary Mesenteric Lymphadenitis 17
References 17

Table 2.1. Main diseases associated with mesenteric lymphadenopathy

1. Malignant diseases
   a. Haematologic (Hodgkin's disease, non-Hodgkin's lymphomas, amyloidosis)
   b. Metastatic (from numerous primary sites)
2. Immunological diseases
   a. Crohn's disease
   b. Ulcerative colitis
   d. Systemic lupus erythematosus
   e. Primary sclerosing cholangitis
   f. Sjögren's syndrome
   g. Primary biliary cirrhosis
3. Infectious diseases
   a. Viral (EBV, CMV, viral hepatitis, herpes simplex, adenovirus, HIV)
   b. Bacterial (*Yersinia paratuberculosis*, Salmonella, Shigella, Campylobacter, brucellosis, tuberculosis, atypical mycobacterial infection)
   c. Parasitic (toxoplasmosis, leishmaniasis, trypanosomiasis, filariasis)
   d. Chlamydial (lymphogranuloma venereum, trachoma)
   e. Fungal (histoplasmosis, coccidioidomycosis)
4. Other disorders
   a. Lipid storage diseases (Gaucher's, Niemann-Pick, Castleman's disease)
   b. Sarcoidosis
   c. Familial Mediterranean fever

## 2.1
## Introduction

With the increasing use of abdominal and bowel ultrasound in the screening and follow-up of bowel diseases, enlargement of the regional mesenteric lymph nodes have become a fairly common clinical finding, particularly in children and young adults. Therefore, since lymphadenopathy may often be an incidental finding in patients being examined for various reasons, the sonographer (and the physician) must decide whether it is a normal finding or a sign of a patient's condition requiring further study. Indeed, mesenteric lymphadenopathy may be a manifestation of various disorders (Table 2.1).

## 2.2
## Normal Mesenteric Lymph Nodes

Regional mesenteric lymph nodes are usually detected as the result of a symptom-directed diagnostic work-up, by a variety of imaging techniques, including ultrasound and colour Doppler ultrasonography, computed tomography (CT) and magnetic resonance imaging (MRI). When they are found, the

G. Maconi, MD
E. Radice, MD
G. Bianchi Porro, MD, PhD
Chair of Gastroenterology, Department of Clinical Sciences, "L. Sacco" University Hospital, Via G.B. Grassi 74, 20157 Milano, Italy

main goal of the diagnostic technique is to suggest whether it is a normal finding or the sign of a past or ongoing abdominal disease, and in this context, to differentiate its benign from malignant nature.

The ultrasonographic criteria of the enlargement of mesenteric lymph nodes has been variably defined as the detection of nodes larger than 4 mm in the short axis (Sivit et al. 1993) and larger than 10 mm in the long axis (Watanabe et al. 1997). This sonographic definition is in agreement with that of a study based on CT studies in an adult population where mesenteric lymphadenitis has been defined as three or more lymph nodes, each 5 mm or greater ≥5 mm in the short axis (Macari et al. 2002). However, this size might not be a reliable normal cut-off value in children where it is much more controversial. A recent study showed that using a threshold of short-axis ≥5 mm for enlarged mesenteric lymph nodes might yield an unacceptably high percentage (54%) of false-positive results and that a better definition of enlarged mesenteric lymph node would be a short axis of >8 mm, which yielded only a 5% false-positive rate (Karmazyn et al. 2005).

Therefore, the sonographic detection of oval, elongated, U-shaped lymph nodes with a short-axis diameter up to 4 mm in adults and 8 mm in children, should be considered a normal finding and should not be misdiagnosed as an early manifestation of a lympho-proliferative disorder.

The size of the nodes alone does not always reflect underlying disease. The number and distribution of lymph nodes is also important. Normal mesenteric lymph nodes may be routinely identified at the mesenteric root and throughout the mesentery, in particular in right iliaca fossa in children (Karmazyn et al. 2005) and at the mesenteric root in adults (Lucey et al. 2005) (Fig. 2.1).

Size, site and number of lymphadenopathy detected by abdominal ultrasound may therefore help in suggesting their nature, or at least in differentiating among their main causes, which may be neoplastic, infectious or inflammatory.

## 2.3
## Neoplastic Conditions

Mesenteric lymphadenopathy may result from metastatic malignancy. The ultrasonographic criteria used to differentiate between benign and malignant cervical nodes may also be adopted to differentiate benign from malignant enlarged mesenteric lymph nodes. Shape, size and echogenicity can been considered for this purpose. Sonography can determine the long (L) axis, short (S) axis, and a ratio of long to short axis. An L/S ratio of <2.0 (namely a round-shaped node) has a sensitivity and a specificity of 95% for distinguishing benign and malignant nodes. This ratio has greater specificity and sensitivity than measurement of either the long or the short axis alone.

The most common malignancy resulting in mesenteric lymphadenopathy is lymphoma. Even if lymphoma may be found in lymphadenopathy in the chest, retroperitoneum, or superficial lymph node chains, mesenteric lymphadenopathy is not uncommon. Enlarged nodes may be seen at the mesenteric root, scattered throughout the peripheral mesentery.

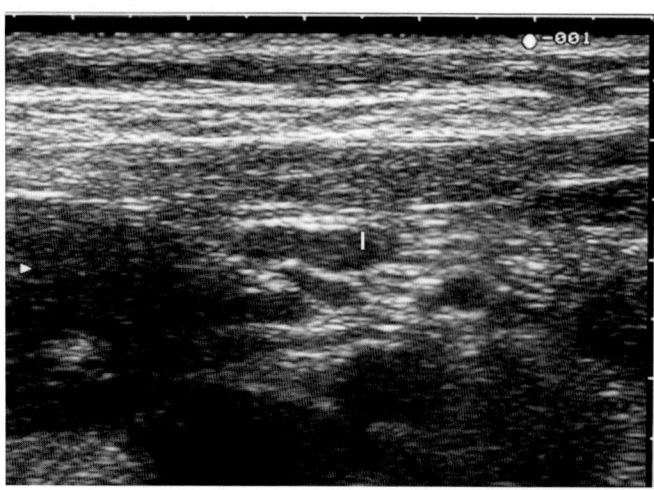

**Fig. 2.1.** Ultrasonographic appearance of normal lymph nodes as an incidental finding in a 23-year-old female patient with constipation

Early in the course of the disease, the lymph nodes may be small, soft and discrete (Fig. 2.2).

As the disease progresses, the enlarged nodes often coalesce and tend to form a conglomerate mass (Fig. 2.3).

Extensive mesenteric lymphadenopathy, due to lymphoma have a characteristic appearance. Mesenteric lymph nodes involved by lymphoma are usually hypoechoic, round and surrounded by hyperechoic mesenteric tissue (Fig. 2.4) (Gorg et al. 1995, 1996a,b).

Mesenteric lymph node involvement by lymphoma is not always associated with lymphomatous involvement of the bowel.

Primary malignancies that most commonly lead to in mesenteric lymphadenopathy include carcinoma of the gastrointestinal tract (in particular, carcinomas of the colon, duodenum and ileum), pancreas and less frequently of the lung and carcinoid (Fig. 2.5). Most primary malignancies involve local lymph nodes before more distant metastases are detected.

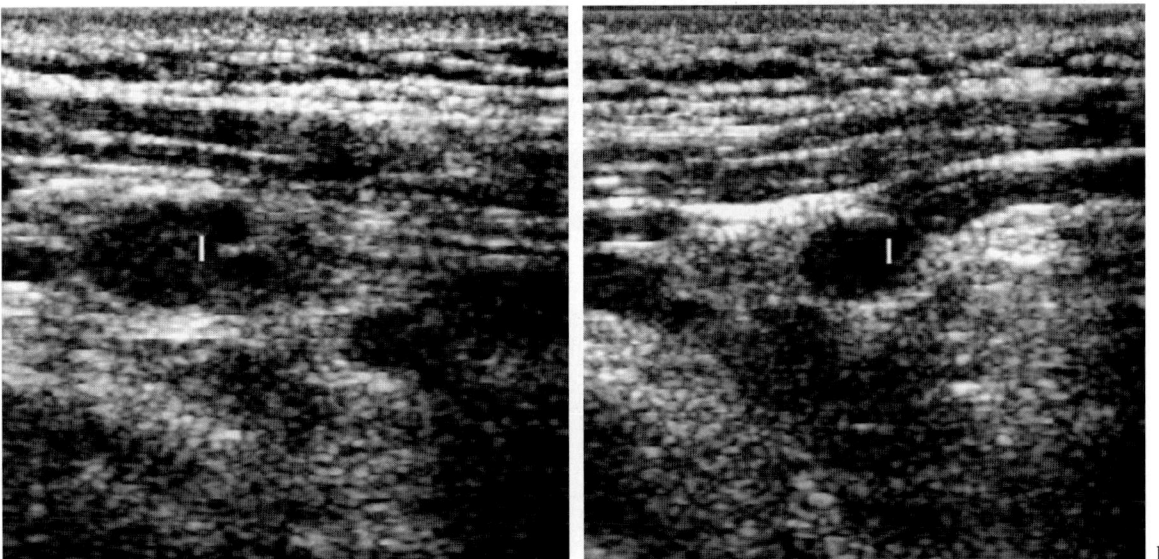

**Fig. 2.2a,b.** Several small, soft and enlarged lymph nodes at mesenteric root, in a 52-year-old patient with early intestinal non-Hodgkin lymphoma

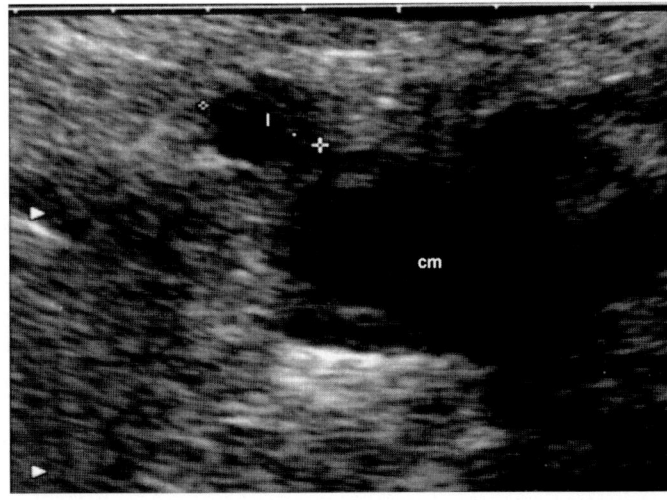

**Fig. 2.3.** Conglomerate abdominal mass formed by multiple coalescent lymph nodes (*cm*) (*l*, lymph node)

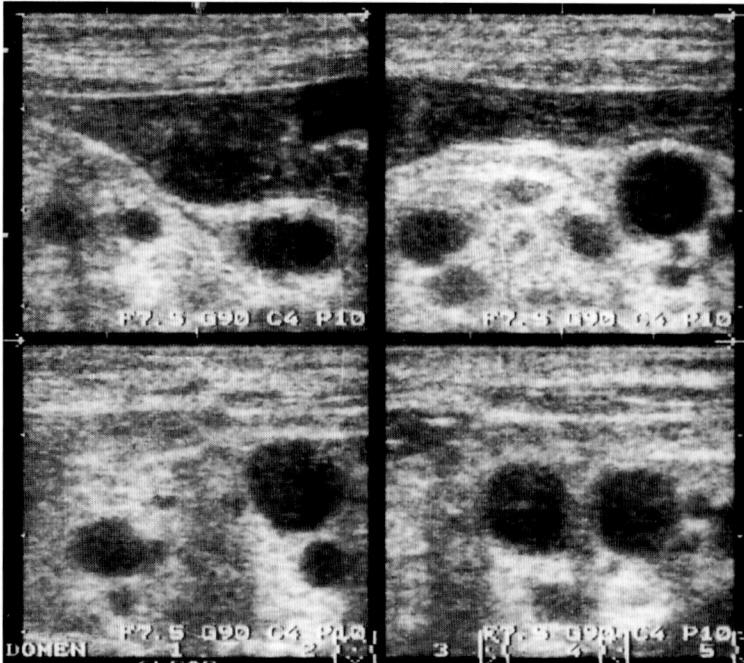

Fig. 2.4. Typical mesenteric lymph node involvement in lymphoma, presenting as hypoechoic, round lesion surrounded by hyperechoic mesenteric tissue

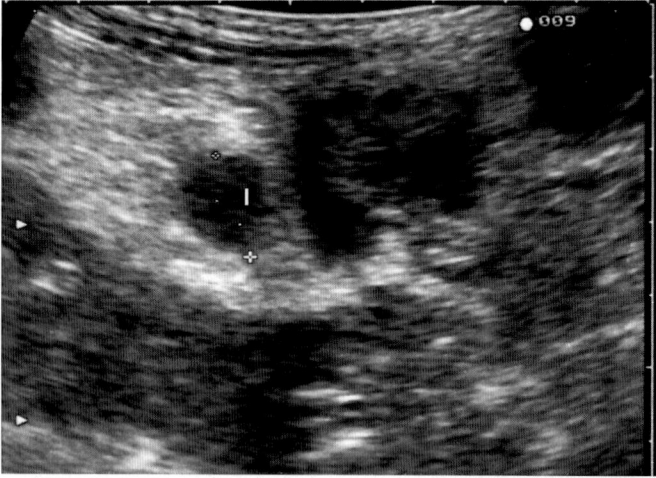

Fig. 2.5. Regional metastatic lymph node (*l*) involvement in patients with gastrointestinal cancer presenting as slight hypoechoic, soft and round lesion

## 2.4
## Inflammatory Conditions

Mesenteric lymphadenopathy may be secondary to an underlying inflammatory process, either a localized inflammatory disease or a systemic inflammatory condition.

Local inflammatory causes, leading to mesenteric lymphadenopathy, are due to local mesenteric inflammation generally due to appendicitis, diverticulitis and cholecystitis.

Appendicitis is frequently associated with lymphadenopathy, most commonly in the mesentery of the right lower quadrant. Although lymph nodes may be identified in the mesentery of the right lower quadrant in the normal population, these are usually small and few in number. Multiple enlarged right lower quadrant lymph nodes, in the presence of an abnormal appendix, are useful in the diagnosis of appendicitis, although lymphadenopathy is not necessarily present to make the diagnosis.

Mesenteric lymphadenopathy may also be seen in cases of diverticulitis. The enlarged nodes are usually identified close to the area of inflamed colon. These reactive nodes associated with diverticulitis are generally small but, unfortunately, not specific. In fact, diverticulitis may mimic perforated colonic carcinoma where adjacent enlarged lymph nodes may also be present.

Mesenteric lymphadenopathy is commonly found in patients with inflammatory bowel disease, both Crohn's disease and ulcerative colitis (MACONI et al. 2005), although it is more common in Crohn's disease. The lymph nodes may be found at the mesenteric root, mesenteric periphery or in the right lower quadrant (Fig. 2.6).

In Crohn's disease, mesenteric lymph nodes are usually described as single or multiple large, hypoechoic oval nodules with homogeneous echogenicity and regular margins, or more rarely as part of a conglomerate mass (MACONI et al. 2005). Therefore, sometimes it may be difficult if not impossible to distinguish between neoplastic and inflammatory conditions of enlarged abdominal lymph nodes.

The prevalence of mesenteric lymphadenopathy in Crohn's disease may vary, mainly in relation to the age of patients and to the duration of disease, lymph nodes being more frequent in young patients and in those with early disease. In particular, enlarged mesenteric lymph nodes can be detected in more than 50% of CD patients under 30 years of age (MACONI et al. 2005; TARJAN et al. 2000) and are also a frequent finding in the presence of septic complications such as fistulas and abscesses. On the contrary, the importance of US assessment of lymph nodes, as a marker of Crohn's disease activity, is still controversial.

Connective tissue diseases, such as systemic lupus erythematosus, systemic sclerosis, or rheumatoid arthritis, may also be related to mesenteric lymphadenopathy (CALGUNERI et al. 2003). In these patients, mesenteric lymphadenopathy is more frequently an occasional US finding and seldom the only manifestation of lymph node involvement.

In many other inflammatory conditions, mesenteric lymphadenopathy is present, and is seldom the only manifestation of the disease such as: coeliac disease (FRAQUELLI et al. 2004), primary sclerosing cholangitis (Fig. 2.7), primary biliary cirrhosis, sarcoidosis and amyloidosis.

In coeliac disease, enlarged lymph nodes are frequently found at mesenteric root level or, less frequently, at the mesenteric periphery. The shape of lymphadenopathies is usually oval or elongated (Fig. 2.8). Cavitation of mesenteric lymph nodes is rarely seen (SCHMITZ et al. 2002).

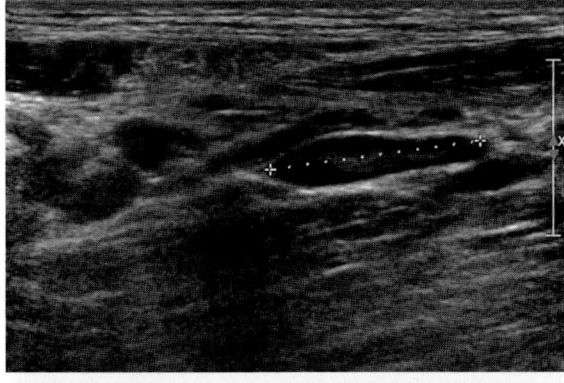
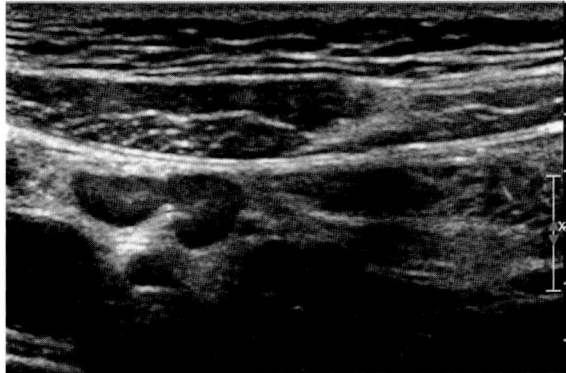
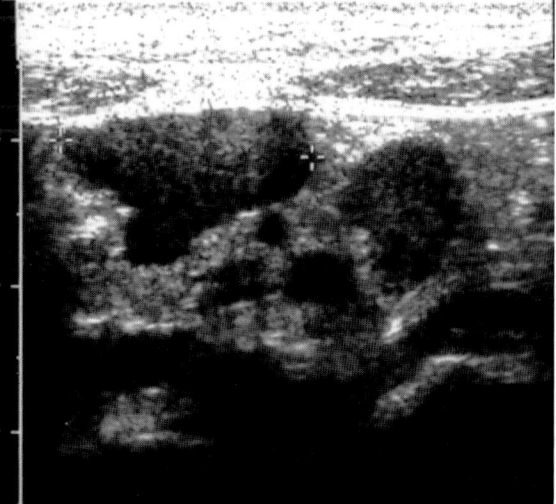

**Fig. 2.6a–c.** Mesenteric lymphadenopathy in a 40-year-old female with Crohn's disease (a,b) and in a 28-year-old male with early ileal and jejunal Crohn's disease (c). US images show multiple peri-intestinal lymphadenopathy in mesentery of right lower quadrant

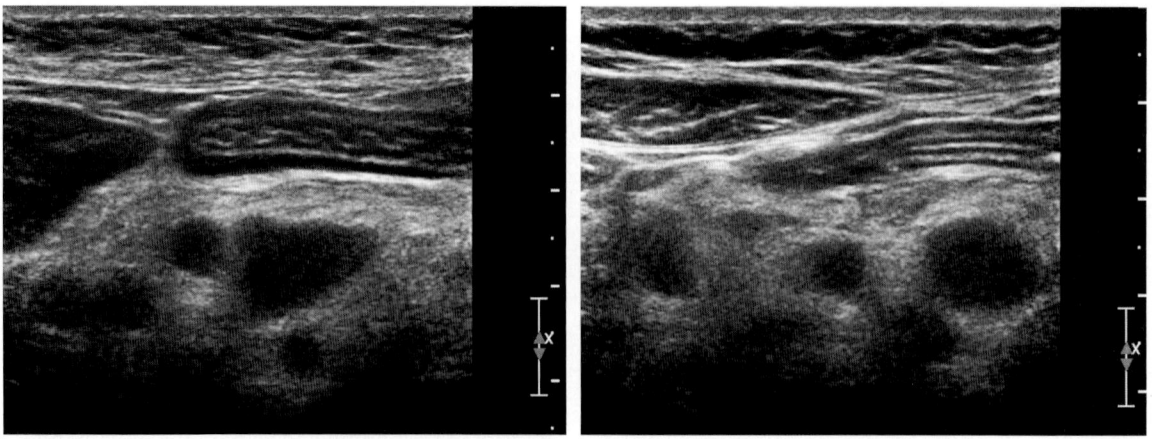

**Fig. 2.7a,b.** Mesenteric lymphadenopathy in a 38-year-old female patient with primary sclerosing cholangitis

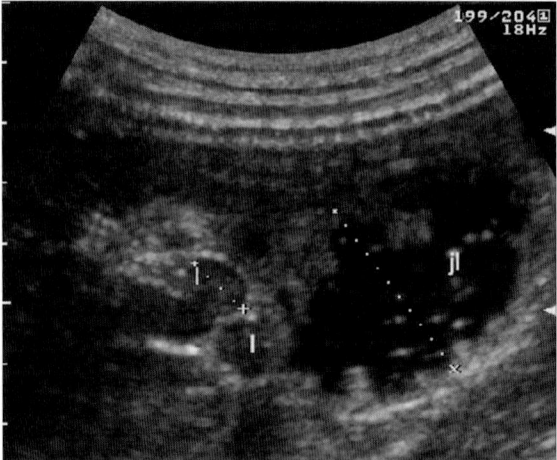

**Fig. 2.8.** Ovoidal or elongated (*a*) lymphadenopathy in patient with coeliac disease

## 2.5
## Infectious Conditions

Intestinal infections, either local or systemic, may result in mesenteric lymphadenopathy.

Enlarged mesenteric lymph nodes are frequently detected in various acute infectious conditions, such as *Yersinia ileitis* and other viral or bacterial infectious forms of enterocolitis and pelvic inflammatory diseases, more commonly in the paediatric population (PUYLAERT 1986; MACARI et al. 2002; RAO et al. 1997).

Infection with *Yersinia enterocolitica* is characterised by small bowel wall thickening in the right lower quadrant in the region of the terminal ileum, and peri-intestinal regional mesenteric lymphadenopathy. The clinical features (diarrhoea, fever and abdominal pain), radiological and ultrasonographic findings are similar to those of Crohn's disease (TROMMER et al. 1998; PUYLAERT et al. 1997). Also in other forms of infectious ileocecitis, caused by *Campylobacter jejuni* or *Salmonella enteritidis*, enlarged regional mesenteric lymph nodes together with thickening of the mucosa and (less frequently) submucosa of the ileum, caecum and ascending colon can be found.

Infection with the human immunodeficiency virus (HIV) may produce isolated lymphadenopathy resulting from direct infection by the virus or from secondary infection (RADIN 1995; TARANTINO et al. 2003). Mesenteric lymphadenopathy in patients with HIV is far more likely to result from an opportunistic infection or even an underlying malignancy than to be caused by direct HIV infection. In this case, the lymph nodes may be enlarged but rarely massive. On the contrary, in HIV positive patients with a CD4 cell count of 50/mL or less, *Mycobacterium avium* complex (MAC) is the main cause of massive mesenteric lymphadenopathy. In HIV patients with mesenteric lymph nodes, in particular if forming a conglomerate mass, MAC infection should always be considered (KOH et al. 2003; TARANTINO et al. 2003) (Fig. 2.9).

Enlarged mesenteric lymph nodes in patients with tuberculosis are generally hypoechoic, round to ovoid, and variable in size. Sometimes, the nodes may be calcified (MALIK and SAXENA 2003; KEDAR 1994). They are frequently found in the right lower quadrant, around the terminal ileum and caecum (Ch. 12).

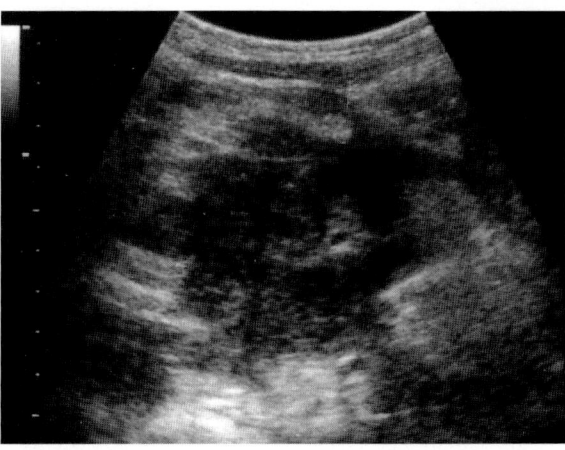 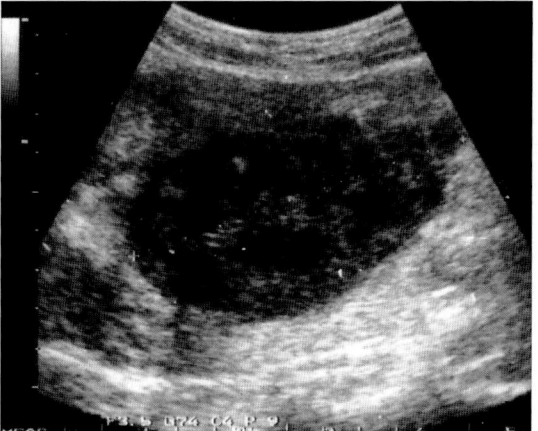

Fig. 2.9a,b. Mesenteric lymph nodes, forming a conglomerate mass, in HIV patient with MAC infection

Other causes of mesenteric lymphadenopathy are Whipple disease (Ch. 10) and familial Mediterranean fever. In particular, mesenteric lymphadenopathy has been reported in up to one-third of patients with familial Mediterranean fever during an acute abdominal attack (Zissin et al. 2003).

## 2.6
## Primary Mesenteric Lymphadenitis

Primary mesenteric lymphadenitis has been defined as right-sided mesenteric lymphadenopathy without an identifiable acute inflammatory process or with a mild (<5 mm) wall thickening of the terminal ileum (Sivit et al. 1993; Vayner et al. 2003; Macari et al. 2002). In most of these cases, an underlying infectious terminal ileitis is thought to be the cause. Mesenteric lymphadenitis is a relatively uncommon cause of acute right lower quadrant pain in adults with a reported variable prevalence between 2% and 14% (Puylaert 1986; Rao et al. 1997). Its clinical presentation is non-specific (abdominal pain, fever, leukocytosis) leading to a clinical and imaging differential diagnosis including appendicitis, infectious ileocecitis, diverticulitis, as well as inflammatory pelvic conditions.

## References

Calguneri M, Ozturk MA, Ozbalkan Z et al (2003) Frequency of lymphadenopathy in rheumatoid arthritis and systemic lupus erythematosus. J Int Med Res 31:345–349

Fraquelli M, Colli A, Colucci A et al (2004) Accuracy of ultrasonography in predicting celiac disease. Arch Intern Med. 64:169–174

Gorg C, Weide R, Gorg K, Restrepo I (1996a) Ultrasound manifestations of abdominal lymphomas. An overview. Ultraschall Med 17:179–184

Gorg C, Weide R, Schwerk WB (1996b) Sonographic patterns in extranodal abdominal lymphomas. Eur Radiol 6:855–864

Karmazyn B, Werner EA, Rejaie B, Applegate KE (2005) Mesenteric lymph nodes in children: what is normal? Pediatr Radiol 35:774–777

Kedar RP, Shah PP, Shivde RS, Malde HM (1994) Sonographic findings in gastrointestinal and peritoneal tuberculosis. Clin Radiol 49:24–29

Koh DM, Burn PR, Mathews G, Nelson M, Healy JC (2003) Abdominal computed tomographic findings of Mycobacterium tuberculosis and Mycobacterium avium intracellulare infection in HIV seropositive patients. Can Assoc Radiol J 54:45–50

Lucey BC, Stuhlfaut JW, Soto JA (2005) Mesenteric lymph nodes: detection and significance on MDCT. AJR Am J Roentgenol 184:41–44

Macari M, Hines J, Balthazar E et al (2002) Mesenteric adenitis: CT diagnosis of primary versus secondary causes, incidence, and clinical significance in pediatric and adult patients. AJR Am J Roentgenol 178:853–858

Maconi G, Di Sabatino A, Ardizzone S et al (2005) Prevalence and clinical significance of sonographic detection of enlarged regional lymph nodes in Crohn's disease. Scand J Gastroenterol 2005; 40:1328–1333

Malik A, Saxena NC (2003) Ultrasound in abdominal tuberculosis. Abdom Imaging 28:574–579

Puylaert JB (1986) Mesenteric adenitis and acute terminal ileitis: US evaluation using graded compression. Radiology 161:691–695

Puylaert JB, Van der Zant FM, Mutsaers JA (1997) Infectious ileocecitis caused by Yersinia, Campylobacter, and Salmonella: clinical, radiological and US findings. Eur Radiol 7:3–9

Radin R (1995) HIV infection: analysis in 259 consecutive patients with abnormal abdominal CT findings. Radiology 197:712–722

Rao PM, Rhea JT, Novelline RA (1997) CT diagnosis of mesenteric adenitis. Radiology 202:145–149

Schmitz F, Herzig KH, Stuber E et al (2002) On the pathogenesis and clinical course of mesenteric lymph node cavitation and hyposplenism in coeliac disease. Int J Colorectal Dis 17:192–198

Sivit CJ, Newman KD, Chandra RS (1993) Visualization of enlarged mesenteric lymph nodes at US examination. Pediatr Radiol 23:471–475

Tarantino L, Giorgio A, de Stefano G, Farella N, Perrotta A, Esposito F (2003) Disseminated mycobacterial infection in AIDS patients: abdominal US features and value of fine-needle aspiration biopsy of lymph nodes and spleen. Abdom Imaging 28:602–608

Tarjan Z, Toth G, Gyorke T, Mester A, Karlinger K, Mako EK (2000) Ultrasound in Crohn's disease of the small bowel. Eur J Radiol 35:176–182

Trommer G, Bewer A, Kosling S (1998) Mesenteric lymphadenopathy in Yersinia enterocolitica infection. Radiologe 38:37–40

Vayner N, Coret A, Polliack G et al (2003) Mesenteric lymphadenopathy in children examined by US for chronic and/or recurrent abdominal pain. Pediatr Radiol 33:864–867

Watanabe M, Ishii E, Hirowatari Y et al (1997) Evaluation of abdominal lymphadenopathy in children by ultrasonography. Pediatr Radiol 27:860–864

Zissin R, Rathaus V, Gayer G, Shapiro-Feinberg M, Hertz M (2003) CT findings in patients with familial Mediterranean fever during an acute abdominal attack. Br J Radiol 76:22–25

# Acute Colonic Diverticulitis and Diverticulosis

Norbert Gritzmann

CONTENTS

3.1 Introduction  19
3.2 **Diverticulosis**  19
3.2.1 Diagnostic Methods  20
3.3 **Diverticulitis**  20
3.3.1 Differential Diagnosis  24
3.4 **Conclusion**  24
References  25

## 3.1 Introduction

The prevalence of colonic diverticulosis is common in developed countries and has been increasing in the past centuries. In autopsy studies from 1910, diverticulosis was found in about 5%, and in the early 1980s diverticula were seen in about 50% of autopsy studies (Farag Soliman et al. 2004).

Prevalence clearly increases with age, varying from <10% in those younger than 40 years, to an estimated 50–66% of patients older than 80 years (Almy and Howell 1980).

There is no apparent gender predilection.

Diverticulosis is usually clinically asymptomatic. About 80–85% of patients with diverticulosis have no symptoms (Cheskin et al. 1990), but it is predisposing for complications such as diverticulitis, perforation, peritonitis, fistulas and even bleeding. For a clear overview presentation of diverticulosis contrast enema has been the diagnostic gold standard for many years.

Diverticulosis can also be diagnosed by colonoscopy. Not only the detection of inflammatory complications, but also a clinical asymptomatic diverticulosis can be seen with sonography. In cases of inflammation, a cross-sectional imaging modality, such as sonography or computed tomography (CT), should be performed to evaluate complications.

## 3.2 Diverticulosis

Particular left-sided colonic diverticula are pseudo-diverticula. They are herniations of the mucosa and submucosa through a weakness in the muscle lining, but do not themselves include the muscle layers surrounding the colon.

They herniate adjacent to the points of penetration of the vasa recta through the bowel wall. Diverticula, therefore, tend to be arranged in rows, situated between the mesenteric and lateral taeniae coli (Burkitt et al. 1974).

Diverticula occur mainly in the distal colon, with as many as 90% of patients having involvement of the sigmoid colon and only 15% having right-sided involvement (Roberts and Veidernheimer 1994).

There are many predisposing factors for getting diverticula. Undoubtedly, these mechanisms act synergistically. The cause of colonic diverticula is related primarily to two main factors: increased intraluminal pressure and weakening of the bowel wall (Truelove 1966). Diminished stool bulk, from insufficient dietary fibre, leads to alterations in gastrointestinal transit time and to elevated colonic pressure.

Diverticula can vary in number from solitary findings to literally hundreds. In size, they are typically 5–10 mm in diameter but can exceed 2 cm. An entity of giant colonic diverticula has been described, with sizes up to 25 cm (Levi et al. 1993).

The frequent appearance of diverticula in cases of Ehlers-Dahnlos syndrome, Marfan syndrome and polycystic kidney disease may cause a congenital weakness of the colonic wall.

In Asia, diverticula can often be found in the right-sided colon. These rare dysontogenetic diverticula

---

N. Gritzmann, MD
Dept. of Radiology and Nuclear Medicine, KH Barmherzige Brüder Salzburg, Kajetanerplatz 1, 5020 Salzburg, Austria

are true diverticula, in which all layers of the colon wall are herniated. These patients are often younger than patients with left-sided diverticulosis.

### 3.2.1
### Diagnostic Methods

Traditionally, contrast enema has been the mainstay in the evaluation of patients suspected of having diverticulosis or acute colonic diverticulitis (Fig. 3.1).

Barium provides better mucosal detail than water-soluble contrast media. The possibility of perforation is a contraindication to its use, for fear of barium peritonitis. In these situations, water-soluble contrast should be used.

Diverticulosis can also be diagnosed by endoscopy (Fig. 3.2); however, when diverticulits is suspected clinically, endoscopy is contraindicated. After the acute phase of inflammation, the colon should be examined to exclude a colon carcinoma. So a complete colonic evaluation should generally be performed 6–8 weeks after the resolution of a diverticulitis. In cases of inflammation, coloscopy is often incomplete and painful for the patient. The risk for perforation is also higher because of the air insufflation.

Sonography can also diagnose diverticulosis of the left hemicolon in many cases (HOLLERWEGER et al. 2002).

Normal diverticula present as hyperechoic protuberances of the colonic wall with acoustic shadowing of variable intensity (Fig. 3.3).

The sonographic appearance depends on the content of the diverticula. In most cases, the diverticula appear hyperechoic because of the air inside. Such echoic diverticula show typical air artefacts up to complete acoustic shadowing.

Hyperechoic diverticula with clear acoustic shadowing are typical of a faecolith inside the diverticulum (Fig. 3.4).

The diverticular wall is thin and often not demonstrable at sonography. Large diverticula may be misdiagnosed as haustrations.

In multi-detector computed tomography (MDCT) the air-filled protuberances are usually easier to diagnose than with sonography. Often it is difficult sonographically to differentiate small faecoliths from air within diverticula.

In a recent study the accuracy of sonography in diagnosing diverticulosis was approximately 60% (HOLLERWEGER et al. 2002).

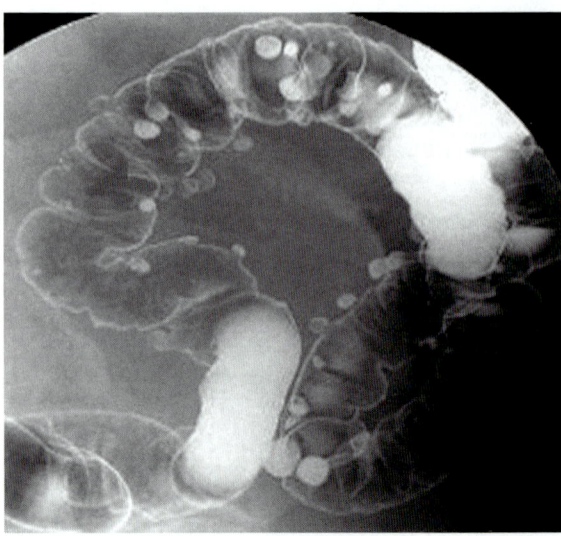

Fig. 3.1. Barium enema shows diverticulosis

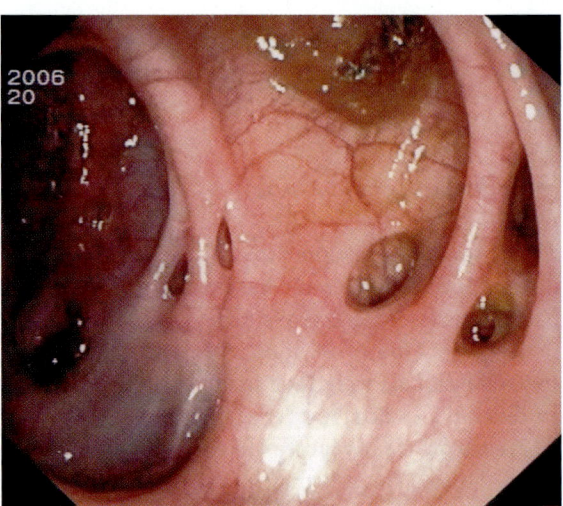

Fig. 3.2. Endoscopy shows diverticula

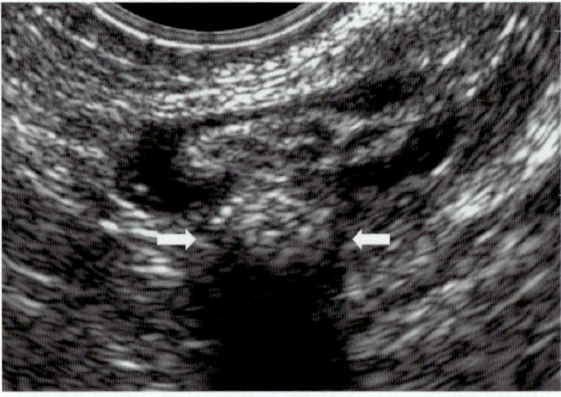

Fig. 3.3. Transvaginal sonography shows a large echogenic diverticulum (*arrows*)

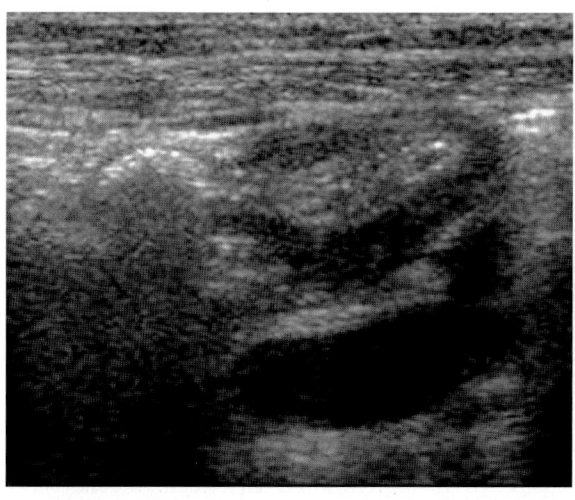 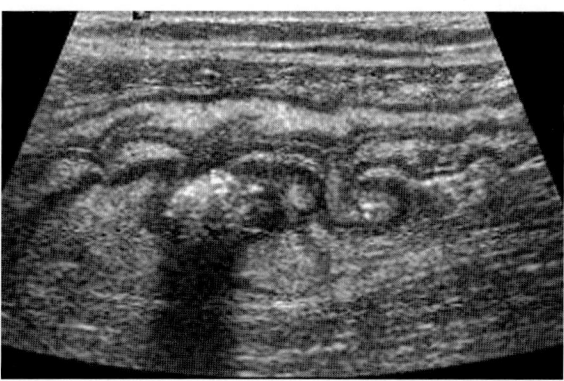

**Fig. 3.4a,b.** Sigmoid colon with echogenic diverticulum. **a** Transverse section with a large echogenic diverticulum. Note the muscular layer of the sigmoid colon (hypoechogenic rim) showing hypertrophy. **b** Longitudinal section shows a diverticulum with an echogenic faecolith inside

## 3.3
## Diverticulitis

Acute colonic diverticulitis is a common cause of acute abdominal symptoms, especially in elderly patients. In turn, diverticulitis develops in 10–25% of the population with diverticulosis (ROBERTS et al. 1995). It is, in virtually all cases, the result of a microperforation of a single diverticulum (Fig. 3.5).

The clinical diagnosis and assessment of acute colonic diverticulitis can be difficult (CHAPPUIS and COHN 1988). The classic pattern of left lower quadrant pain, tenderness, fever, and leukocytosis is suggestive of acute colonic diverticulitis but can be mimicked by numerous acute abdominal conditions. Symptoms such as nausea, vomiting, constipation or diarrhoea lead to a high rate of wrong diagnosis up to 34% of cases.

Dysuria and urinary frequency and urgency may occur if the affected colonic segment lies close to the urinary bladder, and afferent visceral nerves from the inflamed colon, by way of the sacral plexus, may carry referred pain to the scrotum or suprapubic region.

If nearby organs become involved, or if an abscess ruptures into a nearby organ, a fistula may result. Colovesical fistulae are the most frequent type, followed by colovaginal and, less commonly, by colocutaneous fistulae.

Although 85% of cases of diverticulitis occur in the sigmoid and descending colon, diverticula may be found throughout the colon. Right-sided diverticulitis occurs with greater frequency in Asians and tends to follow a more benign course than that which occuring on the left side (WADA et al. 1990).

In acute colonic diverticulitis, ultrasound can evaluate the disease with the same four criteria used with computed tomography (WILSON and TOI 1990): (a) thickening of the bowel wall; (b) diverticula; (c) the echogenicity of these foci varying from hypoechoic (Fig. 3.6a) to predominantly hyperechoic with a surrounding hypoechoic rim (Fig. 3.6b) and hyperechoic with or without internal acoustic shadowing (HOLLERWEGER et al. 2001); and (d) inflammatory pericolonic fat frequently recognised as an adjacent hyperechoic halo. Small air bubbles can be visualised as a sign for microperforation (Fig. 3.6c); therefore, sonographic demonstration of extraluminal hyperechoic foci indicates mesenteric gas.

Longitudinal, linear echogenic tracts are suggestive of fistulous tracts. Thickening of the sigmoid colon along with the roof of the bladder and air within the bladder are signs highly suggestive for a fistula into the bladder.

Sonography can be limited for assessing large and complex abscesses (Fig. 3.7). Overall the accuracy of sonography in diagnosing diverticulitis is more than 90% (HOLLERWEGER et al. 2001).

Transrectal (Fig. 3.8) or endovaginal (Fig. 3.3) sonography can increase the sensitivity of ultrasound when the distal sigmoid or the small pelvis is affected (HOLLERWEGER et al. 2000). This localisation

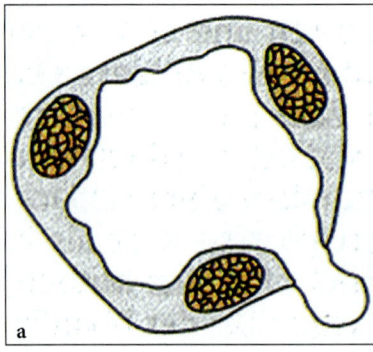 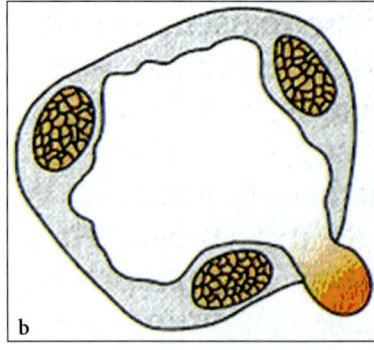 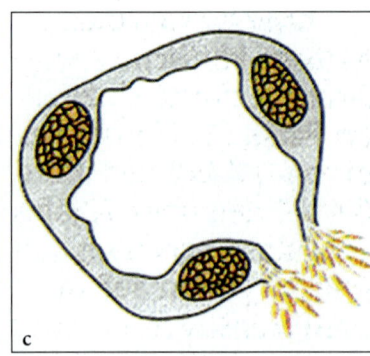

**Fig. 3.5a–c.** Diverticulum (**a**) with inflammation (**b**) and perforation with peridiverticulitis (**c**). In cases of inflammation, the diverticulum becomes obstructed by impacted stool in its neck. This faecolith abrades the mucosa and causes low-grade inflammation, blocking drainage even further. The obstruction may then cause an expansion of the normal bacterial flora, diminished venous outflow with localised ischaemia and altered mucosal defence mechanisms, allowing bacteria to breach the mucosa and extend the process through the full wall, ultimately leading to perforation. (The term "perforated" diverticulitis should be reserved for cases in which a peridiverticular abscess has ruptured into the peritoneal cavity and caused a purulent peritonitis)

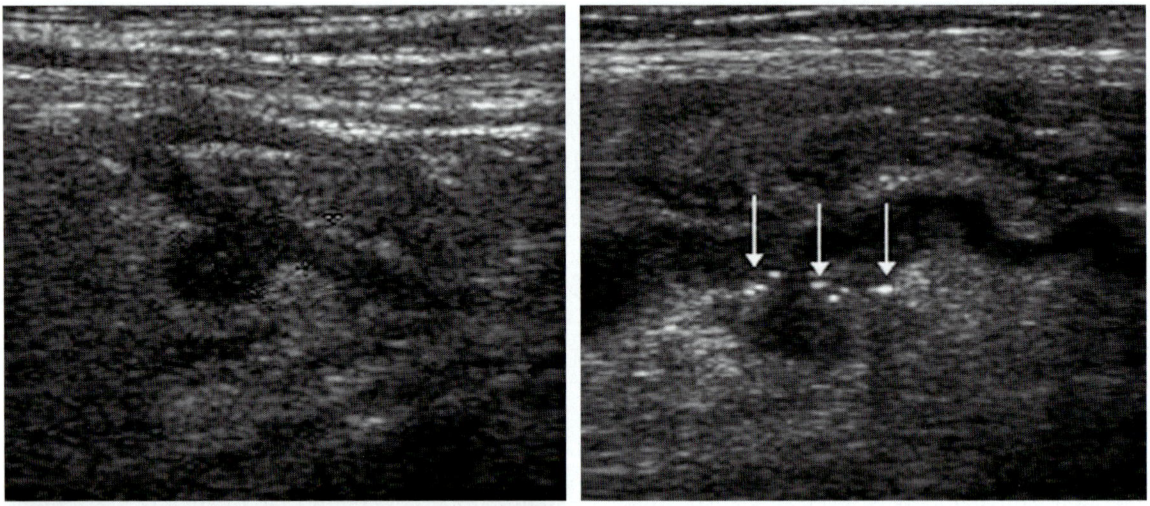

**Fig. 3.6a–c.** Acute colonic diverticulitis. **a** Hypoechoic diverticulum with a surrounding moderate echogenic inflammation. **b** Longitudinal section of the sigmoid colon shows an echo-poor diverticulum with surrounding little air spots (*arrows*) as a sign of microperforation. **c** Extensive inflammatory thickening of the sigmoid colon with an echogenic faecolith in the diverticulum

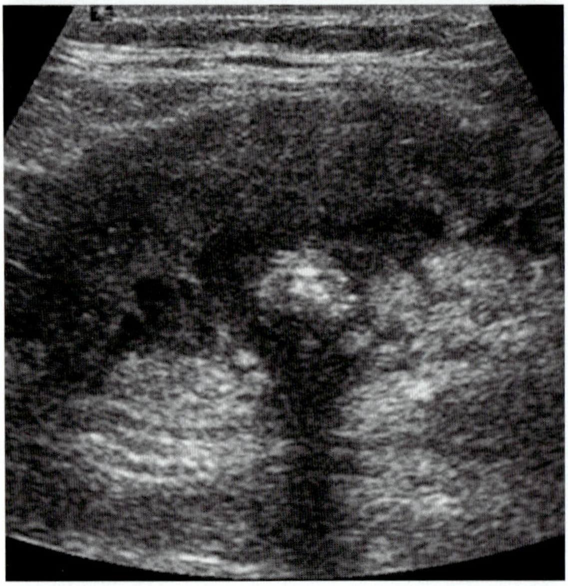

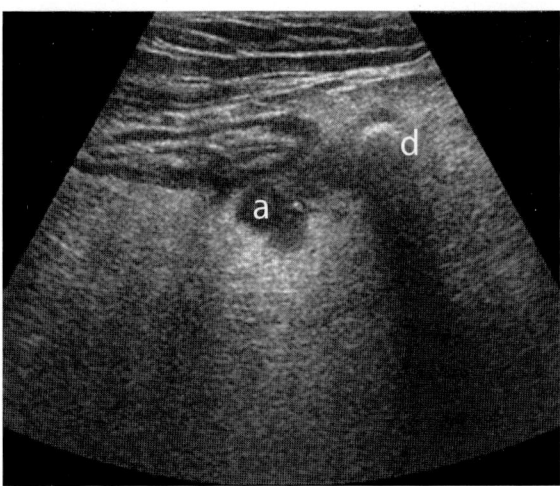

Fig. 3.7. Echoic diverticulum (*d*) with a nearby small peridiverticular hypoechogenic abscess (*a*)

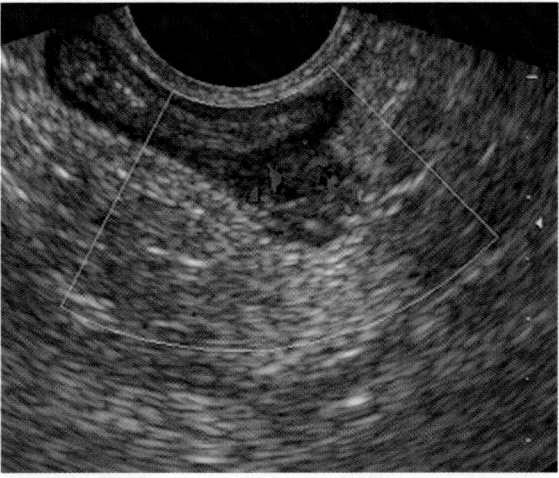

Fig. 3.8. Transrectal scan with 7.5-MHz probe shows a hypoechogenic diverticulum with moderate hypervascularisation and hyperechogenicity of the fat due to moderate inflammation

is frequently obscured by overlaying bowel-loop gas in transabdominal sonography.

Right-sided diverticulitis may be diagnosed sonographically (Fig. 3.9; WADA et al. 1990). Usually, large diverticula are present. In such instances, the main differential diagnosis is appendicitis. The prognosis of right-sided diverticulitis is usually good using conservative treatment. In this context, imaging procedures are important in the differential diagnosis.

At most hospitals, CT has replaced barium enema examination of the colon for diagnosis of suspected diverticulitis. Compared with sonography, the operator dependency is less (AMBROSETTI et al. 1997). One of the reasons is that diverticulitis is primarily an extramural process, and barium enema diagnosis depends on the secondary effects on the barium column caused by the extramucosal manifestations of acute inflammation.

The signs of a moderate diverticulitis in CT are colonic wall thickness >5 mm associated with inflammation of the pericolonic fat (fat stranding). In cases of a pericolonic abscess or other complications, CT should be performed to evaluate the correct extensions of the inflammatory variances.

Intravenous contrast should be given especially when an associated abscess is suspected (Fig. 3.10; BRENGMAN and OTCHY 1998). Care must be taken with interpretation of the results. The patients with colonic carcinoma often have findings similar to those of diverticulitis with conventional CT criteria

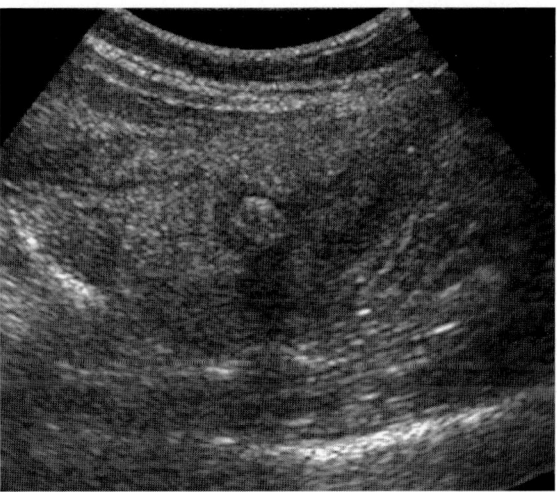

Fig. 3.9. Right-sided diverticulitis. An echogenic diverticulum with surrounding hyperechogenic fat is visualised

such as wall thickening with pericolonic fat involvement (AMBROSETTI et al. 1997). Also with CT the specificity increases when a diverticulum can be found in the inflammatory process. In chronic diverticulitis the degree of stenosis of the colonic lumen can be visualised better with CT.

Bleeding of diverticula is usually difficult to localise by imaging. Angiography may be indicated. Nuclear medicine studies may be performed to localise unclear intestinal bleeding. When diverticulits is suspected clinically, endoscopy is contraindicated. After the acute phase of inflammation, the colon should

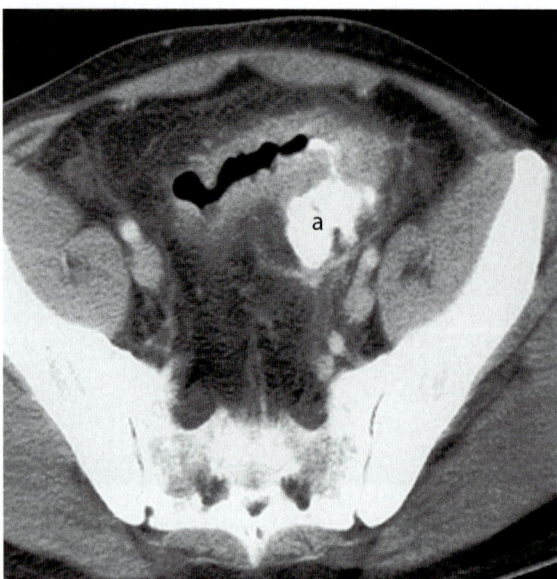

**Fig. 3.10.** A CT scan of a large perisigmoid abscess filled with contrast media (*a*)

be examined to exclude a colon carcinoma. So a complete colonic evaluation should generally performed 6–8 weeks after the resolution of a diverticulitis. In cases of inflammation, coloscopy is often incomplete and painful for the patient. The risk for perforation is also higher because of the air insufflation.

### 3.3.1
### Differential Diagnosis

The differential diagnosis of acute diverticulitis is wide (Gritzmann et al. 2002). One important reason for left lower quadrant pain can be a torsion or necrosis of appendices epiploicae of the left colon. A well-defined point of pain is typical, and is the effect of a local peritonitis.

At sonography the torsion appears as hyperechoic fatty ovoid appendices beside the colon wall. Often these lesions are adherent to the peritoneum.

Any form of colitis, such as pseudomembranous, acute ulcerative colitis or Crohn's colitis can also mimic diverticulitis. Usually, pseudomembranous colitis is associated with antibiotic therapy. In most cases a significant thickening of the colon is found.

Crohn's disease may present with abdominal pain, fever and leucocytosis. Fistulas can complicate both diseases. Apthous ulcers, anorectal involvement and chronic diarrhoea should alert the clinician to this possible diagnosis.

Usually, segmental transmural thickening of the colon and/or the small bowel is seen sonographically. A sub-ileus may be seen.

Colon carcinoma and diverticulitis both affect mainly the distal colon of aging patients in Western countries; both can present with perforation, obstruction or fistula formation. Differentiation obviously has critical prognostic importance. Chronic symptoms of weight loss or bleeding should raise suspicion for carcinoma. In carcinomas usually a circumscribed thickening of the colon is seen. In some cases it is not possible to differentiate diverticulitis from a perforated tumour by imaging methods.

Elderly people with diverticulosis may also have diffuse atherosclerotic vascular disease and thus are also at risk for ischaemic colitis. Ischaemic colitis is found frequently on the left side. Often the thickening is sharp bordered to the normal colon. A thickening with diminished vascularisation is highly suspicious for ischaemic colitis; however, colour signals in a thickened bowel loop do not exclude ischaemia, since non-occlusive ischaemia may be present.

Gynaecological disorders, such as ruptured ovarian cysts, ovarian torsion, ectopic pregnancy or pelvic inflammatory disease, can resemble acute diverticulitis in female patients, but often these patients are younger. Transvaginal sonography may be helpful in obtaining an accurate diagnosis. Stone of the ureter on the left side may simulate diverticulitis.

## 3.4
## Conclusion

Sonography can diagnose diverticulosis with an accuracy of approximately 60%. Most diverticula present as echogenic protrusions in some cases they are hypoechogenic. In most cases, diverticulitis sonographically presents as peridiverticular inflammation. Often microperforations are present. The peridiverticular inflammation of the fat is primarily hyperechogenic, and in advanced cases is hypoechogenic.

Performed by an experienced investigator, sonography shows results comparable to those of CT in diagnosing acute diverticulitis, and an accuracy of more than 90% can be reached. If complications, such as abscess formation or fistulas, are suspected, CT should be performed. In distal sigmoid localisation, transrectal examination provides high-resolution images with a high specificity.

# References

Almy TP, Howell DA (1980) Diverticular disease of the colon. N Engl J Med 302:324–331

Ambrosetti P, Grossholz M, Becker C et al (1997) Computed tomography in acute left colonic diverticulitis. Br J Surg 84:532–534

Brengman ML, Otchy DP (1998) Timing of computed tomography in acute diverticulitis. Dis Colon Rectum 41:1023–1028

Burkitt DP, Walker ARP, Painter NS (1974) Dietary fiber and disease. J Am Med Assoc 229:1068–1074

Chappuis CW, Cohn I (1988) Acute colonic diverticulitis. Surg Clin North Am 68:301–313

Cheskin LJ, Bohlman M, Schuster MM (1990) Diverticular disease in the elderly. Gastroenterol Clin North Am 19:391–403

Farag Soliman M, Wustner M et al (2004) Primary diagnostics of acute diverticulitis of the sigmoid. Sonography versus computed tomography: a prospective study. Ultraschall Med 25:342–347

Gritzmann N, Hollerweger A, Macheiner P, Rettenbacher T (2002) Transabdominal sonography of the gastrointestinal tract. Eur Radiol 12:1748–1761

Hollerweger A, Rettenbacher T, Macheiner P et al (2000) Sigmoid diverticulitis: value of transrectal sonography in addition to transabdominal sonography. Am J Roentgenol 175:1155–1160

Hollerweger A, Macheiner P, Rettenbacher T et al (2001) Colonic diverticulitis: diagnostic value and appearance of inflamed diverticula: sonographic evaluation. Eur Radiol 11:1956–1963

Hollerweger A, Macheiner P, Hubner E et al (2002) Colonic diverticulosis: a comparison between sonography and endoscopy. Ultraschall Med 23:41–46

Levi DM, Levi JU, Roger AL et al (1993) Giant colonic diverticulum: an unusual manifestation of a common disease. Am J Gastroenterol 88:139–142

Roberts PL, Veidernheimer MC (1994) Current management of diverticulitis. Adv Surg 27:189–208

Roberts PL, Abel M, Rosen L et al (1995) Practice parameters for sigmoid diverticulitis: supporting documentation. Dis Colon Rectum 38:126–132

Truelove SC (1966) Movements of the large intestine. Physiol Rev 46:457–512

Wada M, Kikuchi Y, Doy M (1990) Uncomplicated acute diverticulitis of the cecum and ascending colon. Sonographic findings in 18 patients. Am J Roentgenol 155:283–287

Wilson SR, Toi A (1990) The value of sonography in the diagnosis of acute diverticulitis of the colon. Am J Roentgenol 154:1199–1202

# Intestinal Obstruction

Jae Hoon Lim

CONTENTS

4.1 Introduction 27
4.2 Pathology of Bowel Obstruction 27
4.3 Small Bowel Obstruction 28
4.4 Colon Obstruction 32
4.5 Paralytic Ileus 32
References 34

## 4.1
## Introduction

The diagnosis of bowel obstruction used to be made by means of clinical history, physical examination, and plain abdominal radiography; however, abdominal radiographs are not confirmatory or are even confusing, and the cause of obstruction is rarely detected. For the management issue of whether to initiate immediate surgical intervention or to recommend a trial of conservative management, it is mandatory to identify the cause of bowel obstruction. Barium studies are not always satisfactory (Herlinger and Maglinte 1989; Mucha 1987; Dunn et al. 1984). Computed tomography (CT) has been shown to be useful in revealing the level and cause of obstruction (Megibow et al. 1991; Taourel et al. 1995), and recently, multidetector CT scanning has been proven to be very useful (Sinha and Verma 2005a; Sinha and Verma 2005b). Furthermore, multiplanar reformatted imaging may help identify the site, level, and cause of obstruction, and to increase diagnostic confidence (Furukawa et al. 2001) when axial CT findings are indeterminate; therefore, multidetector CT is becoming the first-line diagnostic method in the diagnosis of bowel obstruction (Patak et al. 2005).

Sonography is not considered helpful in most patients with intestinal obstruction. This is easily appreciated if one remembers that the presence of abundant gas in the intestinal tract prevents satisfactory examination of the abdomen, and that adhesions, the most common cause of intestinal obstruction, are not visible on a sonogram (Wilson 1991); however, when the obstructed bowel segments are dilated and filled with fluid, the dilated segments of the bowel loops are well demonstrated and the cause of obstruction can be demonstrated by sonography using the fluid-filled bowel as a sonic window (Fig. 4.1). Judicious use of sonography in evaluating patients with bowel obstruction may be helpful in confirming the presence of obstruction, in determining the level of obstruction, and in identifying of the cause of obstruction (Ko et al. 1993a).

The use of sonography in the era of multi-detector CT scanning is controversial. A CT diagnosis of intestinal obstruction has a decided advantage in terms of accuracy in diagnosis of bowel obstruction and in demonstration of the cause. Furthermore, interpretation of multi-detector CT images is not as operator dependent as sonography; however, sonography is much more widely available than multi-detector CT, much cheaper, and there is no radiation hazard; therefore, sonographic examination may be attempted in patients with normal plain radiographs or gasless abdomen, suspected obstruction in proximal bowel loops, in children, or in pregnant women (Ko et al. 1993b).

## 4.2
## Pathology of Bowel Obstruction

Bowel obstruction is characterized by dilatation of the intestinal segments proximal to the site of obstruction and collapse of the segment distal to the obstruc-

---

J. H. Lim, MD
Department of Radiology and Center for Imaging Science, Samsung Medical Center, Sungkyunkwan University School of Medicine, 50 Ilwon-dong, Kangnam-ku, Seoul 135-710, Korea

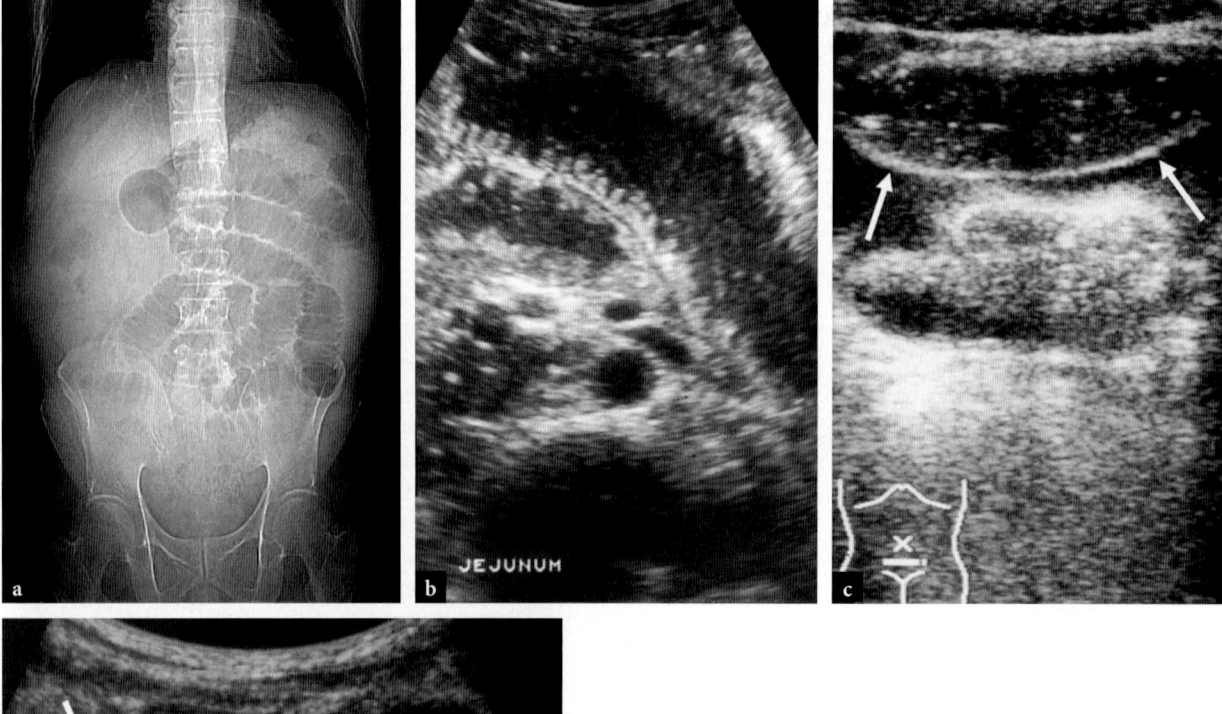

**Fig. 4.1a–d.** Ileal obstruction due to stromal tumor. **a** Abdominal radiograph in supine position shows multiple dilated jejunal loops filled with gas. Dilated ileal loops are not visible because they are filled with fluid. These fluid-filled bowel loops are a good acoustic window through which the dilated bowel loops and the cause of obstruction can be visualized. **b** Sonogram of the jejunum shows dilatation with markedly increased peristalsis, the fluid and tiny gas bubbles moving actively in the dilated bowel lumen. Note thick and compact valvulae conniventes. **c** Sonogram of the ileum shows dilatation with increased peristalsis. Note virtually absent valvulae conniventes (*arrows*). **d** Sonogram of the lower abdomen discloses a lobulated tumor (*short arrows*) arising from the ileum. Note dilated ileal loops (*long arrows*)

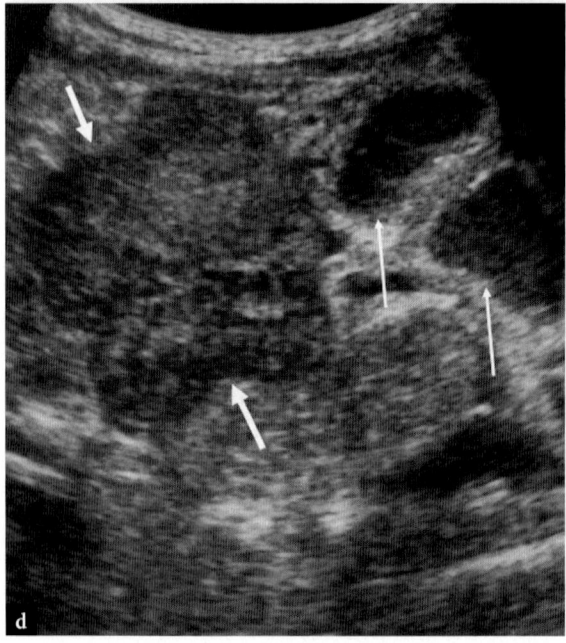

tion. The dilated bowel contains a large amount of fluid, food stuff, or gas. There is increased peristalsis to attempt to pass the luminal content beyond the obstruction site. Bowel obstruction can be due to obturation by blockage of the lumen by bowel content, such as food stuff, bezoar, or gallstone, due to bowel wall abnormality, such as neoplasm or stenosis, and due to extrinsic causes, such as adhesion and hernia. In paralytic ileus, the bowel is dilated and filled with fluid and gas, but there is no peristaltic movement.

## 4.3
## Small Bowel Obstruction

Characteristic sonographic findings of small bowel obstruction is demonstration of dilated bowel loops with active peristalsis (Ko et al. 1993a). Multiple segments of dilated bowel loops can be readily demonstrated when the lumen is filled with fluid. The fluid may be clear or there may be air bubbles or debris. The dilated loops are continuous, the diameter of the bowel lumen being over 2.0 cm and the segments being longer than 10 cm. Valvulae conniventes, or intestinal folds, are prominent and compact along the jejunum and are thin and sparse along the ileum (Fig. 4.1). Sometimes, there is no valvulae conniventes in the distal ileum and the bowel wall is flat. Increased peristalsis of the proximal segment of the bowel can be directly observed. The dilated bowel loop changes in caliber as well as in position, very vigorously, sometimes with some pauses. The fluid and tiny gas bubbles in the involved bowel show to-and-fro or whirling motion (Fig. 4.2). When the lumen is filled with gas, bowel dilatation is not easily recognized and it is difficult to make a diagnosis of bowel obstruction with sonography (Fig. 4.3). Usually, the bowel contains both fluid and gas. Sonographer should try to avoid gas filled lumen by pressing the abdomen with the transducer or change the position of the patient.

The causes of bowel obstruction can be demonstrated (Ko et al. 1993a). Small bowel bezoar is usually caused by persimmons and orange, sometimes by cabbage, sauerkraut, potato peel, or grapefruit.

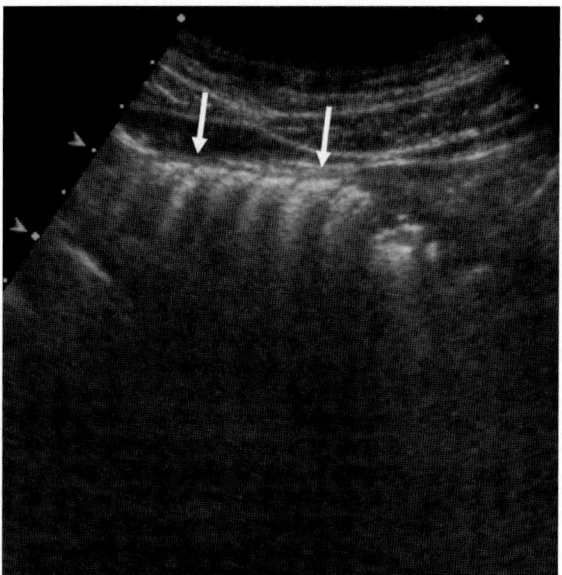

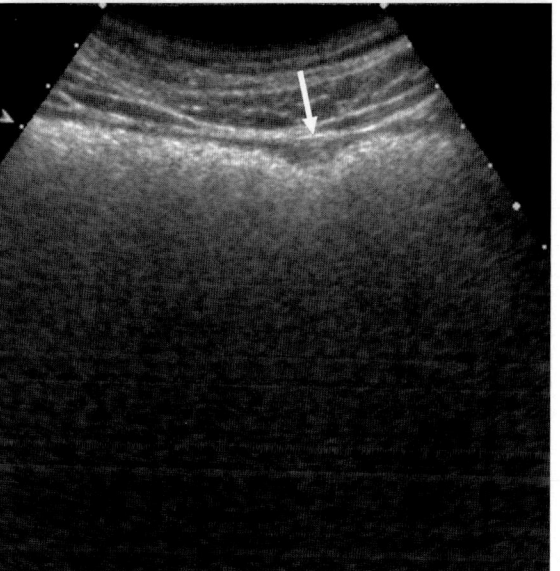

**Fig. 4.3a,b.** Gas-filled distended bowel loops. **a** Sonogram of the gas-filled jejunum shows air trapping in the valvulae conniventes (*arrows*). **b** Sagittal sonogram along the right side of the abdomen shows gas-filled, distended ascending colon. Note a haustral indentation (*arrow*)

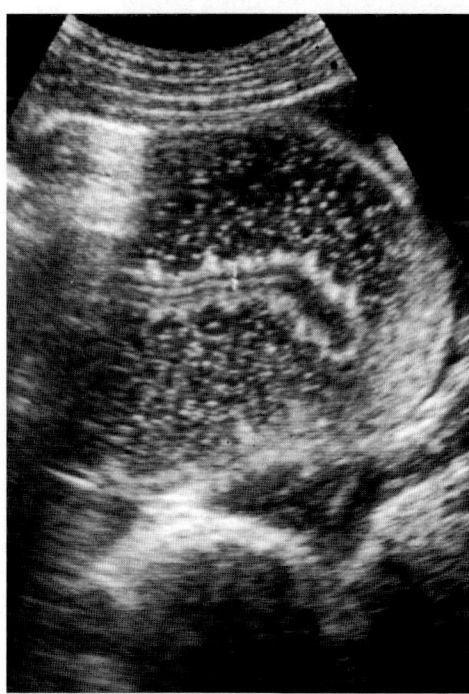

**Fig. 4.2.** Increased peristalsis. Sonogram of the jejunum shows dilated loop with increased peristalsis. The dilated loop shows vigorous change in caliber and position. Tiny gas bubbles in the lumen show to-and-fro and whirling motion

Patients who have had subtotal gastrectomy or gastrojejunostomy are prone to develop bezoars.

Sonographically, bezoars are seen as an intraluminal mass with a hyperechoic arc-like surface casting a clear posterior acoustic shadow (Fig. 4.4; Ko et al. 1993b; TENNENHOUSE and WILSON 1990). Phytobezoar or trichbezoar are the same in sonographic appearances. The obstructed small bowel loops usually contain a large amount of air and bezoars can be overlooked if sonographic examination is not per-

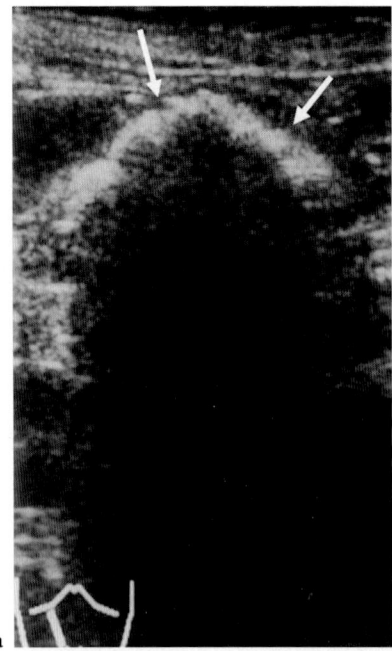 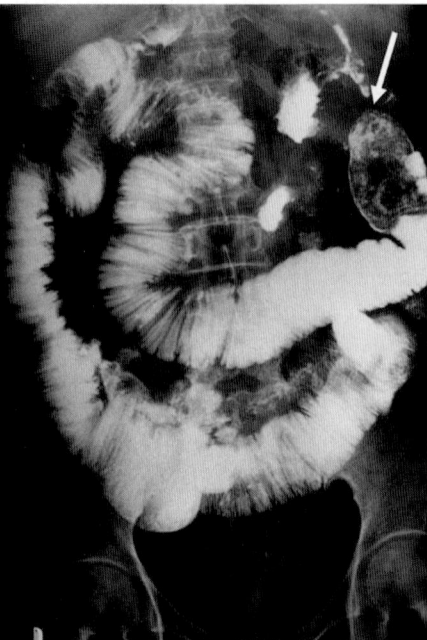

**Fig. 4.4a,b.** Phytobezoar in the jejunum. **a** Sonogram of upper abdomen shows hyperechoic, arc-like echo with clear acoustic shadow within a loop of the jejunum (*arrows*). Bowel loops proximal to the bezoar are dilated and filled with fluid. **b** Small bowel follow-through examination shows a large intraluminal filling defect at the end of the dilated jejunum, representing bezoar (*arrow*)

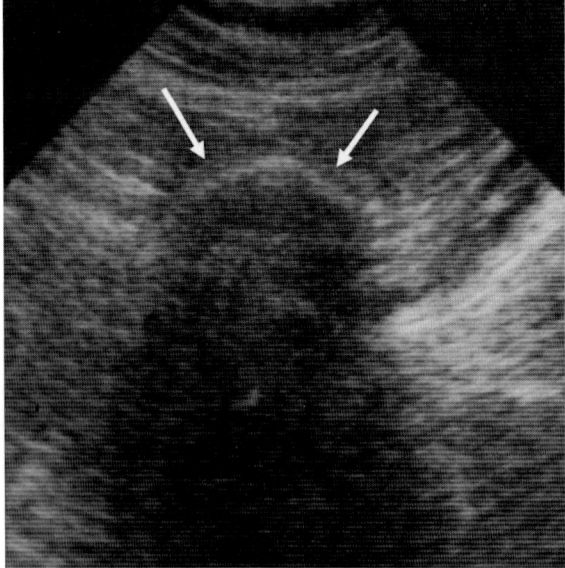 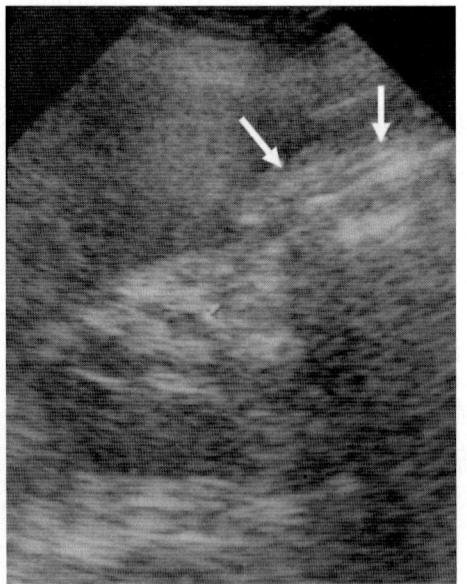

**Fig. 4.5a,b.** Gallstone ileus. **a** Sonogram shows hyperechoic arc-like echo with posterior acoustic shadow within a dilated loop of ileum, representing a large gallstone (*arrows*). **b** Sonogram of the right upper abdomen discloses the gallbladder, which is empty (*arrows*)

formed meticulously. Sonographic findings of gallstone ileus are identical to those of bezoars (Fig. 4.5; Ko et al. 1993a; Davir et al. 1991). Air in the biliary tree or nonvisualization of the gallbladder lumen may be a clue for gallstone ileus.

Small bowel tumor, either primary or metastatic, can be identified as a cause of bowel obstruction (Ko et al. 1993a). At the end of dilated small bowel or between the dilated bowel loops, a tumor can be identified when the tumor is fairly large (Fig. 4.1).

Fluid within the bowel may comes into direct contact with that the mass indicating the mass arises from the bowel. There may be vascular structure in the mass visualized by Doppler study. Small bowel intussusception can be diagnosed by demonstration of bowel-within-bowel by recognizing characteristic multiple concentric rings, caused by invaginating layers of telescoped bowel, seen in cross section of the bowel loop.

Intestinal adhesion, the most frequent cause of bowel obstruction, cannot be demonstrated on sonography. Likewise, internal hernia and congenital fibrotic band can rarely be identified at sonography. Previous history of abdominal operation in patients without a sonographically visible cause of obstruction can lead to a diagnosis of adhesive ileus.

By virtue of demonstrating the vascular flow signal from the vessels of the dilated bowel wall, sonography may be useful in demonstrating the bowel segment at risk of strangulation. The sonographic finding of a thickened bowel wall, valvulae conniventes, and localized ascites within the leaves of the small bowel mesentery, is suggestive of complicated obstruction such as infarction or gangrene, and these cases require rapid surgical decompression (Ko et al. 1993a).

It has been reported that the accuracy of preoperative sonography in establishing the diagnosis of small bowel obstruction was 89% (Ko et al. 1993a). The cause of obstruction, such as tumor, bezoar, gallstone, or recurrent cancer in afferent loop syndrome may be predicted (Ko et al. 1993a; MEISER and MEISSNER 1985). Sonography has definite advantages in the diagnosis of proximal obstruction, such as duodenal or proximal jejunal obstruction (Ko et al. 1993a): in these cases, simple abdominal radiographs are often normal or do not show gas, because frequent vomiting results in lack of air in the obstructed segment (Fig. 4.6). Afferent loop syndrome can be reliably diagnosed with sonography (LEE et al. 1991). The superior mesenteric artery and vein are useful landmarks in the diagnosis of duodenal obstruction such as afferent loop or proximal jejunal obstruction, since the dilated lumen of the third portion of the duodenum crosses the midline anterior to the aorta and behind the superior mesenteric artery and vein (Fig. 4.7). By careful examination, recurrent tumor at the gastric stump as a cause of afferent loop can be diagnosed sonographically (LEE et al. 1991).

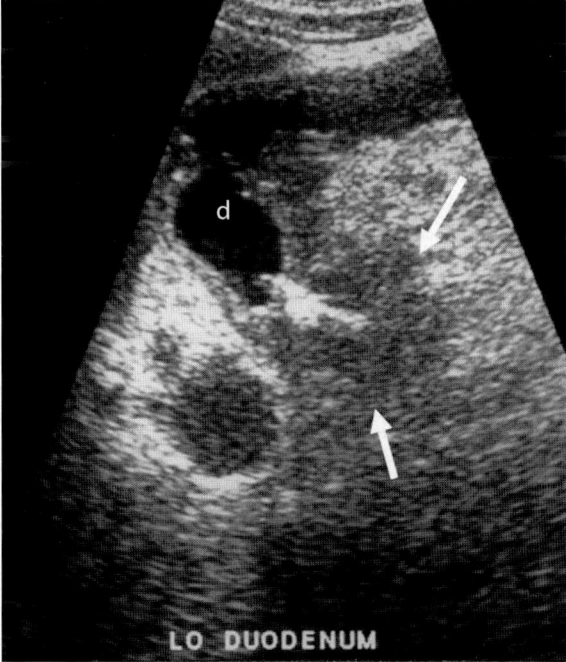
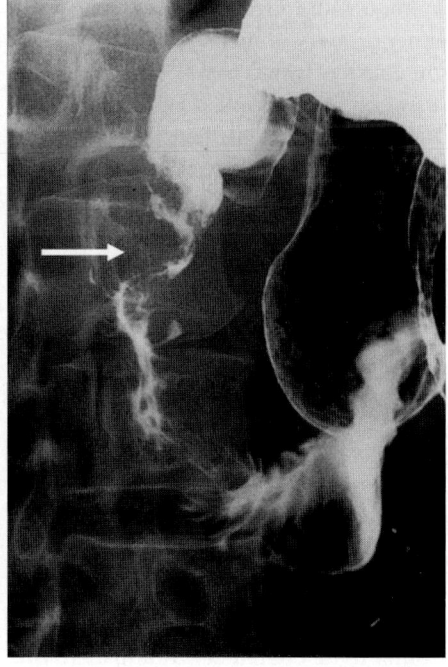

**Fig. 4.6a,b.** Duodenal obstruction by adenocarcinoma. **a** Sagittal sonogram of the right upper abdomen discloses a mass (*arrows*) with dilated first part of the duodenum (*d*). **b** Upper gastrointestinal series shows near-complete obstruction by adenocarcinoma (*arrows*)

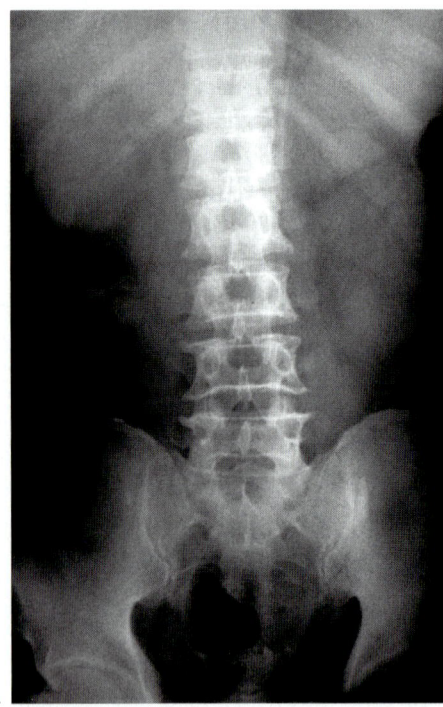
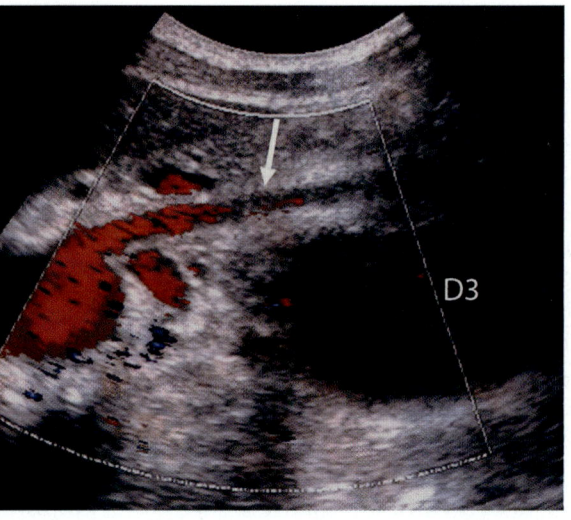

**Fig. 4.7a,b.** Afferent loop syndrome. **a** Supine abdominal radiograph shows virtually absent bowel gas because of frequent vomiting. **b** Sagittal color Doppler sonogram of the upper abdomen shows the dilated third part of the duodenum (*D3*) anterior to the abdominal aorta and posterior to the superior mesenteric artery (*arrows*)

## 4.4
## Colon Obstruction

The most common cause of colonic obstruction is carcinoma, either primary or metastatic, whereas the most common cause of small bowel obstruction is adhesions; therefore, it is necessary to differentiate colonic obstruction from small bowel obstruction. Radiographs of the abdomen may be useful for the diagnosis of colonic obstruction in 60–70% of cases (Gore and Eisenberg 1994). Once colonic obstruction is suspected, contrast enema, is indicated to confirm the obstruction and to determine its level, severity, and cause (Amberg 1994). In the CT era, multidetector row CT examination is the best method for the evaluation of patients with acute abdomen including colon obstruction (Sinha and Verma 2005b; Patak et al. 2005).

Identification of the colon with sonography is relatively difficult because the colon is filled with gas and feces, rather than fluid. As gas and feces are present in various amounts in the normal colon, the diagnosis of obstruction can be made only when the colon is found to be dilated continuously to the level of the lesion (see Fig. 4.3), where abnormal distension ends abruptly, with the colon distal to it free of gas (Wilson 1994). Since the colon is fixed in position, each segment of colon is identified by position.

The causes of colon obstruction can be identified (Kojima et al. 1992). It has been reported that sonography predicted the cause of colon obstruction in 81% (Lim et al. 1994). As the majority of colon obstructions are due to colon cancer or ileocecal intussusception, sonography may reveal an obstructing mass or segmental thickening of the colon wall at the end of the dilated colon (Fig. 4.8; Ko et al. 1993a), or characteristic concentric rings along the sausage-like, invaginated bowel loops in intussusception (Weissberg et al. 1977). Sometimes, a soft tissue mass as a leading point of intussusception can be demonstrated (Fig. 4.9). Sonography is particularly useful in child intussusception (Woo et al. 1992; Verschelden et al. 1992).

## 4.5
## Paralytic Ileus

Paralytic ileus can be reliably diagnosed by sonography by demonstrating very quilt or aperistaltic dilated bowel loops (Fig. 4.10). When the bowel loops are filled with more gas than fluid, sonography may

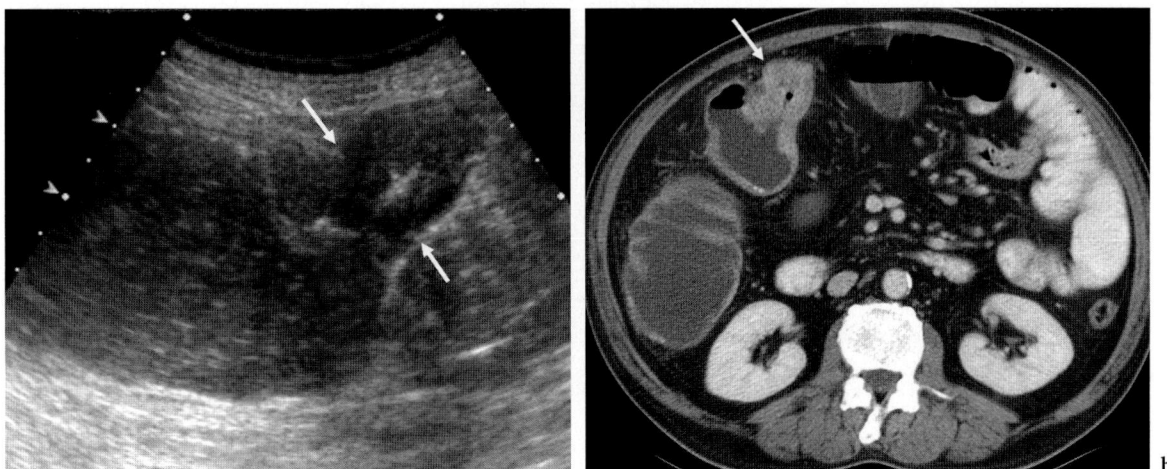

**Fig. 4.8a,b.** Transverse colon obstruction due to adenocarcinoma. **a** Transverse sonogram of the right upper abdomen discloses circumferential thickening of the wall of the transverse colon (*arrows*) and fluid-filled dilated proximal colon. **b** CT image shows encircling thickening of the wall of the transverse colon (*arrow*) due to adenocarcinoma and dilated ascending and transverse colon

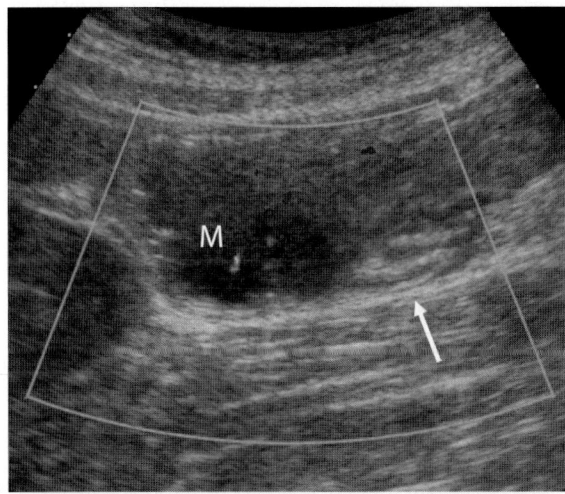

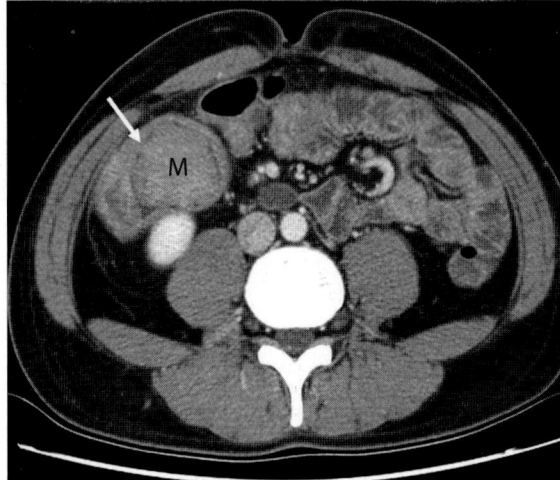

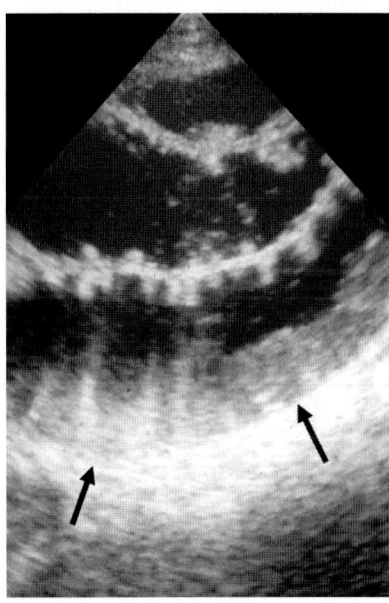

**Fig. 4.10.** Paralytic ileus. Sonogram of the lower abdomen shows dilated jejunum filled with fluid and debris. The dilated loops are essentially static and the bowel contents do not move. Note debris in the dependent part of the dilated loop (*arrows*), indicating no peristaltic movement

**Fig. 4.9a,b.** Ileocolic intussusception due to lymphoma. **a** Sagittal sonogram of the right abdomen shows an oval mass (*M*) in intussusception. Note folded bowel wall at the orifice of intussuscepted bowel (*arrow*). **b** CT image shows a round mass (*M*) surrounded by a thin line of fat invaginated into the ascending colon (*arrow*). Note slightly dilated jejunum and ileum

be of little value. Some difficulty may arise when the obstruction becomes prolonged and the obstructed segment becomes paralytic, and thus may be mistaken for paralytic ileus.

## References

Amberg JR (1994) Overview: the acute abdomen. In: Margulis AR, Burhenne HJ, (eds) Alimentary tract radiology, 5th edn. Mosby, St. Louis, pp 2118–2119

Davir RJ, Sandrasagra FA, Joseph AEA (1991) Ultrasound diagnosis of gallstone ileus. Clin Radiol 43:282–284

Dunn JT, Halls JM, Berne TV (1984) Roentgenographic contrast studies in acute small bowel obstruction. Arch Surg 119:1305–1308

Furukawa A, Yamasaki M, Furuichi K et al (2001) Helical CT in the diagnosis of small bowel obstruction. Radiographics 21:341–355

Gore RM, Eisenberg RL (1994) Large bowel obstruction. In: Gore RM, Levine MS, Laufer I (eds) Textbook of gastrointestinal radiology. Saunders, Philadelphia, pp 1247–1258

Herlinger H, Maglinte DDT (1989) Small bowel obstruction. In: Herlinger H, Maglinte DDT (eds) Clinical radiology of the small intestine. Philadelphia, Saunders, pp 479–509

Ko YT, Lim JH, Lee DH, Lee HW, Lim JW (1993a) Small bowel obstruction: sonographic evaluation. Radiology 188:649–653

Ko YT, Lim JH, Lee DH, Yoon Y (1993b) Small bowel phytobezoars: sonographic detection. Abdom Imaging 18:271–273

Kojima Y, Tsuchiyama T, Niimoto S, Nakagawara G (1992) Adult intussception caused by cecal cancer and diagnosed preoperatively by ultrasonography. J Clin Ultrasound 20:360–363

Lee DH, Lim JH, Ko YT (1991) Afferent loop syndrome: sonographic findings in seven cases. Am J Rogentgenol 157:41–43

Lim JH, Ko YT, Lee DH et al (1994) Determining the site and causes of colonic obstruction with sonography. Am J Roentgenol 163:1113–1117

Megibow AJ, Balthazar EJ, Cho KC, Medwid SW, Birnbaum BA, Noz ME (1991) Bowel obstruction: evaluation with CT. Radiology 180:313–318

Meiser G, Meissner K (1985) Sonographic differential diagnosis of intestinal obstruction: results of a prospective study of 48 patients. Ultraschall Med 6:39–45

Mucha P (1987) Small intestinal obstruction. Surg Clin North Am 67:597–620

Patak MA, Mortele KJ, Ros PR (2005) Multidetector row CT of the small bowel. Radiol Clin North Am 43:1063–1077

Sinha R, Verma R (2005a) Multidetector row computed tomography in bowel obstruction. Part 1. Small bowel obstruction. Clin Radiol 60:1058–1067

Sinha R, Verma R (2005b) Multidetector row computed tomography in bowel obstruction. Part 2. Large bowel obstruction. Clin Radiol 60:1068–1075

Taourel PG, Fabre JM, Pradel JA, Seneterre EJ, Megibow AJ, Bruel JM (1995) Value of CT in the diagnosis and management of patients with suspected acute small bowel obstruction. Am J Roentgenol 165:1187–1192

Tennenhouse JE, Wilson SR (1990) Sonographic detection of a small bowel bezoar. J Ultrasound Med 9:603–605

Verschelden P, Filiatrault D, Garel L et al (1992) Intussusception in children: reliability of US in diagnosis: a preoperative study. Radiology 184:741–744

Weissberg Dl, Scheible W, Leopold GR (1977) Ultrasonographic appearance of adult intussusception. Radiology 124:791–792

Wilson SR (1991) The gastrointestinal tract. In: Rumack CM, Wilson SR, Charboneau JW (eds) Diagnostic ultrasound. Mosby, St. Louis, pp 181–206

Wilson SR (1994) The acute abdomen of gastrointestinal tract origin: sonographic evaluation. In: Margulis AR, Burhenne HJ (eds) Alimentary tract radiology, 5th edn. Mosby, St. Louis, pp 2099–2117

Woo SK, Kim JS, Suh SJ, Paik TW, Choi SO (1992) Childhood intussusception: US-guided hydrostatic reduction. Radiology 182:77–80

# Abdominal Hernias, Volvulus and Intussusception

S. Boopathy Vijayaraghavan

CONTENTS

5.1 **Abdominal Hernias** 35
5.1.1 Inguinal Hernia 35
5.1.2 Femoral Hernia 37
5.1.3 Ventral Hernia 38
5.1.4 Spigelian Hernia 39
5.1.5 Richter's Hernia 39
5.1.6 Complications of Hernia 39
5.1.7 Postoperative Sonography 41
5.1.8 Internal Hernia 41
5.1.9 Diaphragmatic Hernia 43

5.2 **Small Bowel Volvulus** 44

5.3 **Gastric Volvulus** 46

5.4 **Caecal Volvulus** 47

5.5 **Intussusception** 48
5.5.1 Jejunogastric Intussusception 52

References 53

## 5.1 Abdominal Hernias

A hernia is the protrusion of an organ or tissue out of the body cavity in which it normally lies. Abdominal wall hernias are the most common type. They can be congenital or acquired. The aetiological factor may be increased intraabdominal pressure or abdominal weakness. Approximately 75% of all hernias occur in the inguinal region. Approximately 50% of hernias are indirect inguinal hernias, and 24% are direct inguinal hernias. Incisional and ventral hernias account for approximately 10% of all hernias, and femoral hernias for 3%. Unusual hernias account for the remaining 5–10%. The symptoms vary from a visible lump, local pain due to stretching, pain due to pull of the content and that of complications. The hernia may not be seen when the patient is at rest and may require a manoeuvre to make it visible. It can be Valsalva manoeuvre, cough or erect position. The role of sonography consists in the confirmation of the hernia, identification of contents, differentiation of the type, diagnosis of associated conditions and complications and postoperative follow-up.

### 5.1.1 Inguinal Hernia

Inguinal hernia is the most common abdominal hernia. There is bulging of abdominal contents into a defect in the inguinal canal in the lower abdomen. It is more common in males, in whom it can reach up to the scrotum. There are two types of inguinal hernia. In the more common indirect inguinal hernia, the protrusion is through a congenital weakness at the internal ring. In children, it is due to persistence of a patent peritoneal pocket: the persistent processus vaginalis in males and diverticulum of Nuck in females (SCHERER and GROSFELD 1993). In the direct type of inguinal hernia the contents push through a weak spot in the posterior wall of the inguinal canal. The inguinal canal lies between the superficial (external) and deep (internal) inguinal rings. The deep ring lies deep to the mid-inguinal point, which is halfway between the symphysis pubis and the anterior superior iliac spine. In males, the inguinal canal contains the spermatic cord with vas deferens and testicular vessels. In females it contains the suspensory ligament of the ovary (ANDO et al. 1997). Indirect hernia is lateral to the inferior epigastric vessels, whereas the direct one is medial to them.

Sonography of the inguinal region is done at rest and during Valsalva manoeuvre, cough and erect position. Inguinal hernia is diagnosed by the presence of bowel, omentum or other abdominal organs in the inguinal canal, with continuity within the abdomen (Fig. 5.1a; DATTOLA et al. 2002). The contents become

S. Boopathy Vijayaraghavan, MD, DMRD
SONOSCAN Ultrasonic Scan Centre, 15B, Venkatachalam Road, Coimbatore-641 002, Tamil Nadu, India

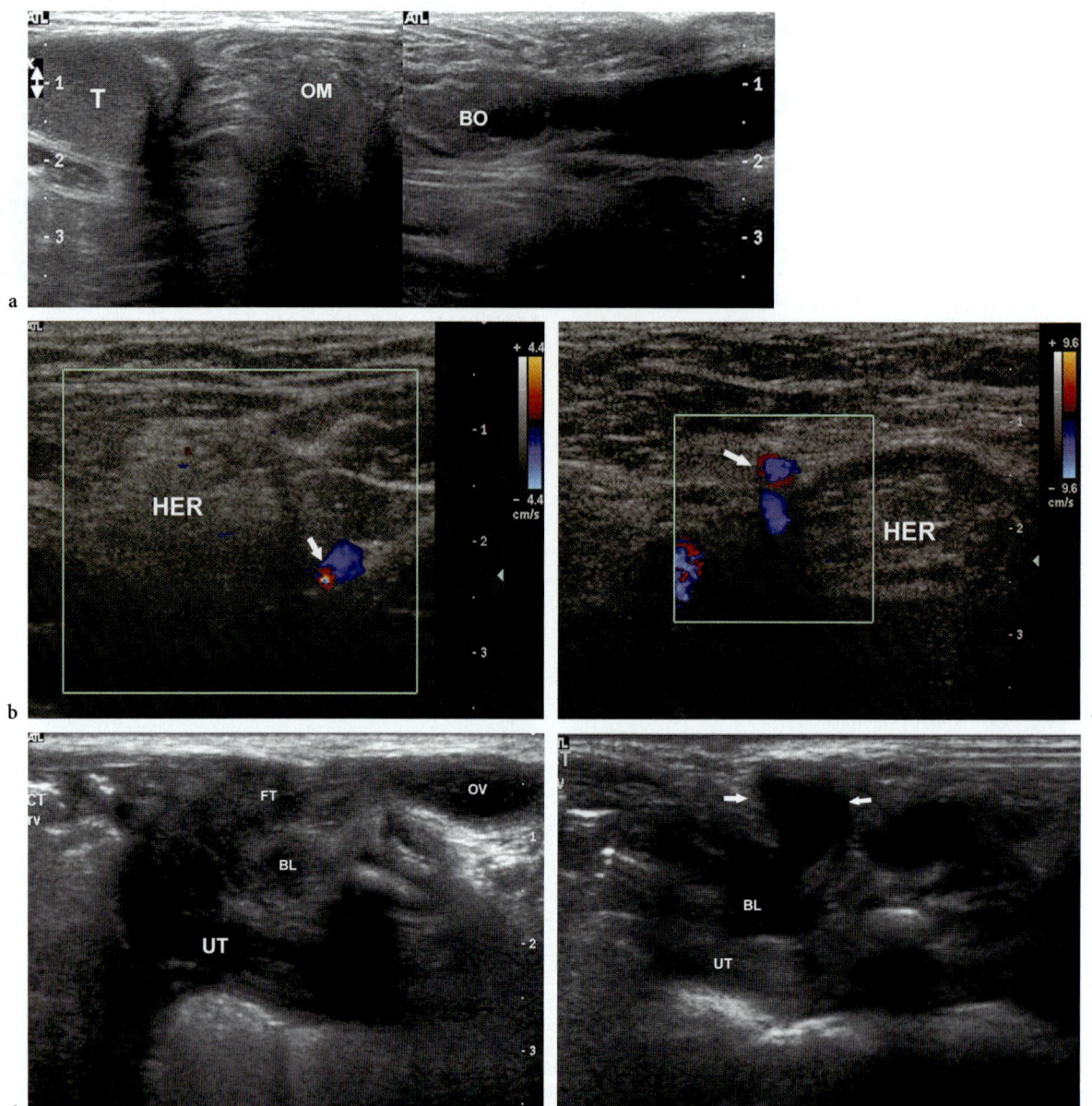

Fig. 5.1a–e. Inguinal hernia. a Oblique scan of inguinoscrotal region shows the inguinal hernia containing omentum (*OM*) and bowel (*BO*). The testis (*T*) is undescended and located in the inguinal canal. b Transverse scan of left inguinal region shows the hernial sac (*HER*) located medial to the inferior epigastric vessels (*arrow*) in direct inguinal hernia. c Indirect inguinal hernia (*HER*) on left side with the neck of sac located lateral to inferior epigastric vessels (*arrow*). d Oblique scan in a premature infant shows the inguinal hernia containing the fallopian tube (*FT*) and ovary (*OV*). e Oblique scan of an infant shows inguinal hernia containing part of the urinary bladder (*arrows*). *BL* urinary bladder, *UT* uterus

prominent when the patient strains, coughs or is in erect position. This feature differentiates the hernia from mimicking conditions such as hydrocele, varicocele and mass. The content of the hernia can be omentum and/or bowel. The omentum is recognized by its characteristic echogenic nature. The bowel is identified by the pattern produced by the contents and air. The small bowel shows peristalsis, whereas the colon lacks it. The bowel is also recognized by tracing it into the abdomen and the type of the bowel can be ascertained by continuity. Colour Doppler study helps to differentiate the direct from the indirect type of inguinal hernia. The neck of the direct inguinal hernia is medial to the inferior epigastric artery, whereas it is lateral to it in indirect inguinal hernia. Firstly, the external iliac artery is sought, and then, by tilting the transducer upward slightly, the inferior epigastric artery is identified. Using another Valsalva manoeuver, the relation between the hernial sac and the inferior epigastric artery is analysed. If the hernial sac appears medial to the inferior epigastric artery, a direct inguinal hernia is diagnosed (Fig. 5.1b). If it appears to be located laterally, an indirect hernia is assumed (Fig. 5.1c; KORENKOV et al. 1999; ZHANG et al. 2001).

The inguinal hernia can be associated with conditions such as hydrocele, varicocele or mass of the cord, like an encysted hydrocele or lipoma, which are readily diagnosed by sonography. In male children an indirect inguinal hernia may be associated with undescended testis. The testis may be lying by the side of the sac in the inguinal canal (Fig. 5.1a), or it may be intraabdominal. This information helps to avoid causing injury to the testis during surgery and to combine orchidopexy during repair. In females the inguinal hernia may contain ovary, fallopian tube, or rarely, the uterus, which are easily identified on sonography (Fig. 5.1d; HUANG et al. 2003). The hernia containing these organs is common in premature infants (GEORGE et al. 2000). Very rarely, the urinary bladder may form the content of a sliding type of inguinal hernia (Fig. 5.1e; CATALANO 1997).

## 5.1.2
## Femoral Hernia

Femoral hernia occurs through a space bounded superiorly by the iliopubic tract, inferiorly by the Cooper's ligament, laterally by the femoral vein and medially by the insertion of the iliopubic tract into Cooper's ligament. It is more common in females than in males. On examination it reveals a mass below the inguinal ligament. On sonography, the femoral hernia is seen posterior to the inguinal ligament and medial to the femoral vein, in contrast to the inguinal hernia, which is anterior to the inguinal ligament (Fig. 5.2; DEITCH and SONCRANT 1981; DATTOLA et al. 2002).

**Fig. 5.2a,b.** Incarcerated femoral hernia. **a** Transverse scan at the level of the femoral vessels of right side shows the neck of the sac containing omentum (*arrows*) medial to the femoral artery (*FA*). The femoral vein is not visualized, as it is compressed. **b** Longitudinal scan shows the echogenic omentum (*OM*) in the sac with fluid (*FL*) due to incarceration

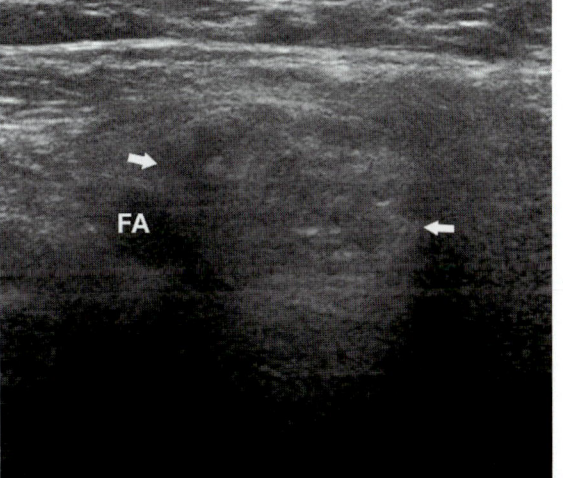

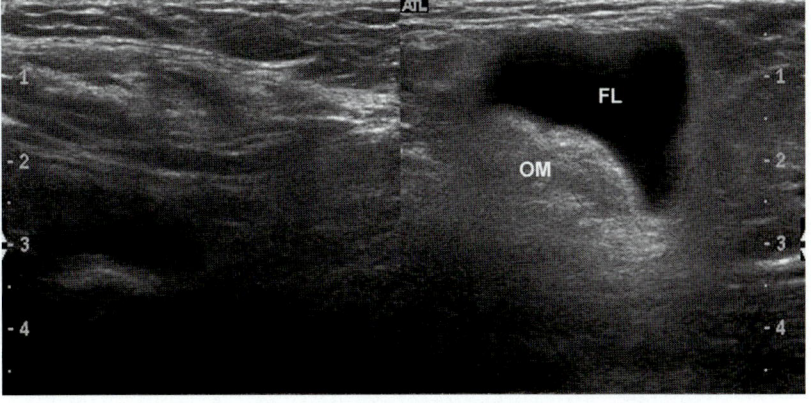

## 5.1.3
## Ventral Hernia

Ventral hernia covers all protrusions through anterior and anterolateral abdominal wall, excluding groin hernias. It is suggested by the patient's clinical history and is well seen on physical examination; however, the patient's history may be atypical and physical examination may be limited in obese patients, in patients with severe abdominal pain or distension, in small hernias or with hernias located in uncommon sites (SPANGEN 1975; MUFID et al. 1997). In certain clinical situations it may be necessary to relate the symptoms to the ventral hernia or, it may be necessary to know whether the ventral hernia is complicated or not. In these situations an imaging investigation becomes necessary. Sonography is a dynamic, non-invasive, easily available and low-cost modality useful in studying the ventral hernia. It is performed at rest and during a manoeuver such as Valsalva, cough or erect position. Sonographic diagnosis of ventral hernia is made when bowel or other abdominal organs or fatty tissue of the abdominal wall is seen protruding out of the abdomen with continuity within the abdomen (RETTENBACHER et al. 2001). The hernial orifice is seen as a defect in the fascia, which is seen as an echogenic line deep to the muscle layer and its location and width can be noted. Sonography reveals the contents, which can be omentum, bowel (Fig. 5.3a) or properitoneal fat (Fig. 5.3b).

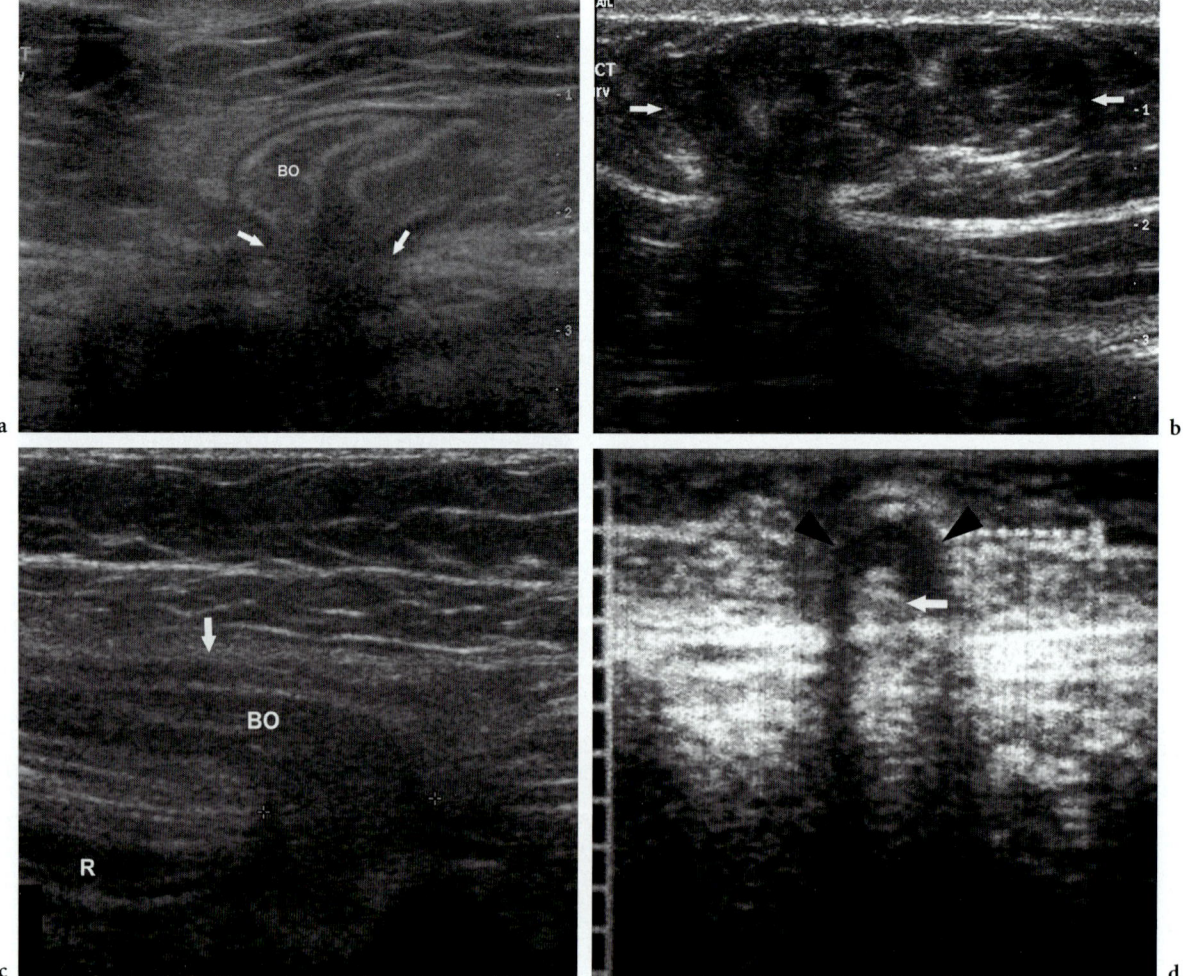

**Fig. 5.3. a** Scan of the anterior abdominal wall with Valsalva manoeuvre shows the ventral hernia containing the bowel loops (*BO*) and the defect in the fascia (*arrows*). **b** Fatty epigastric hernia with herniation of the properitoneal fat (*arrows*). **c** Spigelian hernia shows the defect marked by calipers lateral to the rectus muscle (*R*) and the contents (*BO*) limited anteriorly by the Spigelian fascia (*arrow*). **d** Richter's type umbilical hernia shows fluid-filled hernial sac (*arrowheads*) and irreducible herniation of only a part of the circumference of the bowel (*arrow*), which showed wriggling peristaltic movement in real time

Some ventral hernias are not seen at rest and are brought into view with only one of the manoeuvers. When the hernia is seen at rest, an attempt is made to slide the contents into the abdomen to know if the hernia is reducible. Sonography readily differentiates other conditions that mimic ventral hernia such as lipoma, metastasis, suture granuloma, abscess or endometriosis. Umbilical hernia is a type of ventral hernia that occurs through the weak umbilicus. Fatty epigastric hernia is protrusion of the properitoneal fat through a defect in the linea alba.

## 5.1.4
## Spigelian Hernia

Spigelian hernia is a rare type of ventral hernia in which the abdominal contents protrude through an area of weakness at the junction of linea semilunaris and linea semicircularis (SUTPHEN et al. 1980). The linea semilunaris is a vertical band-like groove that is formed by the union of the medial edges of the aponeuroses of the external oblique, internal oblique, and transverse abdominal muscles. In its upper 75%, the fused aponeurosis of these three muscles splits medially to form the anterior and posterior rectus sheaths. Midway between the umbilicus and symphysis pubis, the aponeurosis of the three lateral abdominal muscles passes medially to cover only the anterior surface of the rectus muscle, leaving the posterior surface of the lower fourth covered only by the transversalis fascia and peritoneum. The line forming the inferior margin of the rectus sheath is called the linea semicircularis. Also, at this level, the fiber bundles of the transverse abdominal and internal oblique muscles are much thinner and more widely spaced, causing further weakening through which omentum and small intestine could potentially protrude. Spigelian hernias occur with equal frequency in men and women and in every age group (MUFID et al. 1997). Spigelian hernias may not appear as distinct masses, making them difficult to diagnose clinically. This is because these hernias always dissect between the layers of the anterior abdominal wall, rather than in the subcutaneous tissues, as other ventral hernias do. Spigelian hernias have been mistaken for abdominal abscesses, seromas, haematomas, ovarian masses, pseudocysts, and malignant omental or peritoneal implants (WECHSLER et al. 1989).

On sonographic examination during the Valsalva manoeuver or erect position, intraabdominal contents, including bowel, mesentery and omentum, are seen to herniate through a defect in the lower quadrant abdominal wall in the space between the rectus muscle medially and the external and internal oblique muscles laterally. The hernia extends medially anterior to the rectus muscle (Fig. 5.3c). The Spigelian fascia, which prevents its extension into the subcutaneous tissue, limits it anteriorly (MUFID et al. 1997). These hernias are also associated with a higher risk of bowel incarceration and strangulation than other abdominal wall hernias.

## 5.1.5
## Richter's Hernia

In Richter's hernia, only part of the circumference of the bowel on the ante-mesenteric border protrudes into a hernia. It can occur with any type of abdominal wall hernia but is more common in femoral hernia. The symptoms and clinical course vary widely, depending on the degree of obstruction, or if strangulation is present. In strangulation, the patient presents with a painful mass, nausea and vomiting. In contrast to other types, there is no abdominal distension as there is no bowel obstruction. On sonography, complicated Richter's hernia is seen as a small segment of bowel showing wriggling movement in the neck of the hernial sac, which contains fluid (Fig. 5.3d). There are no dilated bowel loops in the abdomen (MIDDLEBROOK and EFTEKHARI 1992; HILLER et al. 1994).

## 5.1.6
## Complications of Hernia

The pattern of complications is common for all types of hernia. The complications are irreducibility, obstruction and strangulation. Irreducible (incarcerated) hernia may be due to a narrow neck or adhesion of contents to the sac wall. In obstruction, the intestine in the hernia gets obstructed due to a narrow neck, adhesion or volvulus, but it is viable. Strangulation results when there is compromise to venous drainage and later arterial supply of the contents. In obstructed hernia there is colicky pain, abdominal distension and vomiting. Incarcerated hernia is present at rest; it is irreducible and usually contains some fluid in the sac that can be seen on sonography (Fig. 5.2b; RETTENBACHER et al. 2001). In obstructed hernia the patient has symptoms of intestinal obstruction. There are dilated bowel loops in the abdomen which show active peristalsis. The appearance of the bowel in the hernial sac depends on whether the obstruction is to afferent or efferent loop in the sac. In the more common afferent loop obstruction, the bowel loops in hernial sac remain collapsed and there is transition between the dilated intraabdominal bowel loop and collapsed bowel loop in the hernia (Fig. 5.4a). In efferent loop obstruction, the bowel loop in the hernial sac is dilated. The transition is between dilated loop in hernial sac and collapsed loop in abdomen (Fig. 5.4b). The obstruction may be of closed loop type due to block of both the

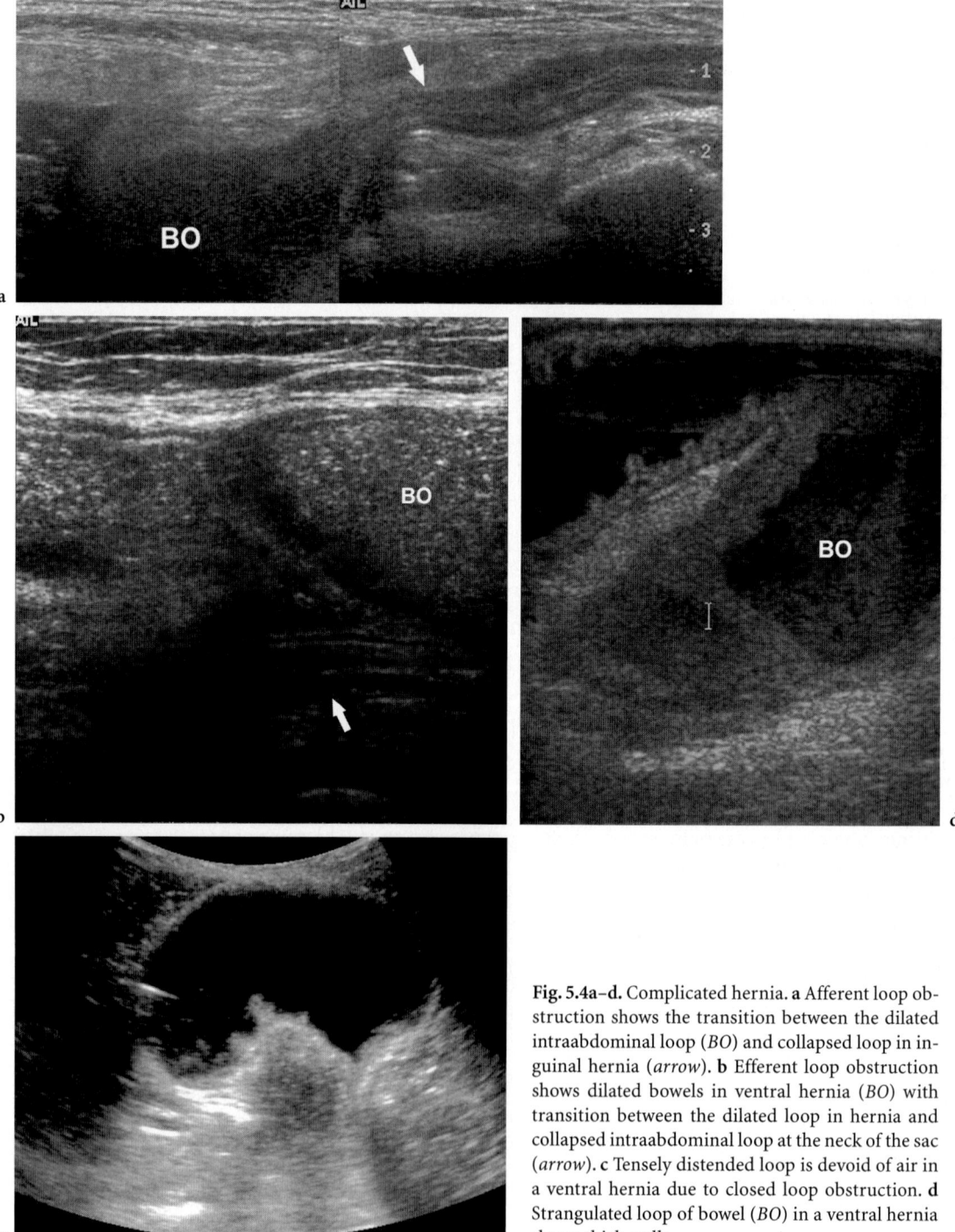

Fig. 5.4a–d. Complicated hernia. a Afferent loop obstruction shows the transition between the dilated intraabdominal loop (*BO*) and collapsed loop in inguinal hernia (*arrow*). b Efferent loop obstruction shows dilated bowels in ventral hernia (*BO*) with transition between the dilated loop in hernia and collapsed intraabdominal loop at the neck of the sac (*arrow*). c Tensely distended loop is devoid of air in a ventral hernia due to closed loop obstruction. d Strangulated loop of bowel (*BO*) in a ventral hernia shows thick walls

afferent and efferent loops at the neck of the hernia, or due to volvulus of the loop in the hernial sac. Here, the loop of bowel in hernial sac is disproportionately more dilated than proximal intraabdominal loops, it is tensely distended and may lack air in its lumen (Fig. 5.4c). The peristalsis is usually absent in this loop as it is tensely distended. In strangulation there is ischaemia of the contents of the hernia. The hernia is tender, with free fluid in the sac. The wall of the aperistaltic bowel is thickened (Fig. 5.4d). On colour Doppler study, no flow is seen in the omentum or bowel, which is strangulated (LIANG et al. 2001). In the case of the bowel, dilated loops of bowel are seen in the abdomen.

## 5.1.7
### Postoperative Sonography

Sonography is useful in postoperative follow-up of the patients with hernia. The prosthetic mesh can be seen as a brightly echogenic reticular line and curled prosthesis (Fig. 5.5a) or a displaced prosthesis can be recognized (PARRA et al. 2004; DATTOLA et al. 2002). Fluid collection (seroma or abscess) is well seen and its relation to prosthesis can be assessed (Fig. 5.5a). If necessary, the fluid can be aspirated under sonographic guidance (PARRA et al. 2004). Adhesion of bowel to the prosthesitic mesh is one of the complications that can lead to bowel obstruction. Sonography can reveal dilated loops and the bowel loop adherent to the mesh (Fig. 5.5b; FURTSCHEGGER et al. 1995). Recurrence of hernia can be confirmed and the location of defect in relation to the mesh can be known. In the case of inguinal hernia, the vascular supply to the testis can be assessed by colour Doppler study, and testicular ischaemia or infarction may be recognized (HOLLOWAY et al. 1998).

## 5.1.8
### Internal Hernia

Internal hernia involves protrusion of a viscus, usually the small bowel, through a normal or abnormal aperture within the peritoneal cavity. Internal hernias are rare, with reported incidence of 0.2–0.9% of autopsies (GHAHREMANI 1984). A substantial proportion of these remain asymptomatic. It is an uncommon cause of small bowel obstruction. About 4% of bowel obstruction is due to internal hernia (FELDMAN et al. 2002). Owing to the risk of strangulation of the contents of the hernia, even small internal hernias are dangerous and may be lethal. This hernia may be either congenital or acquired. Congenital internal hernias include paraduodenal, foramen of Winslow, mesenteric and supravesical hernias. During fetal development the mesentery of the duodenum, ascending colon, and descending colon becomes fixed to the posterior peritoneum. These segments of the bowel become retroperitoneal. Anomalies of mesenteric fixation may lead to abnormal openings through which internal hernias may occur. This is the likely mechanism of paraduodenal and supravesical hernias. Abnormal mesenteric fixation may lead to abnormal mobility of the small bowel and right

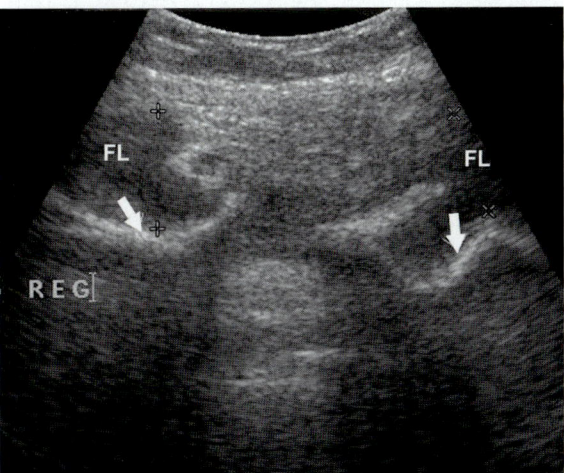
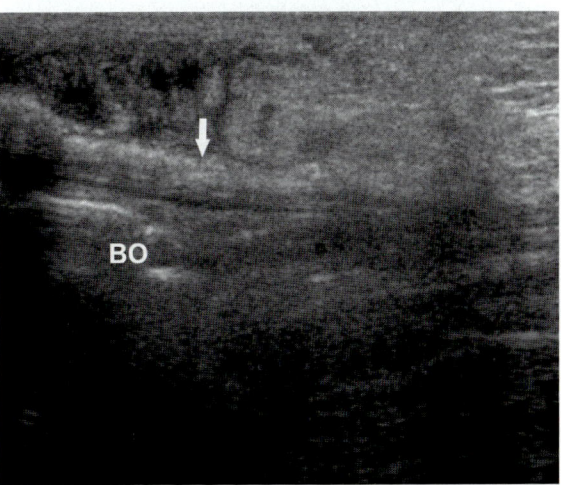

**Fig. 5.5a,b.** Scan of the abdominal wall after hernial repair shows the curled echogenic mesh (*arrows*) with collection of fluid (*FL*) anterior to it in **a**, and bowel (*BO*) adherent to the straight mesh (*arrow*) in **b**

colon, which facilitates herniation. During fetal development, abnormal openings may occur in the pericaecal, small bowel, transverse colon, or sigmoid mesentery, as well as in the omentum, leading to mesenteric hernias. In the case of left paraduodenal hernia, an abnormal foramen (fossa of Landzert) occurs through the mesentery close to the ligament of Treitz, leading under the distal transverse and descending colon and posterior to the superior mesenteric artery. The small bowel may protrude through this fossa. The mesentery of the colon thus forms the anterior wall of a sac enclosing a portion of the small intestine. Mesenteric hernias occur when a loop of intestine protrudes through an abnormal opening in the mesentery of the small bowel or the colon. The most common area for such an opening is in the mesentery of the small intestine, most often, near the ileocolic junction. Various lengths of intestine may herniate, posterior to the right colon, into the right paracolic gutter. Acquired internal hernias may occur as a complication of surgery, or trauma, if abnormal spaces or mesenteric defects are created. Compression of the loops in the internal hernia may lead to obstruction of the herniated intestine. Obstruction may be acute, chronic, or intermittent. Strangulation may occur by compression of vessels at the neck of the sac, or by torsion of the herniated segment. The herniated bowel may also compress arteries in the margins of the mesenteric defect, causing ischaemia of non-herniated intestine.

Any of the various forms of internal hernias may present with symptoms of acute or chronic intermittent intestinal obstruction. The diagnosis is difficult among patients with chronic symptoms and is rarely made preoperatively among patients who present with acute obstruction (GHAHREMANI 1984). About 50% of patients with paraduodenal hernias develop intestinal obstruction, which may be of low grade, chronic, and recurrent, or may be of high grade and acute (ZIMMERMAN and LAUFMAN 1953; NYHUS and CONDON 1989; PERSHAD et al. 1998). In acute bowel obstruction the patients present with colicky abdominal pain with vomiting. The features seen on sonography are: (a) small bowel obstruction, as evidenced by dilated hyperperistaltic loops; (b) zone of transition between dilated and non-dilated bowel; and (c) cluster of collapsed, crowded and compressed small bowel loops, as if enclosed in a bag (Fig. 5.6). This cluster of loops is seen away from the zone of transition: to the left in paraduodenal hernia and to the right in paracecal hernia. These are the features seen when the afferent loop entering the sac is obstructed because of crowding and compression of bowel loops in the sac. When there is obstruction to the efferent loop at the neck, the sac contains dilated loops of small bowel with the zone of transition at the neck of the sac (VIJAYARAGHAVAN 2005). The differential diagnosis for sonographic appearance of internal hernia is abdominal cocoon. In abdominal

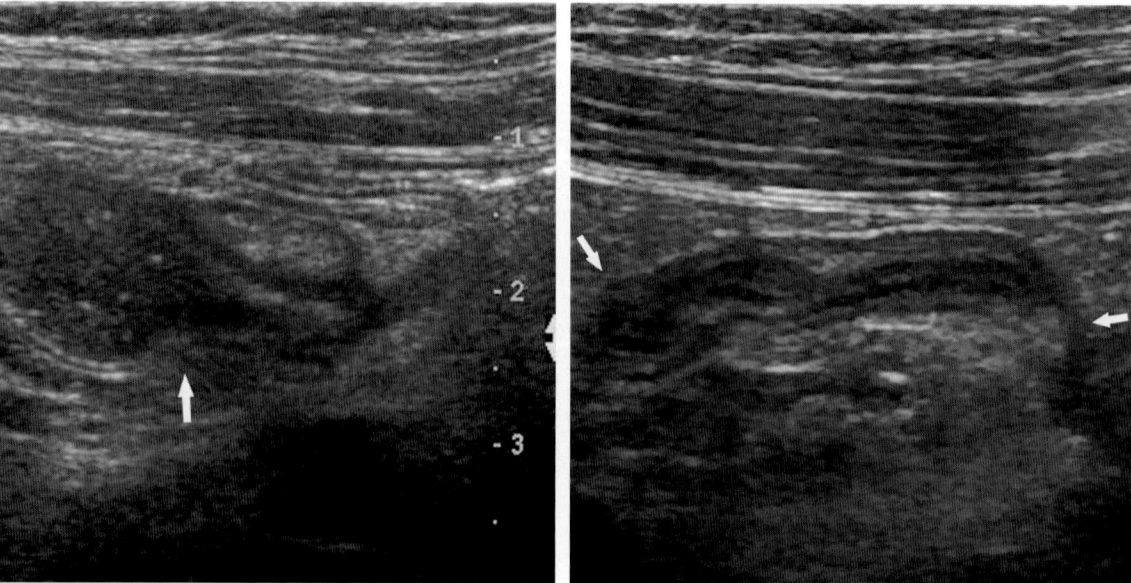

Fig. 5.6a,b. Paraduodenal internal hernia. a Oblique scan above the umbilicus shows the zone of transition (*arrow*) between dilated and non-dilated bowel. b Transverse scan to the left of zone of transition shows the cluster of crowded and compressed loops of bowel as if they are tightly packed within a sac (*arrows*)

cocoon there is no evidence of small bowel obstruction or zone of transition. The loops do not appear to be compressed and show normal peristalsis (VIJAYARAGHAVAN et al. 2003).

## 5.1.9
## Diaphragmatic Hernia

The diaphragmatic hernia is an abnormal protrusion of abdominal organs into the chest through an abnormal opening in the diaphragm or through the oesophageal hiatus. The abnormal opening may be congenital, caused by improper fusion of the various parts of diaphragm during fetal development, or acquired, due to traumatic rupture of the diaphragm. The four basic types of congenital diaphragmatic hernia are the posterolateral Bochdalek hernia, the anterior Morgagni hernia, the hiatus hernia and the rare form of herniation through the central tendon or septum transversum, otherwise called the peritoneopericardial hernia. The left-sided Bochdalek hernia is the commonest of these occurring in approximately 90% of the cases. The congenital diaphragmatic hernia occurs in 1 of every 2000–4000 live births. While congenital diaphragmatic hernia is most commonly a disorder of the newborn period, as many as 10% of patients may present with the condition after the newborn period and even during adulthood. The outcome in patients with late presentation of congenital diaphragmatic hernia is extremely good. During newborn period, the infants exhibit respiratory distress and cyanosis. In later age groups the condition is asymptomatic, or presents with non-specific symptoms.

The diagnosis of left-sided congenital diaphragmatic hernia in the newborn is revealed on a chest X-ray, as it contains air-filled bowels. The right-sided

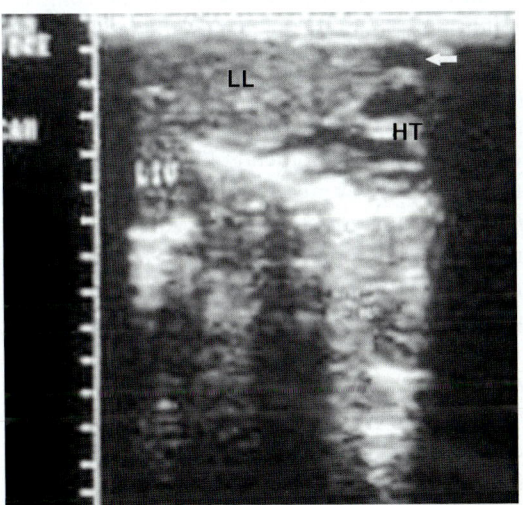
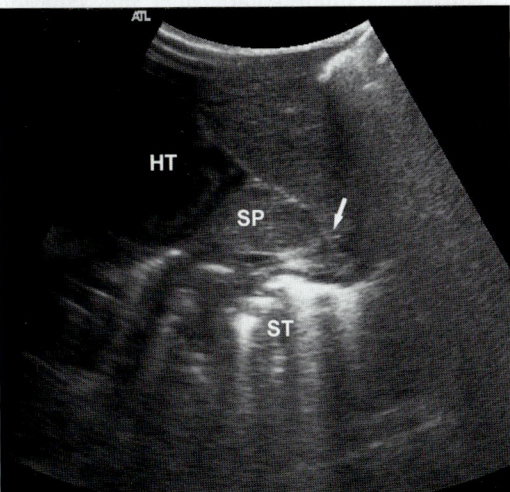
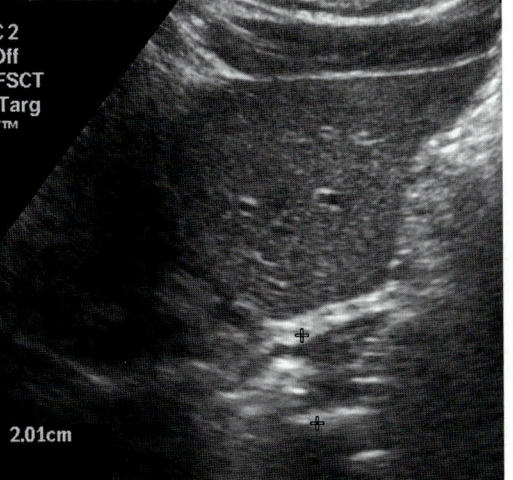

Fig. 5.7. a Oblique scan of epigastrium and precardium shows the left lobe of the liver (*LL*) herniated into the pericardium pushing the heart (*HT*), better outlined by the minimal pericardial fluid (*arrow*). *LIV* intraabdominal liver. b Longitudinal scan of left hypochondrium reveals the defect (*arrow*) in the posterior part of left dome of diaphragm with spleen (*SP*) and air-filled stomach (*ST*) lying in the chest posterior to the heart (*HT*), suggestive of left diaphragmatic hernia of Bochdalek type. c Longitudinal scan of left hypochondrium shows the shortened and thickened intraabdominal oesophagus in gastroesophageal reflux of hiatus hernia

hernia containing solid liver or right kidney may be difficult to diagnose on a chest X-ray. Sonography reveals the defect in the right dome of the diaphragm and the herniated liver or right kidney. In the rare type of peritoneo-pericardial hernia, there is herniation of the left lobe of the liver with, or without colon, into the pericardial sac through a defect of the central tendon of the diaphragm. This hernia also presents in the newborn period as respiratory distress or cyanosis. In such a case an X-ray of the chest will reveal an enlarged cardiac silhouette. Sonography reveals the herniation of left lobe of liver into the pericardial sac containing some pericardial fluid (Fig. 5.7a; Vijayaraghavan 1988). The herniated liver pushes the heart above and laterally. The diaphragmatic hernia of Bochdalek type, presenting in later ages, may be seen on sonography as a defect in the diaphragm with intrathoracic visualization of viscera such as stomach, spleen and bowels, on the left side (Fig. 5.7b), and liver or right kidney on the right side.

In the hiatus hernia the stomach herniates up through the oesophageal hiatus of the diaphragm. There are two types of hiatus hernia. In the sliding type, the gastroesophageal junction and fundus of stomach slide through the hiatus and are situated above the diaphragm. It is associated with gastroesophageal reflux. In the rolling or para-oesophageal type the gastroesophageal junction is in the abdomen, and the fundus of stomach herniates by the side of the oesophagus. Many authors have described the sonographic findings associated with the gastroesophageal reflux caused by the hiatus hernia in children (Naik and Moore 1984; Westra et al. 1990; Le Dosseur et al. 1992). Sonography is performed after the usual feed of formula, milk, water or juice. The transducer is placed in the midline under the xiphisternum and the distal oesophagus is visualized, as it comes out of the diaphragm. The transducer is slightly rotated to obtain the longitudinal section of the intraabdominal portion of the oesophagus and observed for 10 min. The length of the oesophagus is measured from the diaphragm to the cardia and the thickness is measured between the serous layers. The number of episodes of gastroesophageal reflux is also noted. Normal values for these observations have been described for the different age groups of children (Westra et al. 1990; Le Dosseur et al. 1992). Aliotta et al. (1994) have described the thickness of the hiatal portion of the oesophagus in adults indicative of hiatus hernia as 16 mm or more (Fig. 5.7c).

## 5.2
## Small Bowel Volvulus

Small bowel volvulus refers to rotation of the bowel around the mesenteric axis, which often results in a closed-loop obstruction, lymphatic, venous or arterial occlusion (Fig. 5.8a). It is one of the conditions causing small bowel obstruction, which requires prompt diagnosis and treatment to avoid poor outcome, as it can progress rapidly to gangrene of bowel. It is a rare but life-threatening emergency. It is more common in Africa (24–60/100,000) and Asia, compared with Western countries (1.7–5.7/100,000; Gulati et al. 1973; Cathcart et al. 1981; Schwartz and Ellis 1989; Parkes 1997). The small bowel volvulus can be primary or secondary depending on whether a predisposing factor is present or not. Predisposing condition may be congenital or acquired. Malrotation of midgut, a persistent omphalalomesenteric duct and mesenteric cyst are some of the congenital conditions. Some of the acquired conditions are adhesion, ascariasis and a mesenteric cyst or tumour. In malrotation of midgut, there is arrest of the rotation and fixation phase of embryonic development, which results in developmental failure of peritoneal fixation and a narrow mesenteric pedicle. The narrow mesenteric pedicle predisposes to volvulus because of increased mobility. Increase in the weight of the distal aspect of mesentery due to a mesenteric cyst or tumour, a mass of ascaris worms and dilated loop of bowel in a closed-loop obstruction can predispose to volvulus. The third factor, which predisposes volvulus, is restriction of the bowel at a fixed point, which acts as a fulcrum for rotation. The point of fixation may be at the apex of the volvulus, as seen in persistent omphalalomesenteric duct and adhesion of bowel to abdominal wall or it may be at the base, as seen in adhesions between two loops of bowel with volvulus occurring at this site. Volvulus in malrotation of midgut typically presents in the neonatal period but can also occur at a later age and even in adults. The volvulus due to other causes may occur at any age. The clinical presentation of volvulus of small bowel can be non-specific and includes bilious vomiting, abdominal pain and distension. Some patients may have chronic or intermittent symptoms.

Early diagnosis of small bowel volvulus is crucial for better outcome of management as it can prevent complications. The vascular occlusion can lead to ischaemia and gangrene of the bowel. The closed-loop obstruction may lead to tense distension of the bowel with secondary perforation and resulting peritonitis. Sonography has the advantages of easy availability, relative lack of need for patient preparation and absence of ionizing radiation. The sonographic findings described previously, such as dilated thick-walled bowel loops to the right of spine with increased peritoneal fluid (LEONIDAS et al. 1991) and dilated duodenum (HAYDEN et al. 1984), are non-specific. The "whirlpool" sign, proposed by PRACROS et al. (1992), is specific for midgut volvulus, as it directly indicates the anatomic alteration caused by the volvulus and is not seen in other conditions. FISHER (1981) was the first to describe the whirlpool sign as a CT finding of midgut volvulus. The twisted loops of bowel and branching mesenteric vessels create surrounding strands of soft tissue attenuation

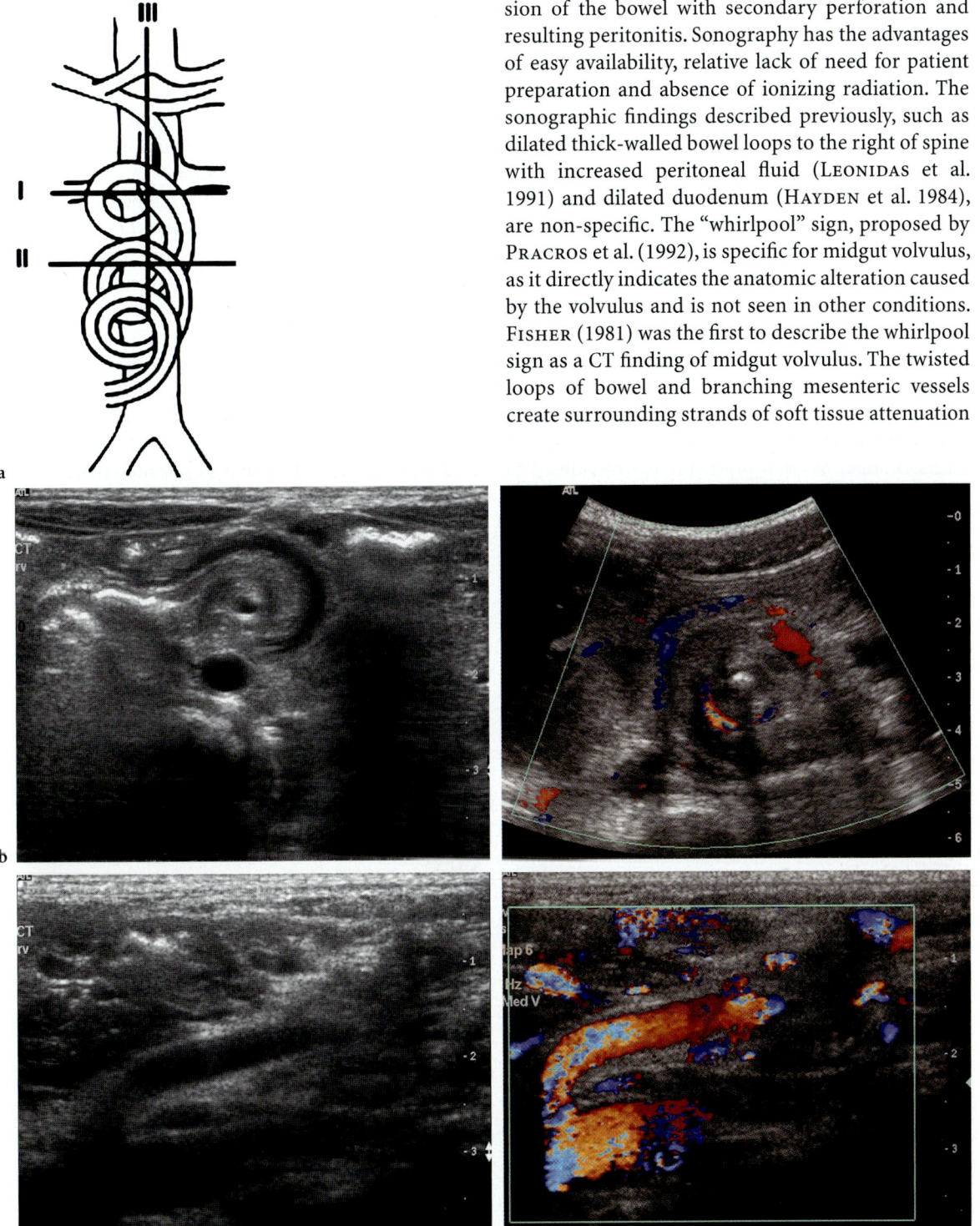

**Fig. 5.8a–e.** Small bowel volvulus in malrotation of midgut. **a** Line diagram shows the rotation of vessels and planes of section. **b** Transverse section through plane I shows the mass of whirlpool with its axis formed by superior mesenteric artery seen as a hypoechoic dot. **c** Similar section through plane II with color Doppler shows the mass of whirlpool with the superior mesenteric vessels going around the central echogenic axis formed by wrapped-up omentum. **d** Longitudinal section through superior mesenteric artery (plane III) shows the truncated superior mesenteric artery sign. **e** The same appearance on colour Doppler study

within the background of mesenteric fat attenuation, giving the appearance of whirlpool or hurricane on a weather map. On gray-scale sonography the whirlpool sign, as it is classically described for volvulus in malrotation, is seen as a round mass of incomplete concentric rings of alternative echogenic and hypoechoic bands in the transverse scan of the epigastrium below the pancreas (Fig. 5.8b; Pracros et al. 1992). On real-time scanning, when the transducer is moved down, the characteristic whirlpool appearance is seen where the echo-poor band of superior mesenteric vessels is seen to wrap in the clockwise direction, around the central axis. The same findings are more definitively seen on colour Doppler study (Fig. 5.8c). The size of the mass, the number of concentric rings and number of turns on downward movement of the transducer will depend on the number of turns present in the volvulus. The appearance of the central axis of the mass varies. In the upper part of the mass, the central axis is formed by the superior mesenteric artery, which appears as a hypoechoic dot (Fig. 5.8b). In the lower part of the mass, the axis appears as a brightly echogenic dot, sometimes with a shadow (Fig. 5.8c). This is produced by the wrapped-up mesentery. The superior mesenteric artery is not seen in the lower part as it deviates in its course, to wrap around the central axis. The same feature is seen on longitudinal scan of superior mesenteric artery as a truncated superior mesenteric artery sign (Sze et al. 2002), with only the proximal part of the superior mesenteric artery being visible (Fig. 5.8d,e). This is because of the fact that in volvulus, the superior mesenteric artery deviates laterally after a varying length of straight course proximally. This is in accordance with the corkscrew appearance of the superior mesenteric artery on angiography, which has been described as the "barber pole" sign (Buranasiri et al. 1973; Griska and Popky 1980). In volvulus of malrotation, in addition to the whirlpool sign, there is alteration of the relationship between the superior mesenteric artery and the vein. The vein is normally to the right of the artery. In malrotation the vein is seen either anterior to, or to the left of, the artery.

In volvulus, due to other causes, the location and axis of the mass with whirlpool appearance can vary. In a mesenteric cyst with volvulus of most of the small bowel, the mass is seen below the pancreas, as seen in volvulus of malrotation (Vijayaraghavan et al. 2004). Alternatively, when the volvulus involves only a segment of small bowel, the mass is located close to the umbilicus, just above or to the right of it. The best image of the mass is seen in slightly oblique scans and not on true transverse scans, as the axis of volvulus may be oblique. In a newborn, who had an atresia of small bowel secondary to intrauterine volvulus due to persistent omphalomesenteric duct, the mass of whirlpool was seen to the right of umbilicus. Rarely, the mass may be very small and the concentric rings are not well appreciated if the segment of bowel involved is very small. In such a situation the movement of the transducer along the axis brings about the typical whirlpool sign. On CT scan the mass of whirlpool sign has to be in the axial plane to be seen. Since oblique scans are possible with ultrasound, even obliquely placed masses of whirlpool are well seen on sonography. This fact, along with the dynamic study of movement of transducer to elicit the whirlpool sign, increases the sensitivity of ultrasound. The causative lesions of the volvulus-like mesenteric cyst, or ball of worms, will be seen. The complications of volvulus, such as closed-loop obstruction, gangrene of bowel or penumoperitoneum (Vijayaraghavan et al. 2004), are seen, if present. In some patients the closed-loop obstruction may be the only feature seen on sonography to suggest a segmental volvulus. In the closed-loop obstruction a loop of dilated small bowel is seen filled with only fluid devoid of air (Fig. 5.9; Cho et al. 1989), whereas the proximal dilated loops contain fluid and air.

## 5.3
## Gastric Volvulus

Gastric volvulus is an abnormal degree of rotation of one part of the stomach around another varying from 180–360°, leading to a closed-loop obstruction and possible strangulation (Cameron and Howard 1987). It is a rare surgical emergency. It can be primary or secondary, depending upon the absence or presence of predisposing conditions, such as congenital or traumatic diaphragmatic hernia (Kohli et al. 1997; Pelizzo et al. 2001), diaphragmatic eventration (Oh et al. 2000), wandering spleen (Pelizzo et al. 2001) or asplenia–polysplenia syndromes (Aoyama and Tateishi 1986). Four types of gastric volvulus have been reported based on the axis of rotation of the stomach:

1. In the more common organoaxial volvulus (59%), the stomach rotates on its longitudinal axis connecting the cardia and the pylorus. There is rever-

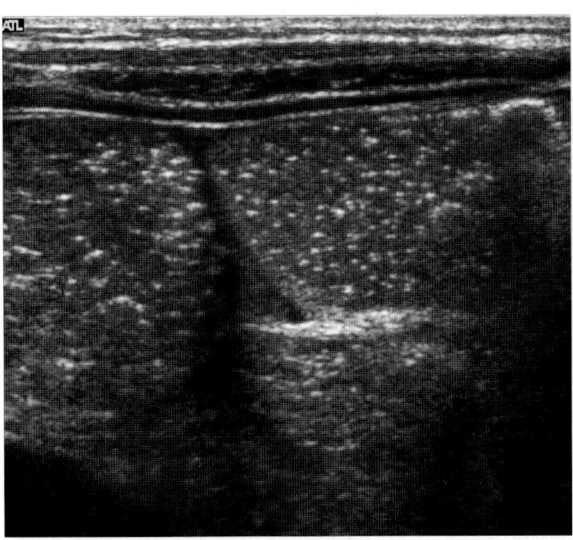 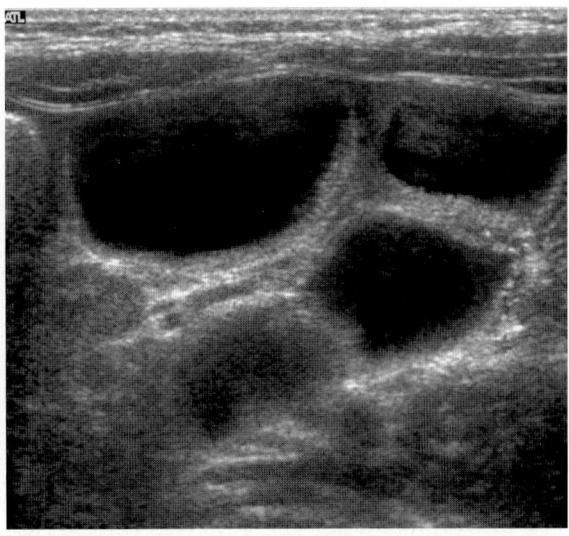

**Fig. 5.9a,b.** Closed-loop obstruction in segmental small bowel volvulus. **a** The proximal dilated loops of bowel show intraluminal fluid with microbubbles of air seen as echogenic dots. **b** Section through the loops of closed loop show the lumen filled with clear fluid devoid of air

sal of greater and lesser curvatures with two fluid-filled closed compartments. This type is more commonly associated with strangulation.
2. The second type is mesenteroaxial volvulus (29%), where the stomach rotates about a vertical axis perpendicular to the cardiopyloric line passing through the middle of lesser and greater curvatures.
3. The third type shows features of both organoaxial and mesenteroaxial volvulus (2%).
4. The last type is unclassified (10%; SHIVANAND et al. 2003). The aetiology is unclear. It is believed that the major factor leading to gastric volvulus is the laxity of the four gastric ligaments: gastrophrenic, gastrohepatic, gastrosplenic, and gastrocolic, which anchor the stomach (WASTELL and ELLIS 1971; DEITEL 1973; CARTER et al. 1980; LLANEZA and SALT 1986). The gastric volvulus may be acute or chronic. Acute volvulus is often a surgical emergency. It presents a clinical triad of violent retching with inability to vomit, acute severe epigastric pain with upper abdominal distension and inability to pass a nasogastric tube, as described by BORCHARDT in 1904. On plain X-ray and barium meal study, the stomach is seen as two fluid-filled compartments. The stomach is thoracoabdominal in position when the gastric volvulus is associated with diaphragmatic hernia or eventration.

On sonography, there are two dilated fluid-filled compartments of stomach which is thoracoabdominal in position, with a constriction between the upper and lower parts resembling a "peanut", henceforth called the "peanut sign" (Fig. 5.10a; MATSUZAKI et al. 2001). The continuity of oesophagus with stomach and stomach with duodenum cannot be demonstrated (Fig. 5.10b,c). The spleen is seen in the epigastrium between the left lobe of liver and stomach (Fig. 5.10d), because it is carried with the rotating stomach. Chronic gastric volvulus is usually asymptomatic or produces non-specific abdominal symptoms. Most often it is discovered as an incidental finding on barium study or CT scan (CHIECHI et al. 1992).

## 5.4 Caecal Volvulus

Volvulus of the caecum is torsion of the caecum around its own mesentery, which often results in a closed-loop obstruction. It can occur only in the small percentage (11–25%) of the population who have a developmental failure of peritoneal fixation with resultant increased mobility of the caecum (MONTES and WOLF 1999). It accounts for 11% of all intestinal volvulus. It usually occurs in patients who are 30–60 years old. There may be history of previous abdominal surgery, violent cough, atony of the colon, extreme exertion, unpressurized air travel

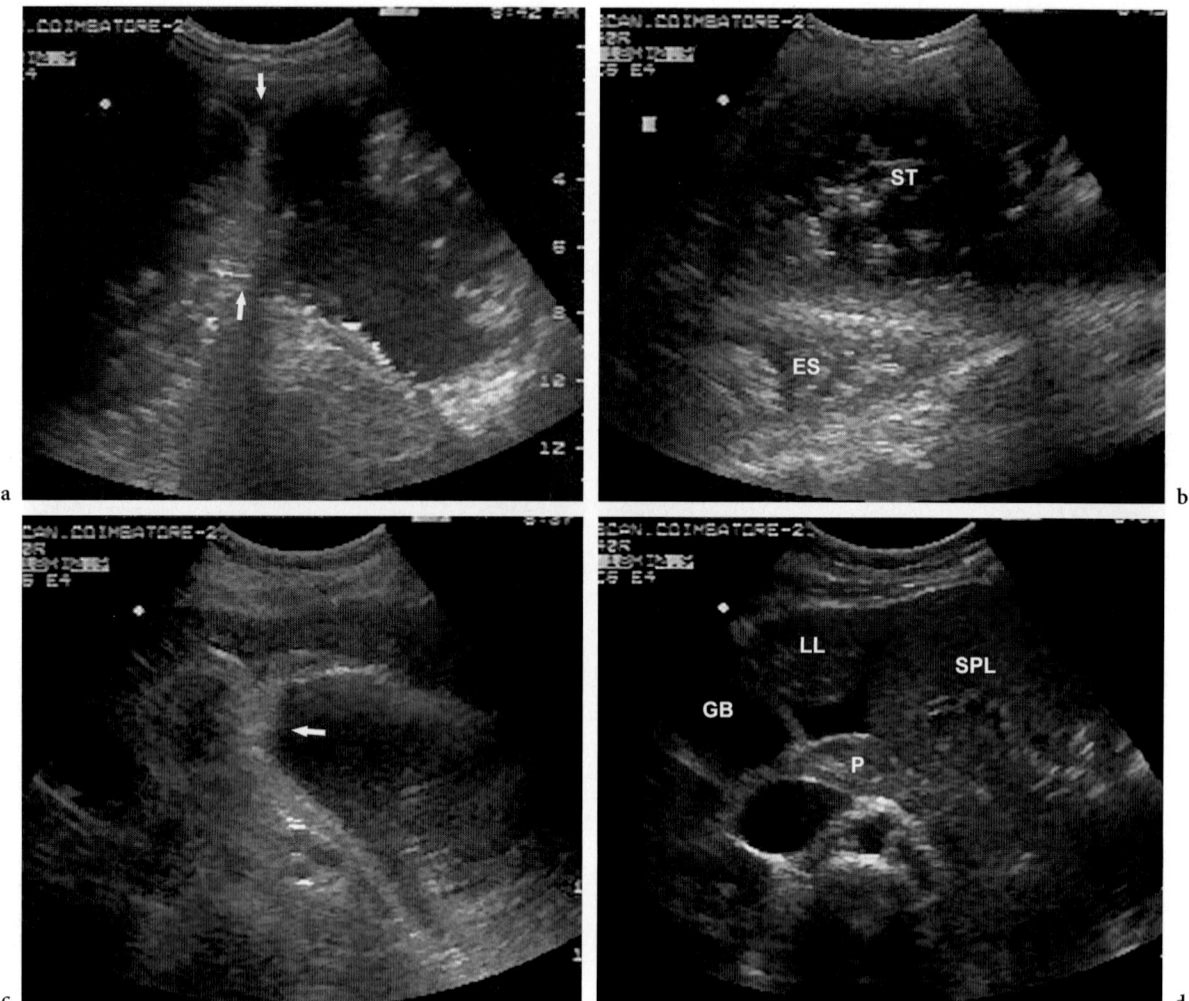

Fig. 5.10a–d. Gastric volvulus. a Oblique scan through the left lower intercostal space shows the peanut sign with the stomach seen as two fluid-filled compartments with a constriction between them (*arrows*). b Longitudinal scan shows lack of continuity between fluid-filled lower oesophagus (*ES*) and stomach (*ST*). c Oblique scan of epigastrium showing the blind ending lower compartment of stomach with lack of continuity with duodenum (*arrow*). d Transverse scan of epigastrium shows the spleen (*SPL*) located between left lobe of liver (*LL*) and body of pancreas (*P*) with some free fluid between. *GB* gallbladder

or third-trimester pregnancy. Patients usually present with nausea, vomiting, constipation and acute abdominal pain. In caecal volvulus, the caecum turns in clockwise direction and also inverts, occupying the left upper quadrant of the abdomen (FIELD 1994; PERRET and KUNBERGER 1998). The terminal ileum is usually twisted along with the caecum. This results in closed loop obstruction, causing massive dilatation of caecum and a small part of terminal ileum, which lie in the left upper quadrant. There is also small bowel obstruction. The CT signs of caecal volvulus are well described (MOORE et al. 2001). Similar features are seen on sonography. The small bowel loops are dilated and show peristalsis indicating obstruction. The caecum, identified by its relation to the appendix, is seen as a grossly dilated bowel in left upper quadrant medial to the spleen (Fig. 5.11). The dilatation is disproportionately large compared with the dilated small bowels. The ascending colon is seen to be collapsed and normal.

## 5.5 Intussusception

Intussusception is defined as the invagination of a proximal segment of bowel (intussusceptum) into an adjacent distal segment (intussuscepiens). It is

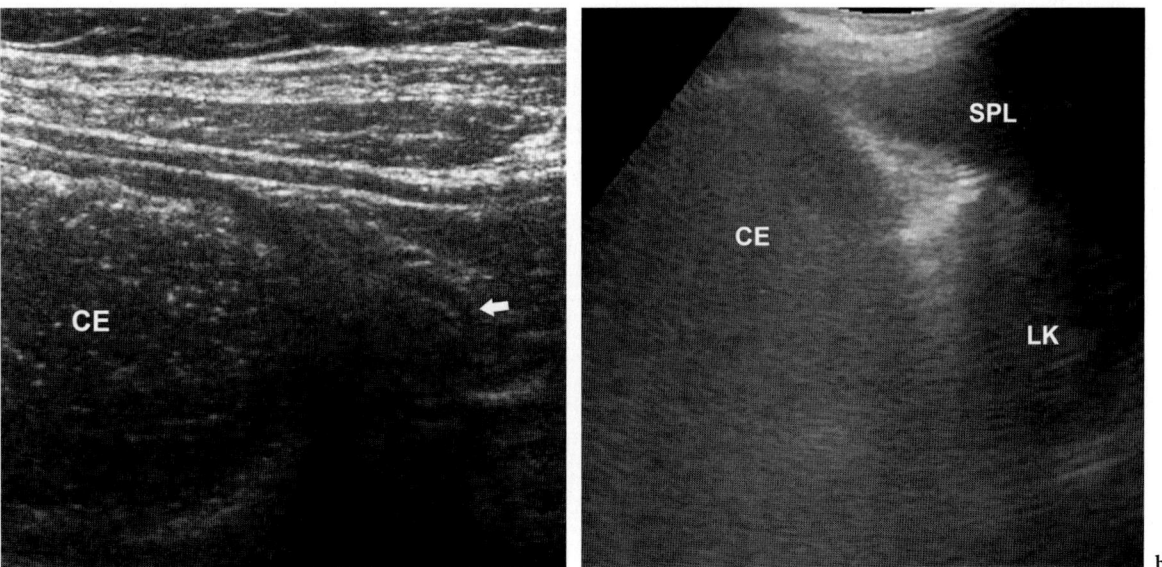

**Fig. 5.11a,b.** Caecal volvulus. **a** Oblique scan of left hypochondrium shows a huge dilated caecum (*CE*) with cross section of appendix close to it (*arrow*). **b** Transverse scan of left flank shows the location of dilated caecum (*CE*) medial to spleen (*SPL*). *LK* left kidney

common in children and rare in adults. While there is no cause or lead point in children, there is an identifiable lesion as the lead point in 75–85% of adults with intussusception (YEH and RABINOWITZ 1982; SWISCHUK et al. 1985). The causative lesion of small bowel is usually benign (52–61%), and 50% of those of colon prove to be malignant (WEILBAECHER et al. 1971; WEISSBERG et al. 1977). Intussusception is the most common cause of bowel obstruction in children. The clinical presentation is usually acute in children. They present with abdominal pain or incessant cry in very young, vomiting and passage of blood and mucus (red currant jelly) in stools (BOWERMAN et al. 1982). On clinical examination, a mass is usually located. Even though no identifiable causative lesion is seen in most of the children, hypertrophied lymph follicles in distal ileum are thought to initiate the intussusception; hence, ileocolic intussusception is the common type. In adults, the presentation is usually chronic and intermittent with abdominal pain and vomiting. There are three types of intussusception depending on the segment of bowel involved: (a) enteroenteric or small bowel intussusception (small bowel into small bowel); (b) ileocolic (ileum into stationary ileoceacal valve); and (c) colocolic (the colon into colon). As the intussusception progresses, the mesentery is caught between the entering and returning bowels. This leads to a cycle of venous obstruction, oedema and eventually ischaemic necrosis of the bowel.

On sonography intussusception is seen as a mass showing the multiple concentric rings sign or doughnut sign on short axis. The multiple concentric rings sign is specific for this condition (SKAANE and SKJENNALD 1989), with a reported accuracy of up to 100% (WANG and LIU 1988) and is not seen in any other pathology (Fig. 5.12a). The various layers of the bowels forming the intussusception are seen well differentiated when the oedema is less pronounced, which results in the formation of this multiple concentric rings sign on transverse scan. In longitudinal scan, these layers are seen as multiple parallel hypoechoic and hyperechoic stripes resembling a sandwich (Fig. 5.12b). When the oedema of the bowel becomes marked the differentiation of layers is lost resulting in a doughnut sign (Fig. 5.12c). But careful scan of the segment slightly proximal to the oedematous portion may reveal the characteristic concentric rings sign on transverse scan and multiple stripes sign in longitudinal scan in most patients (MONTALI et al. 1983). This manoeuvre is significant since the doughnut sign is a non-specific one, seen in most of the pathological conditions of the bowel. With improved resolution of the scanners most of the intussusceptions show the characteristic multiple concentric rings sign. Even though there is no differential diagnosis when the multiple concentric rings sign and multiple stripes sign are seen, care must be taken to exclude transient intussusception of small bowel. This is more so when the patient is asymptomatic and the lesion is seen centrally as in small bowel intussusception. The transient intussusception is usually (a) of short segment, (b) of small size, (c) lacking wall swelling, (d) located in central abdomen, (e) non-obstructive, (f) with persistent wall motion, and (g) without a lead point lesion (Fig. 5.12d,e; Kim 2004). Classically, the lesion is seen to move along the length of the bowel with peristalsis. The most important feature is that it is transient and a repeat scan after an interval of time fails to show the lesion; however, it is known that spontaneous reduction of an intussusception with all classical features, including oedematous walls, can happen (Kornecki et al. 2000). Rarely, small bowel intussusception can be asymptomatic and the author has seen two masses of small bowel intussusception in an asymptomatic patient with Peutz-Jeghers syndrome. Even rarer is the double intussusception (Kazez et al. 2004). On sonography, the double intussusception shows three circles, called the "triple-circle sign" (Fig. 5.12f).

Ileocolic intussusception, seen in children, is the commonest type. It is idiopathic and seen in children up to about 4 years. Enteroenteric or small bowel intussusception is the next common type. Here the mass of intussusception is seen in the centre of the abdomen, whereas in the ileocolic and colocolic types, it is along the periphery, where the colon is located. If the small bowel intussusception starts in distal ileum, it can become ileocolic. There is a lead-point lesion in most of the small bowel intussusceptions. This can be a polyp, lipoma, lymphoma, Meckel's diverticulum and haematoma of Henoch-Schonlein purpura. In some patients the lead-point lesion can be seen on sonography. One study has reported identification of a lead-point lesion in two-thirds and a specific diagnosis in nearly one-third of the patients (Navarro et al. 2000). The appearance of the lead-point lesion varies from a pedunculated hypoechoic mass in adenomatous polyp (Fig. 5.13a), echogenic mass in inflammatory polyp (Fig. 5.13b), sessile echogenic mass in lipoma, and a sessile echo-poor wall thickening in lymphoma. Colour Doppler study is useful in delineating the mass lesion at the tip of the intussusception (Fig. 5.13b). A cystic mass is seen as the lead point in an inverted Meckel's diverticulum (Daneman et al. 1997) or appendix (Fig. 5.13c; Koumanidou et al. 2001). A similar cystic mass may be seen as a false cystic lead point produced by fluid trapped within the intussuscepted mesentery (Kenney 1990). A lead-point lesion is always seen in colocolic intussusception and most of them are malignant.

Sonography is also useful in the treatment of childhood intussusception, the majority of which are idiopathic. Even though barium enema and air enema were used in the past to reduce intussusception, hydrostatic reduction under sonographic control has evolved as the method of choice in recent years. Very high success rates, up to 95.5%, have been reported without any complications, in a large series of 337 patients (Wang and Liu 1988). It has an added advantage of lack of radiation exposure. In this technique after confirmation of presence of intussusception, hydrostatic reduction is attempted with introduction of an enema of tapwater (Wood et al. 1992), saline (Wang and Liu 1988; Kim 2004), or Hartmann's solution (Riebel et al. 1993). The height of the enema bag is raised gradually from 80 cm (60 mm Hg) to a maximum of 155 cm (120 mm Hg). The progress of reduction of intussusception is followed by sonography. Complete reduction is confirmed by disappearance of the mass, reflux of fluid into terminal ileum and visualization of fluid-filled ileal loops. If complete reduction is not achieved by maintaining the pressure for 5 min, the colon is drained and the same procedure is repeated after a rest of 3–5 min. When complete reduction has been achieved, sonography is repeated after an interval to rule out recurrence. The hydrostatic reduction is not attempted if certain risk factors are seen on initial sonography. These are patients older than 12 years, patients in shock, in presence of peritonitis, bowel perforation, gross abdominal distension and sonographic features of small bowel intussusception, and in recurrent intussusception of more than two episodes. Colour Doppler signs predicting the ischaemia of the intussusceptum have been reported with contradictory results (Lagalla et al. 1994; Kong et al. 1997; Hanquinet et al. 1998), but absence of flow on colour Doppler study is not a contraindication for hydrostatic reduction (Lagalla et al. 1994). The success rate of reduction is affected by left-sided location of intussusception, presence of

**Fig. 5.12a–f.** Intussusception. **a** Short-axis scan of the transverse colon shows the intussusception with the concentric rings sign. **b** Long-axis scan shows the multiple stripes sign. **c** Doughnut sign of intussusception in short axis scan of transverse colon. **d** Transverse and **e** longitudinal scan of a transient intussusception. **f** Triple-ring sign of a double intussusception

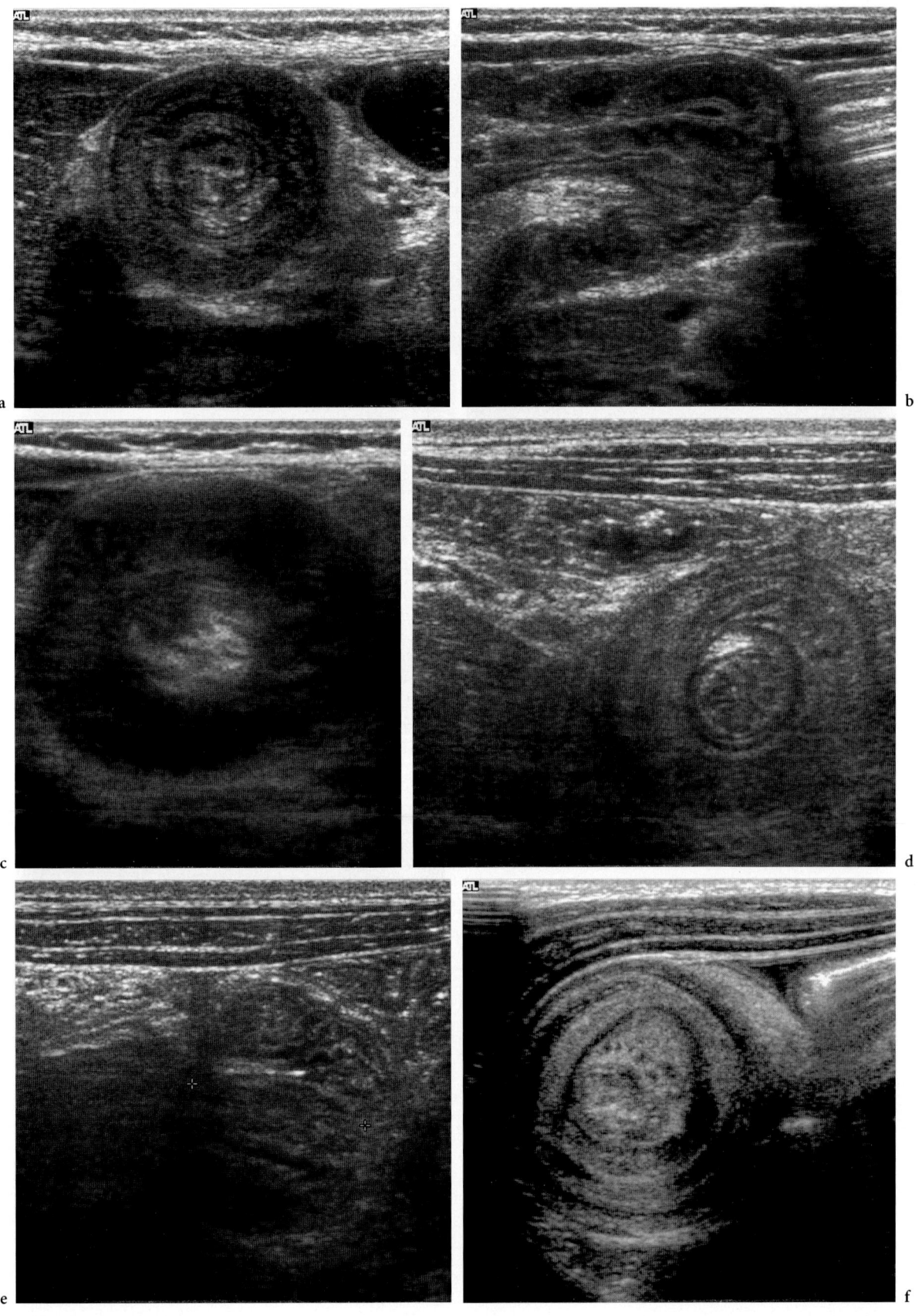

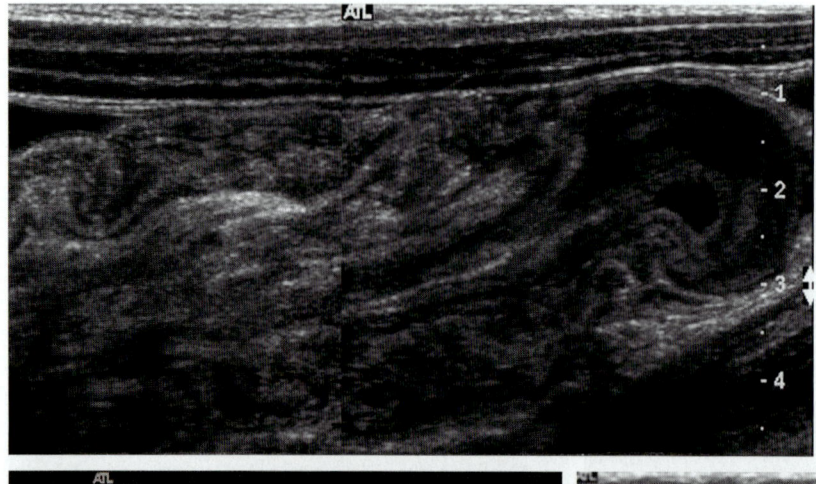

Fig. 5.13. Lead-point lesion in intussusception. a Adenomatous polyp. b Inflammatory polyp. c Inverted Meckel's diverticulum seen as cystic mass

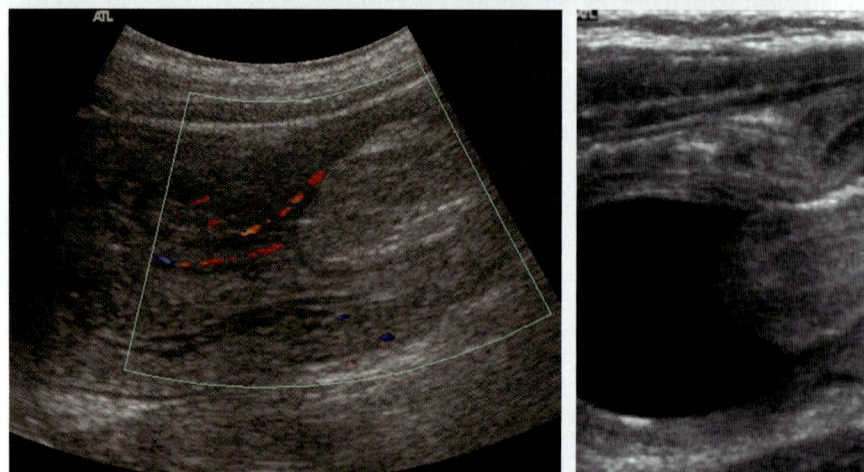

entrapped fluid in the intussusception and level of experience of the sonologist (CRYSTAL et al. 2002).

### 5.5.1
### Jejunogastric Intussusception

Jejunogastric intussusception is invagination of the jejunum into stomach after a gastrojejunostomy. It is usually seen 10–30 years after the initial surgery (WHEATLEY 1989; SU et al. 2001). It results in efferent loop obstruction producing epigastric pain and vomiting. If treatment is delayed, it can produce haemetemesis and necrosis of the invaginated loop (BRYNITZ and RUBINSTEIN 1986; HAMMOND et al. 2001). Sonography is the investigation of choice, as it reveals with ease a dilated fluid-filled stomach and the intussuscepted oedematous, typically sausage- or banana-shaped mass of invaginated jejunum in the lumen of stomach (Fig. 5.14).

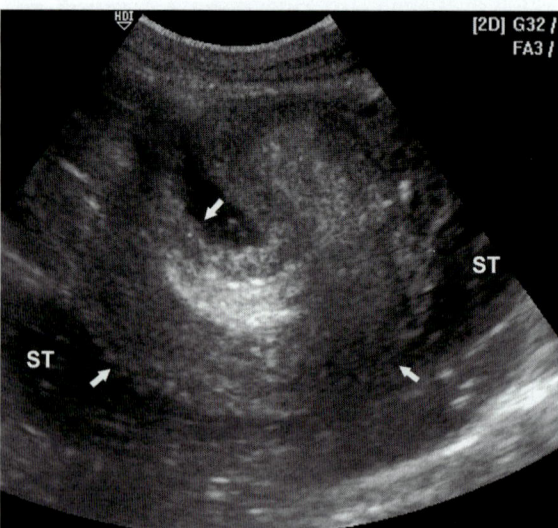

Fig. 5.14. Oblique scan of left hypochondrium shows the fluid-distended stomach (*ST*) with a banana-shaped mass of jejunogastric intussusception (*arrows*)

# References

Aliotta A, Rapaccini GL, Pompili M, et al (1994) Ultrasonographic signs of sliding, gastric, and hiatal hernia: their prospective evaluation. J Ultrasound Med 13:665–669

Aliotta A, Rapaccini GL, Pompili M, et al. (1995) Ultrasonographic signs of sliding gastric hiatal hernia and their prospective evaluation. J Ultrasound Med 14:457–61

Ando H, Kaneko K, Ito F, Seo T, Ito T (1997) Anatomy of the round ligament in female infants and children with an inguinal hernia. Br J Surg 84:404–405

Aoyama K, Tateishi K (1986) Gastric volvulus in three children with asplenic syndrome. J Pediatr Surg 21:307–310

Borchardt M (1904) Zur pathologic and therapie des magenvolvulus. Arch Klin Chir 74:243

Bowerman RA, Silver TM, Jaffe MH (1982) Real-time ultrasound diagnosis of intussusception in children. Radiology 143:527–529

Brynitz S, Rubinstein E (1986) Hematemesis caused by jejunogastric intussusception. Endoscopy 18:162–164

Buranasiri SI, Baum S, Nusbaum M, Tumen H (1973) The angiographic diagnosis of midgut malrotation with volvulus in adults. Radiology 109:555–556

Cameron AE, Howard ER (1987) Gastric volvulus in childhood. J Pediatr Surg 22:944–947

Carter R, Brewer LA III, Hinshaw DB (1980) Acute gastric volvulus. A study of 25 cases. Am J Surg 140:99–106

Catalano O (1997) US evaluation of inguinoscrotal bladder hernias: report of three cases. Clin Imaging 21:126–128

Cathcart RS III, Williamson B, Gregorie HB Jr, Glasow PF (1981) Surgical treatment of midgut nonrotation in the adult patient. Surg Gynecol Obstet 152:207–210

Chiechi MV, Hamrick-Turner J, Abbitt PL (1992) Gastric herniation and volvulus: CT and MR appearance. Gastrointest Radiol 17:99–101

Cho KC, Hoffman-Tretin JC, Alterman DD (1989) Closed-loop obstruction of the small bowel: CT and sonographic appearance. J Comput Assist Tomogr 13:256–258

Crystal P, Hertzanu Y, Farber B, Shabshin N, Barki Y (2002) Sonographically guided hydrostatic reduction of intussusception in children. J Clin Ultrasound 30:343–348

Daneman A, Myers M, Shuckett B, Alton DJ (1997) Sonographic appearances of inverted Meckel diverticulum with intussusception. Pediatr Radiol 27:295–298

Dattola P, Alberti A, Dattola A, Giannetto G, Basile G, Basile M (2002) Inguino-crural hernias: preoperative diagnosis and post-operative follow-up by high-resolution ultrasonography. A personal experience. Ann Ital Chir 73:65–68

Deitch EA, Soncrant MC (1981) The value of ultrasound in the diagnosis of nonpalpable femoral hernias. Arch Surg 116:185–187

Deitel M (1973) Chronic or recurring organoaxial rotation of the stomach. Can J Surg 16:195–205

Feldman M, Friedman LS, Sleisenger MH (2002) Sleisenger and Fordtran's Gastrointestinal and liver disease, 7th edn, vol 2. Saunders, Philadelphia

Field S (1994) Alimentary tract radiology, 5th edn, vol 1. Mosby, St. Louis

Fisher JK (1981) Computed tomographic diagnosis of volvulus in intestinal malrotation. Radiology 140:145–146

Furtschegger A, Sandbichler P, Judmaier W, Gstir H, Steiner E, Egender G (1995) Sonography in the postoperative evaluation of laparoscopic inguinal hernia repair. J Ultrasound Med 14:679–684

George EK, Oudesluys-Murphy AM, Madern GC, Cleyndert P, Blomjous JG (2000) Inguinal hernias containing the uterus, fallopian tube, and ovary in premature female infants. J Pediatr 136:696–698

Ghahremani GG (1984) Internal abdominal hernias. Surg Clin North Am 64:393–406

Griska LB, Popky GL (1980) Angiography in mid-gut malrotation with volvulus. Am J Roentgenol 134:1055–1056

Gulati SM, Grover NK, Tagore NK, Taneja OP (1973) Volvulus of the small intestine in India. Am J Surg 126:661–664

Hammond N, Miller FH, Dynes M (2001) Intussusception into the enteroanastomosis after Billroth II gastrectomy and Roux-en-Y jejunostomy: sonographic and CT findings. Am J Roentgenol 177:624–626

Hanquinet S, Anooshiravani M, Vunda A, Le Coultre C, Bugmann P (1998) Reliability of color Doppler and power Doppler sonography in the evaluation of intussuscepted bowel viability. Pediatr Surg Int 13:360–362

Hayden CK Jr, Boulden TF, Swischuk LE, Lobe TE (1984) Sonographic demonstration of duodenal obstruction with midgut volvulus. Am J Roentgenol 143:9–10

Hiller N, Alberton Y, Shapira Y, Hadas-Halpern I (1994) Richter's hernia strangulated in a spigelian hernia: ultrasonic diagnosis. J Clin Ultrasound 22:503–505

Holloway BJ, Belcher HE, Letourneau JG, Kunberger LE (1998) Scrotal sonography: a valuable tool in the evaluation of complications following inguinal hernia repair. J Clin Ultrasound 26:341–344

Huang CS, Luo CC, Chao HC, Chu SM, Yu YJ, Yen JB (2003) The presentation of asymptomatic palpable movable mass in female inguinal hernia. Eur J Pediatr 162:493–495

Kazez A, Ozel SK, Kocakoc E, Kiris A (2004) Double intussusception in a child: the triple-circle sign. J Ultrasound Med 23:1659–1661

Kenney IJ (1990) Ultrasound in intussusception: a false cystic lead point. Pediatr Radiol 20:348

Kim JH (2004) US features of transient small bowel intussusception in pediatric patients. Korean J Radiol 5:178–184

Kohli A, Vig A, Azad T (1997) Intrathoracic gastric volvulus: acute and chronic presentation. J Indian Med Assoc 95:522–523

Kong MS, Wong HF, Lin SL, Chung JL, Lin JN (1997) Factors related to detection of blood flow by color Doppler ultrasonography in intussusception. J Ultrasound Med 16:141–144

Korenkov M, Paul A, Troidl H (1999) Color duplex sonography: diagnostic tool in the differentiation of inguinal hernias. J Ultrasound Med 18:565–568

Kornecki A, Daneman A, Navarro O, Connolly B, Manson D, Alton DJ (2000) Spontaneous reduction of intussusception: clinical spectrum, management and outcome. Pediatr Radiol 30:58–63

Koumanidou C, Vakaki M, Theofanopoulou M, Nikas J, Pitsoulakis G, Kakavakis K (2001) Appendiceal and appendiceal-ileocolic intussusception: sonographic and radiographic evaluation. Pediatr Radiol 31:180–183

Lagalla R, Caruso G, Novara V, Derchi LE, Cardinale AE (1994) Color Doppler ultrasonography in pediatric intussusception. J Ultrasound Med 13:171–174

Le Dosseur P, Beaudet S, Dacher J et al (1992) Etude du reflux gastro-oesophagien chez l'enfant. Rev Im Med 4:153

Leonidas JC, Magid N, Soberman N, Glass TS (1991) Midgut volvulus in infants: diagnosis with US. Work in progress. Radiology 179:491–493

Liang RJ, Wang HP, Huang SP, Wu MS, Lin JT (2001) Color Doppler sonography for ventral hernias in patients with acute abdomen: preliminary findings. J Clin Ultrasound 29:435–440

Llaneza PP, Salt WB 2nd (1986) Gastric volvulus. More common than previously thought? Postgrad Med 80:279–283, 287–288

Matsuzaki Y, Asai M, Okura T, Tamura R (2001) Ultrasonography of gastric volvulus: "peanut sign". Intern Med 40:23–27

Middlebrook MR, Eftekhari F (1992) Sonographic findings in Richter's hernia. Gastrointest Radiol 17:229–230

Montali G, Croce F, Pra L de, Solbiati L (1983) Intussusception of the bowel: a new sonographic pattern. Br J Radiol 56:621–623

Montes H, Wolf J (1999) Cecal volvulus in pregnancy. Am J Gastroenterol 94:2554–2556

Moore CJ, Corl FM, Fishman EK (2001) CT of cecal volvulus: unraveling the image. Am J Roentgenol 177:95–98

Mufid MM, Abu-Yousef MM, Kakish ME, Urdaneta LF, Al-Jurf AS (1997) Spigelian hernia: diagnosis by high-resolution real-time sonography. J Ultrasound Med 16:183–187

Naik DR, Moore DJ (1984) Ultrasound diagnosis of gastro-oesophageal reflux. Arch Dis Child 59:366–367

Navarro O, Dugougeat F, Kornecki A, Shuckett B, Alton DJ, Daneman A (2000) The impact of imaging in the management of intussusception owing to pathologic lead points in children. A review of 43 cases. Pediatr Radiol 30:594–603

Nyhus LM, Condon RE (1989) Hernia, 3rd edn. Lippincott, Philadelphia

Oh A, Gulati G, Sherman ML, Golub R, Kutin N (2000) Bilateral eventration of the diaphragm with perforated gastric volvulus in an adolescent. J Pediatr Surg 35:1824–1826

Parkes G (1997) Primary small bowel volvulus in rural Nepal. Trop Doct 27:156–158

Parra JA, Revuelta S, Gallego T, Bueno J, Berrio JI, Farinas MC (2004) Prosthetic mesh used for inguinal and ventral hernia repair: normal appearance and complications in ultrasound and CT. Br J Radiol 77:261–265

Pelizzo G, Lembo MA, Franchella A, Giombi A, D'Agostino F, Sala S (2001) Gastric volvulus associated with congenital diaphragmatic hernia, wandering spleen, and intrathoracic left kidney: CT findings. Abdom Imaging 26:306–308

Perret RS, Kunberger LE (1998) Case 4: Cecal volvulus. Am J Roentgenol 171:855, 859–860

Pershad J, Simmons GT, Chung D, Frye T, Marques MB (1998) Two acute pediatric abdominal catastrophes from strangulated left paraduodenal hernias. Pediatr Emerg Care 14:347–349

Pracros JP, Sann L, Genin G, Tran-Minh VA, Morin de Finfe CH, Foray P, Louis D (1992) Ultrasound diagnosis of midgut volvulus: the "whirlpool" sign. Pediatr Radiol 22:18–20

Rettenbacher T, Hollerweger A, Macheiner P, Gritzmann N, Gotwald T, Frass R, Schneider B (2001) Abdominal wall hernias: cross-sectional imaging signs of incarceration determined with sonography. Am J Roentgenol 177:1061–1066

Riebel TW, Nasir R, Weber K (1993) US-guided hydrostatic reduction of intussusception in children. Radiology 188:513–516

Scherer LR III, Grosfeld JL (1993) Inguinal hernia and umbilical anomalies. Pediatr Clin North Am 40:1121–1131

Schwartz SI, Ellis H (1989) Maringot's abdominal operations, 9th edn, vol 1. Aleton and Large, Norwalk, Connecticut

Shivanand G, Seema S, Srivastava DN et al (2003) Gastric volvulus: acute and chronic presentation. Clin Imaging 27:265–268

Skaane P, Skjennald A (1989) Ultrasonic features of ileocecal intussusception. J Clin Ultrasound 17:590–593

Spangen L (1975) Ultrasound as a diagnostic aid in ventral abdominal hernia. J Clin Ultrasound 3:211–213

Su MY, Lien JM, Lee CS, Lin DY, Tsai MH (2001) Acute jejunogastric intussusception: report of five cases. Chang Gung Med J 24:50–56

Sutphen JH, Hitchcock DA, King DC (1980) Ultrasonic demonstration of Spigelian hernia. Am J Roentgenol 134:174–175

Swischuk LE, Hayden CK, Boulden T (1985) Intussusception: indications for ultrasonography and an explanation of the doughnut and pseudokidney signs. Pediatr Radiol 15:388–391

Sze RW, Guillerman RP, Krauter D, Evans AS (2002) A possible new ancillary sign for diagnosing midgut volvulus: the truncated superior mesenteric artery. J Ultrasound Med 21:477–480

Vijayaraghavan SB (1988) Diaphragmatic eventration into the pericardial sac: sonographic diagnosis. J Clin Ultrasound 16:510–512

Vijayaraghavan SB (2006) Sonographic features of internal hernia. J Ultrasound Med 25:105–110

Vijayaraghavan SB, Palanivelu C, Sendhilkumar K, Parthasarathi R (2003) Abdominal cocoon: sonographic features. J Ultrasound Med 22:719–721

Vijayaraghavan SB, Ravikumar VR, Srimathy G (2004) Whirlpool sign in small-bowel volvulus due to a mesenteric cyst. J Ultrasound Med 23:1375–1377

Wang GD, Liu SJ (1988) Enema reduction of intussusception by hydrostatic pressure under ultrasound guidance: a report of 377 cases. J Pediatr Surg 23:814–818

Wastell C, Ellis H (1971) Volvulus of the stomach. A review with a report of 8 cases. Br J Surg 58:557–562

Wechsler RJ, Kurtz AB, Needleman L et al (1989) Cross-sectional imaging of abdominal wall hernias. Am J Roentgenol 153:517–521

Weilbaecher D, Bolin JA, Hearn D, Ogden W 2nd (1971) Intussusception in adults. Review of 160 cases. Am J Surg 121:531–535

Weissberg DL, Scheible W, Leopold GR (1977) Ultrasonographic appearance of adult intussusception. Radiology 124:791–792

Westra SJ, Wolf BH, Staalman CR (1990) Ultrasound diagnosis of gastroesophageal reflux and hiatal hernia in infants and young children. J Clin Ultrasound 18:477–485

Wheatley MJ (1989) Jejunogastric intussusception diagnosis and management. J Clin Gastroenterol 11:452–454

Wood SK, Kim JS, Suh SJ, Paik TW, Choi SO (1992) Childhood intussusception: US-guided hydrostatic reduction. Radiology 182:77–80

Yeh H, Rabinowitz J (1982) Ultrasonography of gastrointestinal tract. Semin Ultrasound CT MR 3:331

Zhang GQ, Sugiyama M, Hagi H, Urata T, Shimamori N, Atomi Y (2001) Groin hernias in adults: value of color Doppler sonography in their classification. J Clin Ultrasound 29:429–434

Zimmerman LM, Laufman H (1953) Intraabdominal hernias due to developmental and rotational anomalies. Ann Surg 138:82–91

# Ischemic Colitis

Etienne Danse

CONTENTS

6.1 Introduction 55
6.2 Imaging Findings 55
6.3 Sonographic Findings 56
6.4 Computed Tomography Findings 56
6.5 Proposed Strategy 57
References 58

## 6.1 Introduction

Ischemic colitis is the most usual form of acute intestinal ischemia and is most commonly associated with a low mortality level, under 10% (Martson et al. 1966; Boley 1990; Robert et al. 1993; Toursarkissian and Thompson 1997; Danse et al. 2004; Balthazar et al. 1999). Diagnosis is based on the association of clinical data, endoscopic findings, radiological data, and histology (Martson et al. 1966; Boley 1990; Robert et al. 1993; Toursarkissian and Thompson 1997). There are mainly two distinct forms of ischemic colitis: the transient form with spontaneous resolution, and the severe form. Two types of severe forms of ischemic colitis are to be considered: (a) ischemic colitis associated with a delayed stenosis caused by colonic wall fibrosis; and (b) ischemic colitis complicated by an early perforation caused by gangrenous evolution (Martson et al. 1966; Boley 1990; Robert et al. 1993; Longo et al. 1997). Ischemic colitis is usually related to a good prognosis in the transient form and when there is a delayed stenosis. The gangrenous form, which is unusual, is frequently associated with a fatal outcome. Any segment of the colon can be affected, from the ileo-cecal valve to the rectum, but there is a predisposition for the left colon, due to its reduced vascular network.

Early identification of prognostic factors is helpful for an optimal therapy (Martson et al. 1966; Longo et al. 1992; Toursarkissian and Thompson 1997; Longo et al. 1997). These factors are present in 50% of the patients and include age, duration of the symptoms, underlying diseases (cardiovascular diseases and diabetes mellitus), abdominal aortic surgery, and hypovolemic shock. These factors are frequently related to the severe forms of ischemic colitis (Longo et al. 1992; Longo et al. 1997; Danse et al. 2000a,b). It was also demonstrated that lactate dehydrogenase (LDH) levels and leukocyte count are significantly higher in severe forms of ischemic colitis (Danse et al. 2000a).

Endoscopy is helpful for the recognition of suggestive findings for ischemic colitis; however, endoscopy is not demonstrative for the identification of the severity of the ischemic colitis if we consider its limitation for the correct delineation of the disease extension along the colon. Indeed, endoscopy is classically limited to a recto-sigmoidoscopy in the emergency context, in order to avoid perforation during the procedure. Additionally, biopsy samples are limited to the superficial layers of the colonic wall (the mucosa and a part of the submucosa). For these reasons, sonography and computed tomography (CT) can contribute to the diagnosis of ischemic colitis. These techniques are also helpful for the delineation of the disease extension along the colon, and for recognition of severity factors (Balthazar et al. 1999; Federle et al. 1984; Jeffrey et al. 1994; Bozkurt et al. 1994; Philpotts et al. 1994; Ranschaert et al. 1994; Chou 2002).

## 6.2 Imaging Findings

Radiological findings suggestive of ischemic colitis were initially described on contrast enema (Boley

E. Danse, MD, PhD
Dept. of Radiology, St-Luc University Hospital, Université Catholique de Louvain, 10, Av Hippocrate, 1200 Brussels, Belgium

1990; Danse et al. 1997; Danse et al. 2000a; Danse et al. 2001). The role of conventional radiology for the recognition of severity factors is limited to its ability to show the extension in length of the colonic wall changes (Martson et al. 1966; Robert et al. 1993; Toursarkissian 1997). Sonography and CT can be useful for the recognition of intestinal wall changes and insufficiency of the splanchnic arterial network. Sonography is combined with a color flow imaging of the colonic wall and the main splanchnic vessels (Danse et al. 1997; Danse et al. 2001). CT is usually performed with intravenous contrast iodine injection. This approach allows identification of the wall vascularization and its alteration. Sonographic and CT findings include evaluation of the wall thickening, presence or absence of the wall stratification, detection of gas into the colonic wall (colonic pneumatosis) and the pericolic changes (Balthazar et al. 1999; Danse et al. 2000a; Federle et al. 1984; Bozkurt et al. 1994; Philpotts et al. 1994; Ranschaert et al. 1994; Danse et al. 2004; Teefey et al. 1996). Sonography and CT can also show signs for a prediction of the severity of ischemic colitis (Danse et al. 2000a; Chou 2002; Wiesner et al. 2001; Ripolles et al. 2005).

## 6.3
## Sonographic Findings

Sonography can contribute to the visualization of colonic wall changes in cases of ischemic colitis. We have to look for colonic wall thickening (>5 mm), presence of stratification, identification of the mural flow, as well as delimitation of the disease extension along the colonic wall and its localization (most frequently on the left colon; Danse et al. 2004). The wall thickening is easy to detect. In ischemic colitis, it is usually slightly more pronounced that in inflammatory bowel disease, but it is in the same range as in infectious colites (from 8 to 9 mm; Danse et al. 2000a; Jeffrey et al. 1994; Bozkurt et al. 1994; Teefey et al. 1996). It can mimic the nodular thickening observed in pseudomembranous colitis (Danse et al. 2004; Ranschaert et al. 1994). The increased mural thickness is caused by submucosal hematoma due to reperfusion injuries. Disappearance of the wall stratification is not systematic (dedifferentiation) but more frequently noted than in other acute colonic disease (Fig. 6.1). If absence of mural flow is noted with color Doppler, this is a clearly suggestive sign of ischemia (Danse et al. 2004; Teefey et al. 1996; Quillin and Siegel 1994; Hata et al. 1992; Siegel et al. 1997; Shirahama et al. 1999). Nevertheless, absence or reduced mural flow are reported only in 20–50% of the patients with a final diagnosis of ischemic colitis (Fig. 6.2; Danse et al. 2000a; Ripolles et al. 2005).

When sonography is considered as the initial diagnostic method for ischemic colitis, it is associated with a sensitivity of 93% for the adequate recognition of suggestive sonographic signs (Ripolles et al. 2005). Additionally, disappearance of the wall stratification and absence of mural flow are indicators of the severity of ischemic colitis with a sensitivity of 82% and a specificity of 92% (Danse et al. 2000a; Jeffrey et al. 1994; Danse et al. 2004; Cheung et al. 1992). Hyperechogenicity of the pericolic fatty tissue can be detected with sonography in patients with ischemic colitis. This sign has to be considered as a severity factor of ischemia as well as the absence of mural flow (Fig. 6.3; Ripolles et al. 2005). Predisposing factors can be detected with sonography when stenoses and/or occlusion of the main splanchnic arteries are visualized (celiac trunk, superior and inferior mesenteric arteries; Danse et al. 2001). Splanchnic vascular insufficiency requires stenosis or occlusion of at least two of the three splanchic arteries. Significant stenosis of the celiac trunk is present when the maximal systolic velocity is higher than 1.5 m/s. Superior and inferior mesenteric arteries are considered as significantly stenosed if the maximal systolic velocity is higher than 2.75–3 m/s (Bowersox et al. 1991). Sonography has been recently reported as useful for the follow-up of patients by showing disappearance of the colonic wall changes (Ripolles et al. 2005).

## 6.4
## Computed Tomography Findings

Thickening of the colonic wall related to ischemic colitis is visible with CT, within the same values as sonography (8–9 mm; Horton et al. 2000; Philpotts et al. 1994). The CT findings observed in ischemic colitis are of three types: (a) heterogeneous thickening with hypoperfused areas combined with pericolic fat stranding (40–60% of the patients); (b) homogeneous thickening without any change of the pericolic fat tissue (33–37% of the cases); and (c) colonic pneumatosis within a thin colonic wall (6–21% of the cases; Balthazar et al. 1999). Ascites is pres-

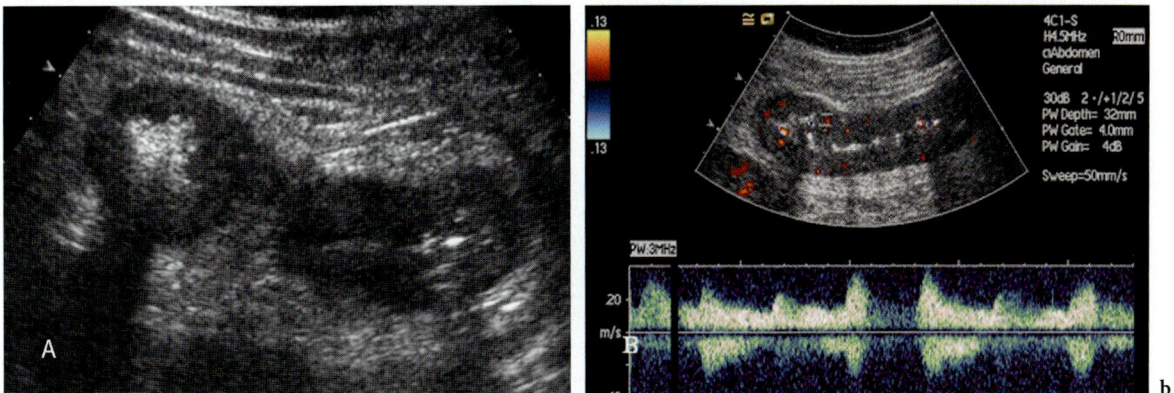

**Fig. 6.1a,b.** Ischemic colitis in a young female (drug addict). **a** Sonogram of the left colon shows diffuse hypoechoic thickening of the colonic wall, without stratification. **b** Preserved mural flow is demonstrated with color Doppler sonography

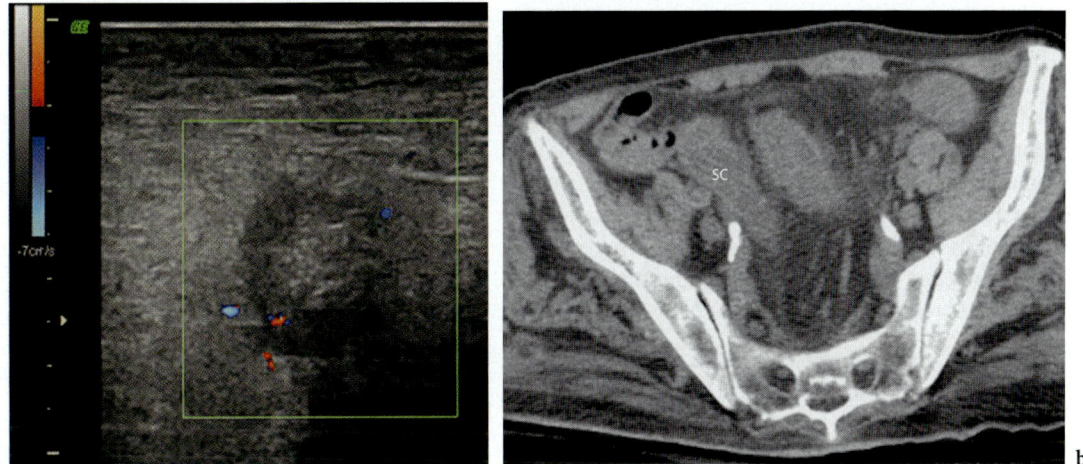

**Fig. 6.2a,b.** Ischemic colitis in an 82-year-old patient. **a** Transverse view of the sigmoid colon shows thickening of the colon, with wall stratification and discrete mural flow detected with color Doppler sonography. The pericolic fat tissue is slightly infiltrated. **b** A CT scan of the pelvis of the same patient shows diffuse thickening of the sigmoid colon (SC)

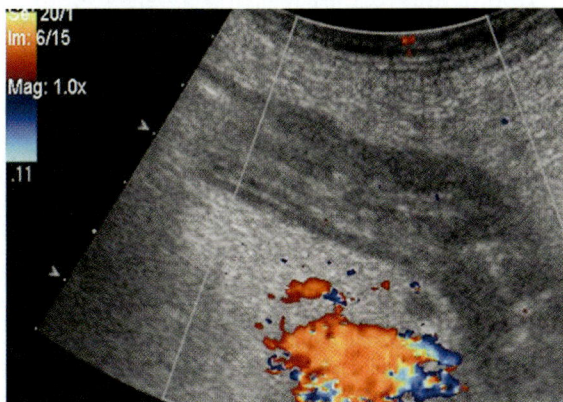

**Fig. 6.3.** Ischemic colitis with preserved wall stratification but without mural flow. Infiltration of the pericolic fat tissue. Resection was performed in emergency, revealing extended necrosis of the left colon

ent in <30% of the patients (BALTHAZAR et al. 1999; PHILPOTTS et al. 1994). Severity factors of ischemic colitis at CT are the presence of a thin colonic wall, with pneumatosis and reduced or absent colonic wall enhancement when iodine contrast injection is performed (BALTHAZAR et al. 1999).

## 6.5
## Proposed Strategy

When there is a strong suspicion of ischemic colitis, recto-sigmoidoscopy is performed and can be completed with an abdominal color Doppler study. The role of sonography is to detect the extension of the colitis, and to detect suggestive signs of ischemic colitis (colonic wall thickening of the left colon without identifiable mural flow). Prognosis factors, including wall stratification, pericolic fatty tissue hyperechogenicity, and ascites, are sought by means of sonography. Suggestive predisposing factors, such as stenoses and/or occlusion of the main splanchnic arteries, can also be detected with color Doppler sonography. When sonography is normal or inconclusive, CT is then performed, with intravenous contrast injection, if possible; however, ischemic colitis is a frequent, initially unsuspected, condition. The radiologist is often the first physician to suggest intestinal ischemia when he/she identifies a segmental or diffuse colonic wall thickening with sonography or CT, in patients for whom cross-sectional imaging studies are required for acute non-specific abdominal pain. In these cases, when a colonic wall change is noted with sonography or CT, the radiologist can suggest ischemic colitis on the basis of the localization of the affected segment, the absence of mural flow or enhancement, visualization of an infiltration of the pericolic fat tissue, pneumatosis, and stenoses or occlusions of the splanchnic arteries. In these initially unsuspected cases, endoscopy is needed to confirm the ischemic changes of the colonic wall (DANSE et al. 2005).

## References

Balthazar EJ, Yen BC, Gordon RB (1999) Ischemic colitis: CT evaluation of 54 cases. Radiology 211:381–388
Boley JS (1990) Colonic ischemia: 25 years later. Am J Gastroenterol 85:931–934
Bowersox JC, Zwolak RM, Walsh DB et al (1991) Duplex ultrasonography in the diagnosis of celiac and mesenteric artery occlusive disease. J Vasc Surg 14:780–788
Bozkurt T, Richter F, Lux G (1994) Ultrasonography as a primary diagnostic tool in patients with inflammatory disease and tumors of the small intestine and the large bowel. J Clin Ultrasound 22:85–91
Cheung AH, Wang KY, Jiranek GC et al (1992) Evaluation of a 20-MHz ultrasound transducer used in diagnosing porcine small bowel ischemia. Invest Radiol 27:217–223
Chou CK (2002) CT manifestations of bowel ischemia. AJR Am J Roentgenol 178:87–91
Danse E (2004) Imagerie des urgences abdominales non traumatiques de l'adulte. Encyclopédie Médico-Chirurgicale 33:705
Danse EM, Laterre PF, Van Beers BE et al (1997) Early diagnosis of acute intestinal ischemia: contribution of color Doppler sonography. Acta Chir Belg 97:173–176
Danse EM, Van Beers BE, Jamart J et al (2000a) Prognosis of ischemic colitis: comparison of color Doppler sonography with early clinical and laboratory findings. AJR Am J Roentgenol 175:1151–1154
Danse EM, Van Beers BE, Materne R (2000b) Small bowel wall changes in acute mesenteric ischemia: sonographic findings. Ultrasound Med Biol 26:A128
Danse EM, Hammer F, Matondo H et al (2001) Ischémie mésentérique chronique d'origine artérielle: mise en évidence de réseaux de vicariance par échographie Doppler couleur ("Doppler couleur"). J Radiol 82:1645–1649
Danse E, Jamart J, Hoang P et al (2004) Focal bowel wall changes detected with colour Doppler ultrasound: diagnostic value in acute non-diverticular diseases of the colon. Br J Radiol 77:917–921
Danse E, Dewit O, Goncette L et al (2005) Que faire en cas d'affection aiguë du colon? Une échographie, un scanner, des clichés conventionnels ou une endoscopie? SFR Paris octobre 2005, Formation Médicale Continue 23:241–253
Federle MP, Chun G, Jeffrey RB, Rayor R (1984) Computed tomographic findings in bowel infarction. AJR Am J Roentgenol 142:91–95
Hata J, Haruma K, Suenaga K et al (1992) Ultrasonographic assessment of inflammatory bowel disease. Am J Gastroenterol 87:443–447
Horton KM, Corl FM, Fishman EK (2000) CT evaluation of the colon: inflammatory disease. Radiographics 20:399–418
Jeffrey RB, Sommer G, Debatin JF (1994) Color Doppler sonography of focal gastrointestinal lesions: initial clinical experience. J Ultrasound Med 13:473–478
Longo WE, Ballantyne GH, Gusberg RJ (1992) Ischemic colitis: patterns and prognosis. Dis Colon Rectum 35:726–730
Longo WE, Ward D, Vernava AM, Kaminski DL (1997) Outcome of patients with total colonic ischemia. Dis Colon Rectum 40:1448–1454
Martson A, Pheils MT, Thomas ML, Morson BC (1966) Ischaemic colitis. Gut 7:1–15
Philpotts LE, Heiken JP, Westcott MA, Gore RM (1994) Colitis: use of CT findings in differential diagnosis. Radiology 190:445–449
Quillin SP, Siegel MJ (1994) Gastrointestinal inflammation in children: color Doppler ultrasonography. J Ultrasound Med 13:751–756
Ranschaert E, Verhille R, Marchal G, Rigauts H, Ponette E (1994) Sonographic diagnosis of ischemic colitis. J Belge Radiol 77:166–168
Ripolles T, Simo L, Martinez-Perez MJ et al (2005) Sonographic findings in ischemic colitis in 58 patients. AJR Am J Roentgenol 184:777–785
Robert JH, Mentha G, Rohner A (1993) Ischaemic colitis: two distinct patterns of severity. Gut 34:4–6
Shirahama M, Ishibashi H, Onohara S, Dohmen K, Miyamoto Y (1999) Color Doppler ultrasound for the evaluation of bowel wall thickening. Br J Radiol 72:1164–1169
Siegel MJ, Friedland JA, Hildebolt CF (1997) Bowel wall thickening in children: differentiation with US. Radiology 203:631–635
Teefey SA, Roarke MC, Brink JA et al (1996) Bowel wall thickening: differentiation of inflammation from ischemia with color Doppler and duplex US. Radiology 198:547–551
Toursarkissian B, Thompson RW (1997) Ischemic colitis. Surg Clin North Am 77:461–470
Wiesner W, Mortelé KJ, Glickman JN, Ji H, Ros P (2001) Pneumatosis intestinal and portomesenteric venous gas in intestinal ischemia: correlation of CT findings with severity of ischemia and clinical outcome. AJR Am J Roentgenol 177:1319–1323

# Chronic Inflammatory Bowel Diseases

# Crohn's Disease

Giovanni Maconi, Elisa Radice, and Gabriele Bianchi Porro

CONTENTS

7.1 Introduction 61
7.2 Pathological Features 61
7.3 Ultrasonographic Features of Bowel Walls 62
7.3.1 Bowel Wall Thickening 62
7.3.2 Bowel Wall Echo Pattern 64
7.3.3 Bowel Wall Vascularity 64
7.3.4 Elasticity and Peristalsis 65
7.3.5 Mesenteric Hypertrophy and Mesenteric Lymph Nodes 65

7.4 Abdominal Complications of Crohn's Disease 66
7.4.1 Stenosis and Intestinal Occlusion 66
7.4.2 Sinus Tracks and Fistulae 66
7.4.3 Intra-abdominal Abscesses and Inflammatory Masses 68
7.4.4 Perforation 70

References 70

**Table 7.1.** Indications for bowel US in CD

- Early evaluation of patients with suspected CD
- Evaluation of site and extension of CD
- Differential diagnosis between chronic inflammatory colitis
- Diagnosis of CD abdominal complications
  - Stenosis and intestinal occlusion
  - Internal and external fistulae
  - Intra-abdominal abscesses
  - Perforation and toxic megacolon
- Assessment of CD activity
- Post-operative follow-up and prediction of CD recurrence

## 7.1 Introduction

Abdominal ultrasound (US), thanks to its accuracy, good repeatability and non-invasiveness is currently employed in many chronic inflammatory conditions, not only for purely diagnostic purposes, but also for management of the disease. In Crohn's disease (CD) patients, US has become the first-line imaging procedure for early diagnosis of the disease (Parente et al. 2004a), and more frequently for the follow-up, to detect intra-abdominal complications (strictures, fistulae and abscesses), to assess activity and monitor the course of disease, as a prognostic index of recurrence (Table 7.1).

G. Maconi, MD
E. Radice, MD, PhD
G. Bianchi Porro, MD, PhD
Chair of Gastroenterology, Department of Clinical Sciences, "L. Sacco" University Hospital, Via G.B. Grassi 74, 20157 Milano, Italy

## 7.2 Pathological Features

Crohn's disease is a chronic granulomatous inflammatory condition of the alimentary tract of unknown origin. Although there are no pathognomonic features of the disease, it is characterised by a segmental and transmural inflammation of the intestinal wall, particularly ileum (30%), colon (20%) or both the large and small bowel (50%). Macroscopically, the bowel wall often appears greatly thickened, and hypo-elastic or stiff with luminal narrowing (Fig. 7.1).

Mucosal abnormalities consist of longitudinal and aphthous ulcerations, which, in advanced disease, may penetrate into the submucosa and muscularis leading the serosa and outside, creating fissures and fistulas. These may invade the adjacent loops, organs, skin or end blindly in the mesentery, sometimes resulting in intra-abdominal or retroperitoneal abscesses. The mesentery is often thickened and fatty, surrounding the thickened walls and containing enlarged lymph nodes.

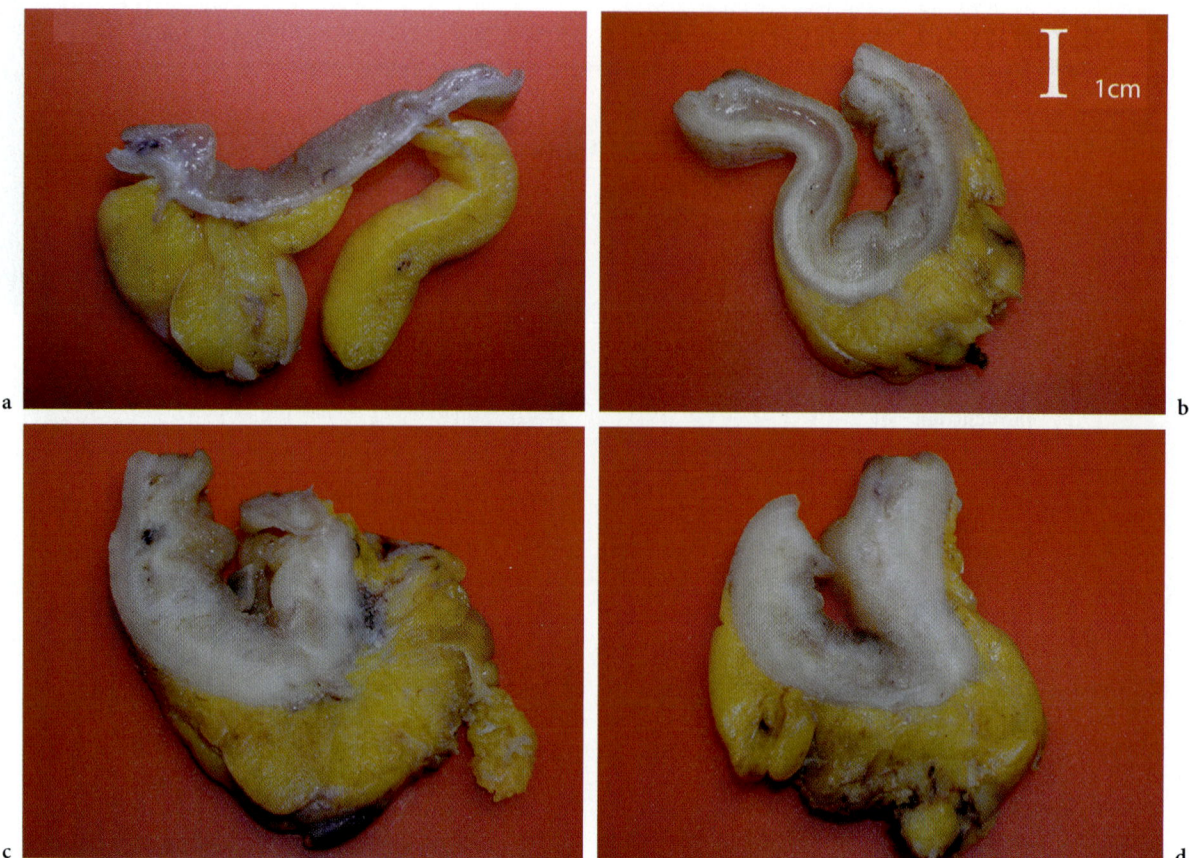

**Fig. 7.1a–d.** Opened transverse sections of a normal ileal wall (**a**); thickened bowel wall in a CD patient with loose (*left side*) and markedly inflamed (*right side*) submucosa (**b**); markedly thickened bowel wall with fibrosis and loss of stratification (**c,d**). (Courtesy of Dr. Paolo Fociani, Department of Pathology, 'L.Sacco' University Hospital, Milan)

## 7.3
## Ultrasonographic Features of Bowel Walls

The US manifestations of CD reflect the pathological features, consisting of abnormalities of bowel wall or representing its intra-abdominal complications. The abnormalities of bowel wall include bowel wall thickening, alterations of bowel wall echo pattern, hyperaemia, loss of elasticity and peristalsis, mesentering hypertrophy and mesenteric lymph nodes. Intra-abdominal complications of CD typically include stenoses and obstruction, fissures and fistulae, as well as inflammatory masses (phlegmon or abscesses).

### 7.3.1
### Bowel Wall Thickening

US examination in CD patients frequently reveals stiff and thickened bowel walls, usually >4 mm (which is considered the limit of normal bowel wall for the ileum and colon) up to 15 mm. The wall thickness of a diseased segment is measured in a transverse section from the central hyperechoic line of the lumen (representing interface between content of the lumen and the mucosa) to the outer hyperechoic margin of the wall (representing the serosa) (Fig. 7.2). Literature usually considers the maximum bowel wall thickness that can be reproduced along the bowel wall for at least 2–4 cm.

The abnormal thickening of bowel walls is the most widely and commonly US finding reported in the literature to diagnose CD. In a recent meta-analysis aiming at evaluating the impact of different cut-off values of bowel wall thickening (3 mm vs 4 mm) in determining the presence of CD, Fraquelli et al. (2005) showed that when a >3-mm cut-off level was observed for abnormality, sensitivity and specificity were 88% and 93%, respectively, whilst when a cut-off level of >4 mm was used, sensitivity was 75% and specificity 97%.

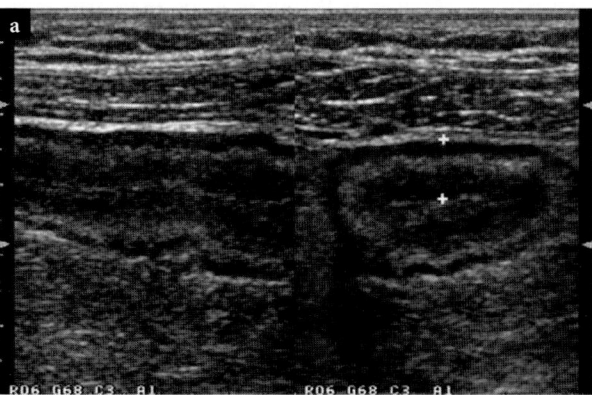 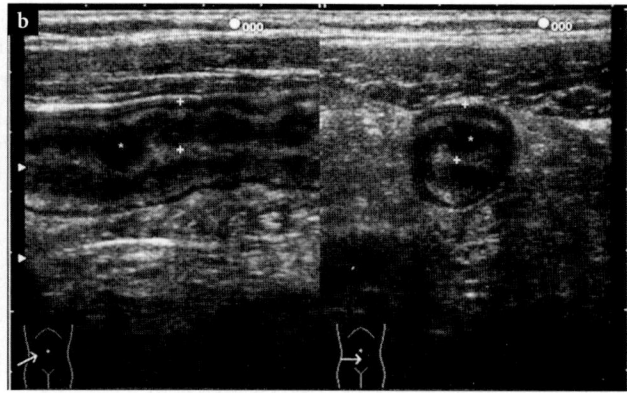

**Fig. 7.2a,b.** Longitudinal (*left*) and transverse (*right*) sections of a thickened bowel wall characterised by stratified echo pattern showing the markers (+) on the inner hyperechoic line (lumen) and outer hyperechoic margin (serosa) of the thickened wall. (*Asterisk*, gross nodularity of the mucosa)

However, these remarkable data also show that intestinal US, even in expert hands, may result in false negative and false positive findings. False negative findings may occur in obese patients or when CD is characterized by only superficial lesions, such as rare aphthous ulcers or mucosal erosions (Maconi et al. 1996a). False positive findings rely on the fact that thickening of the bowel walls is not specific for CD, being present also in infectious, neoplastic and other inflammatory diseases (Truong et al. 1998). Therefore, when US is used as a first imaging diagnostic procedure, the diagnosis of CD is suggested when wall thickening involves the terminal ileum, is circumferential and segmental. However, the definitive diagnosis – when possible, and always for colonic lesions – should rely on endoscopic and histological examinations of pathological tissues. US may represent a useful tool, prior to other invasive or expensive diagnostic investigations, which can be postponed in the case of negative US findings.

However, in known CD patients the accuracy of US in detecting bowel wall thickness has been usefully employed in localizing CD lesions within the bowel (particularly ileal lesions, which can be detected in more than 90%) and in assessing the length of small bowel involvement (Brignola et al. 1993; Maconi et al. 1996a; Parente et al. 2003, 2004a).

The clinical significance of the degree of bowel wall thickening in known CD patients is controversial. Several studies attempted to establish a relationship between maximum bowel wall thickness and clinical (Crohn's disease activity index, CDAI) and biochemical (erythrocyte sedimentation rate, C reactive protein) parameters of CD activity. However, almost all the results of these studies produced weak correlations, although somewhat significant, thus leaving the role of bowel US in the assessment of CD activity, in clinical practice, still controversial (Maconi et al. 1996a; Futagami et al. 1999; Haber et al. 2000, 2002; Mayer et al. 2000).

In known CD patients, the US assessment of bowel wall thickening has been used to identify postoperative recurrences following resection, to assess the efficacy of conservative surgical treatment, and to obtain predictive data on the risk of recurrences in these patients. Post-operative endoscopic recurrences of CD may be correctly identified using bowel US in more than 80% of patients (Di Candio et al. 1986; Andreoli et al. 1998). Moreover, the potential of US to accurately define transmural inflammatory changes during the course of CD, offers the possibility to assess the behaviour of diseased bowel walls following conservative surgery (namely strictureplasty and miniresection), which has become the new standard surgery of intestinal stenoses in CD patients. It has been shown that the behaviour of US thickening of bowel walls 6–12 months after conservative surgery is a strong predictor of the outcome of the disease. In fact, in patients showing an improvement or return to normality of the bowel wall thickening, the clinical and surgical recurrence rate have been significantly lower than in those maintaining the same level of bowel wall thickening (Maconi et al. 2001). Likewise, it has been shown in a series of 174 unselected CD patients, that bowel wall thickness >7 mm at US was the major risk factor (OR=19) for intestinal resection within the following 12 months (Castiglione et al. 2004).

Therefore, bowel US appears to offer a useful alternative to invasive procedures, such as ileo-colonoscopy or contrast radiology, in the post-surgical follow-up of CD patients, in particular for those CD patients who have undergone conservative surgery in whom endoscopy is not suitable to identify CD patients at high risk of clinical and surgical relapse, thus offering the opportunity to tailor the appropriate post-surgical medical treatment.

### 7.3.2
### Bowel Wall Echo Pattern

The affected segment in CD should be analysed with respect not only to wall thickness but also to bowel wall echo pattern. The bowel wall may maintain the regular stratification (Fig. 7.2) or may be characterised by a partial or complete loss of layering. Sometimes, bowel segments with alternate persistence and loss of stratification, may be observed.

In stratified echo pattern, the thickened walls display a variable enlargement of the mucosal, submucosal or muscular layers. Often the layer corresponding to the submucosa is thicker than others (Fig. 7.3a). The echo-stratification may be interrupted by hypoechoic areas (some with hyperechoic spots) corresponding to deep ulcers (Fig. 7.3b), or may completely disappear (Fig. 7.3c). In this case, the walls are often characterized by large, deep longitudinal ulcers associated with intense inflammation and neovascularization (KUNIHIRO et al. 2004).

The clinical and pathological significance of bowel echo pattern and, in particular, its importance in defining CD activity has been investigated in two studies, one of which was in patients with stenosis. Both these studies, where in vivo US images were compared with the in vitro histopathological findings of related resected specimens of the bowel, showed that the loss of stratification (hypoechoic echo pattern) correlated with the severity of inflammation and that persistence of stratification in bowel wall of strictures suggested a high degree of fibrosis within the submucosa and *muscularis mucosae* (HATA et al. 1994; MACONI et al. 2003a).

### 7.3.3
### Bowel Wall Vascularity

The increased vascularity is often observed in bowel wall with decreased echogenicity. This is likely due

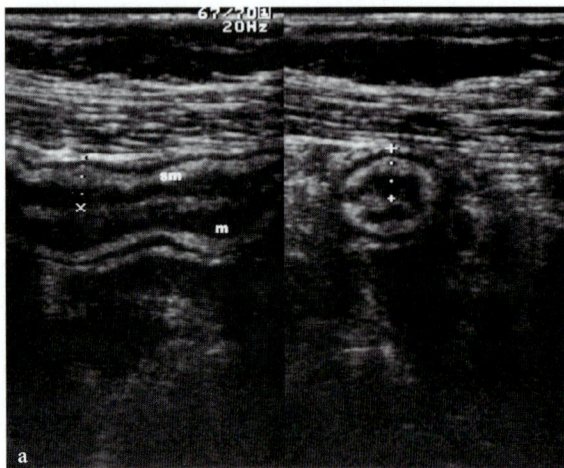

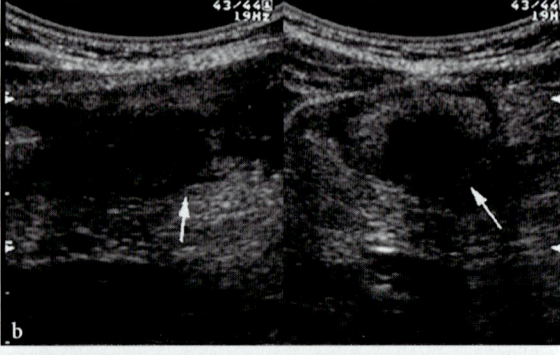

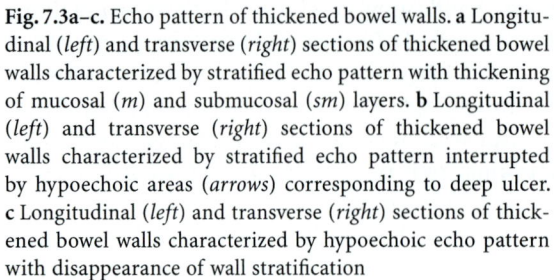

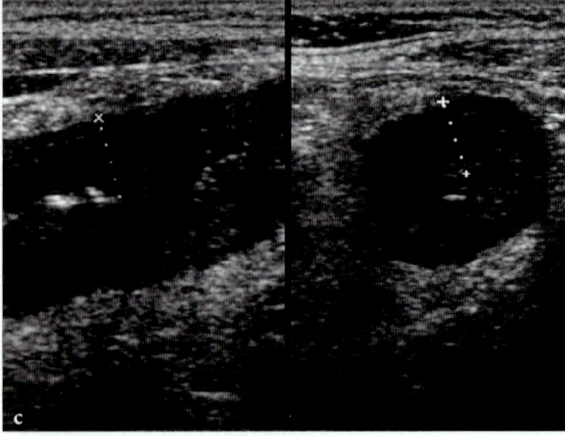

**Fig. 7.3a–c.** Echo pattern of thickened bowel walls. **a** Longitudinal (*left*) and transverse (*right*) sections of thickened bowel walls characterized by stratified echo pattern with thickening of mucosal (*m*) and submucosal (*sm*) layers. **b** Longitudinal (*left*) and transverse (*right*) sections of thickened bowel walls characterized by stratified echo pattern interrupted by hypoechoic areas (*arrows*) corresponding to deep ulcer. **c** Longitudinal (*left*) and transverse (*right*) sections of thickened bowel walls characterized by hypoechoic echo pattern with disappearance of wall stratification

to hyperaemia and neovascularization related to the increased inflammatory response (MACONI et al. 2003a; DI SABATINO et al. 2004). Therefore, vascularity within the thickened bowel walls, assessed by power colour Doppler US, has been used as an index of CD activity (Fig. 7.4).

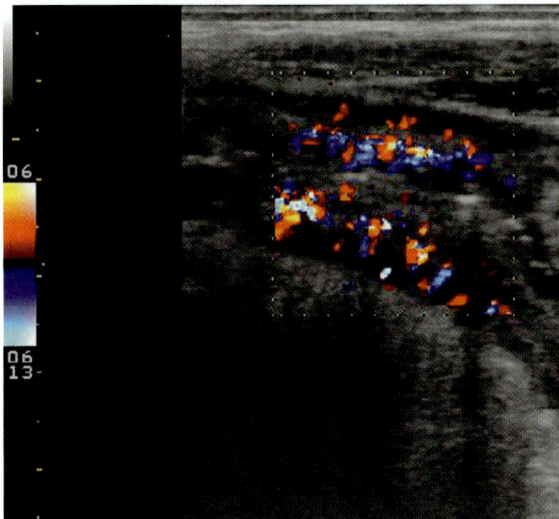

**Fig. 7.4.** The increased vascularity within the bowel wall shown by colour Doppler US

Vascularity has been evaluated using a simple scoring system according to the semi-quantitative (and subjective) intensity of colour signals and/or by analysis of Doppler curves (measurement of resistive index) obtained from vessels detected within the bowel walls. However, neither of these parameters correlated well with clinical or biochemical activity in most studies, whereas a significant correlation was often found between vascularity and endoscopic/radiological activity (SPALINGER et al. 2000; ESTEBAN et al. 2001; HABER et al. 2002; HEYNE et al. 2002; SCHOLBACH et al. 2004; NEYE et al. 2004; YEKELER et al. 2005).

To increase the sensitivity of Doppler US in detecting vascularity of diseased bowel walls, US contrast agents have been introduced. This issue will be widely discussed elsewhere (see Ch. 20).

### 7.3.4
### Elasticity and Peristalsis

Thickened bowel walls in CD are variably associated with reduction or absence of peristalsis in the small bowel and loss of haustra coli in the colon (SARRAZIN and WILSON 1996; DI MIZIO et al. 2004). Although this manifestation is quite subjective and difficult to quantitatively assess, it has been regarded as a relevant sign in most US studies, probably because it is associated with intestinal stenosis. To date, small bowel enteroclysis is considered the most reliable diagnostic tool to show elasticity of the diseased intestinal loops and to accurately detect intestinal strictures. The use of oral contrast agents may be useful for a more accurate US assessment of this feature.

### 7.3.5
### Mesenteric Hypertrophy and Mesenteric Lymph Nodes

This abnormality, also commonly termed as creeping fat or fibrofatty proliferation in the mesentery, appears at US as a hyperechoic, sometimes inhomogeneous area surrounding thickened bowel walls (Fig. 7.5). It is found in up to 40% of CD patients (GOLDBERG et al. 1983) and has been regarded as a frequent cause of bowel loop separation at conventional X-ray studies. Accuracy, prevalence, and clinical significance of US assessment of this condition remain largely unknown.

Enlarged mesenteric lymph nodes appear at US as oval, homogeneous, hypoechoic nodules with regular

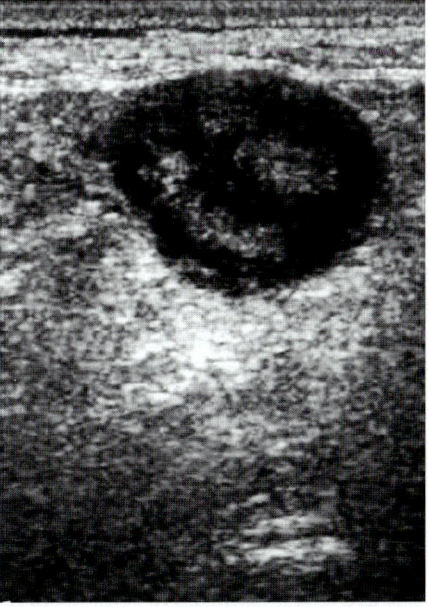

**Fig. 7.5.** Mesenteric hypertrophy, appearing at US as hyperechoic, sometimes inhomogeneous area surrounding thickened bowel walls

margins (Fig. 7.6). This is a frequent finding in CD patients. Its prevalence and clinical significance is discussed elsewhere (see Ch. 2).

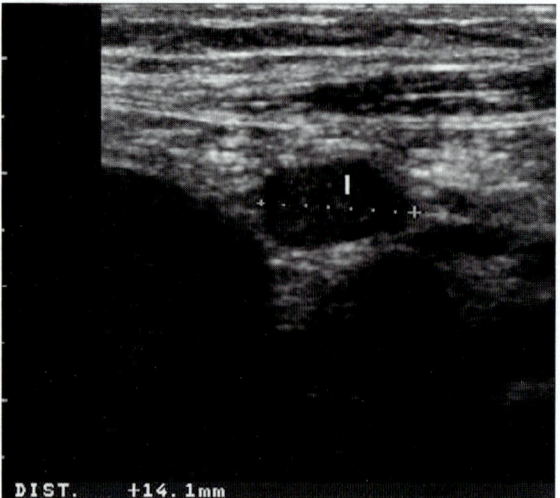

**Fig. 7.6.** Enlarged mesenteric lymph node (*l*) appearing at US as oval, homogeneous hypoechoic nodule with regular margin

## 7.4
## Abdominal Complications of Crohn's Disease

The clinical course of CD is often characterized by abdominal complications such as stenosis, fistulae or abscesses, and rarely by free perforation.

### 7.4.1
### Stenosis and Intestinal Occlusion

Stenosis develops in 21% of patients with ileal CD and in 8% of those with ileocolic disease (FENOGLIO-PREISER et al. 1989; SIMPKINS and GORE 1994). It is the most frequent cause of surgery. The diagnostic gold standard of this complication is contrast radiography, which reveals all the occluded sites, the degree of intestinal narrowing and the length of the stenotic segments.

Bowel stenosis can be revealed by US as thickened bowel walls, associated with narrowed lumen and increased diameter of the proximal loop >2.5–3 cm. Acute stenoses are often associated with a variable amount of liquid and gas within the lumen of the proximal loop and with increased peristalsis (Fig. 7.7a) (Ko et al. 1993). In chronic, incomplete, stenoses the amount of air within the proximal loop prevails, and peristalsis is usually weak (Fig. 7.7b).

Using this definition, US correctly diagnoses stenosis in 70%–79% of unselected CD patients and in >90% of patients with severe intestinal stenoses requiring surgery, with false-positive diagnoses limited to 7% (MACONI et al. 1996b; GASCHE et al. 1999; PARENTE et al. 2002, 2004b). Results may be even better using an oral contrast agent (see Ch. 21).

US assessment of the echo pattern of the bowel wall of the strictures may also offer an insight into the histological features, discriminating between fibrotic and inflammatory strictures (MACONI et al. 2003a). Loss of stratification of the bowel wall at the level of the stricture suggests its inflammatory nature with a low degree of fibrosis, whilst the presence of stratification suggests a higher degree of fibrosis of the stenosis (Fig. 7.8).

### 7.4.2
### Sinus Tracks and Fistulae

Fistulae occur in 17%–82% of CD patients. They are a transmural extension of the disease, often resulting from intestinal stenosis (OBERHUBER et al. 2000), which ends blindly in the surrounding mesentery or connects intestinal loops or adjacent organs. Depending on their site and extension, abdominal fistulae are commonly subdivided into external or internal (enteroenteric, enteromesenteric).

Fistulae may appear on US as hypoechoic ducts or hypoechoic areas between intestinal loops or between loops and other structures such as the bladder (enterovesical fistula) or the skin (enterocutaneous fistulae) (Fig. 7.9). Sometimes, fistulae display internal echoic spots due to the presence of air, debris or intestinal material (MACONI et al. 1996b; GASCHE et al. 1999).

At present, there is no reliable technique for the diagnosis of this complication. Using surgical findings as a reference standard, we showed that the accuracy of US and X-ray studies in detecting internal fistulae was comparable with a sensitivity of 71.4% for US and 69.6% for X-ray studies, and a specificity of 95.8% for both. We also showed that the combination of these two techniques significantly improved preoperative diagnostic performance (sensitivity 97.4% and specificity 90%) and that in selected severe cases of CD, with clinical suspicion of septic complications (i.e., abdominal mass or fever), sensitivity of US is even higher (88.5%), thus confirming the high sen-

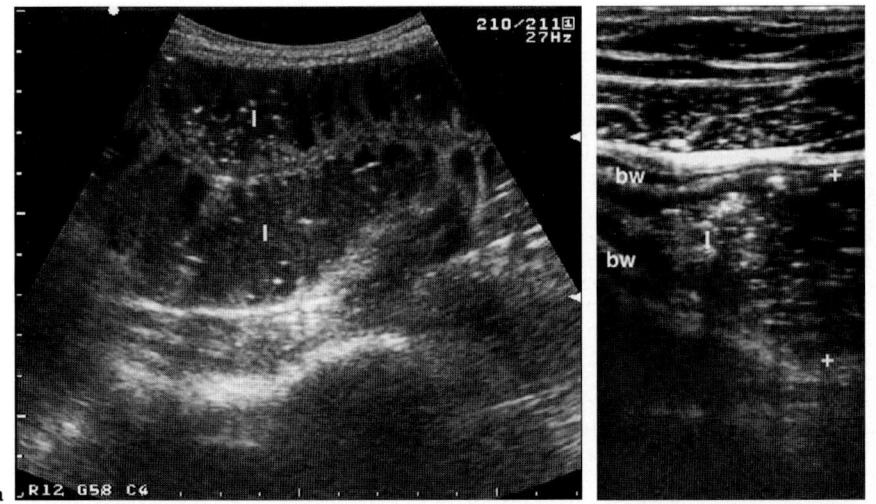

**Fig. 7.7a,b.** Stenosis at US presented as thickened bowel wall, with narrowing of lumen associated with pre-stenotic dilatation > 3 cm in diameter, and often associated with liquid content and air in the lumen. **a** Acute stenosis associated with a variable amount of liquid and gas within the lumen (*l*) of the proximal loop and with increased peristalsis. **b** Chronic, incomplete stenosis characterised by stratified bowel wall echo pattern, showing of gas within the proximal loop and weak peristalsis (*bw*, bowel wall; *l*, lumen)

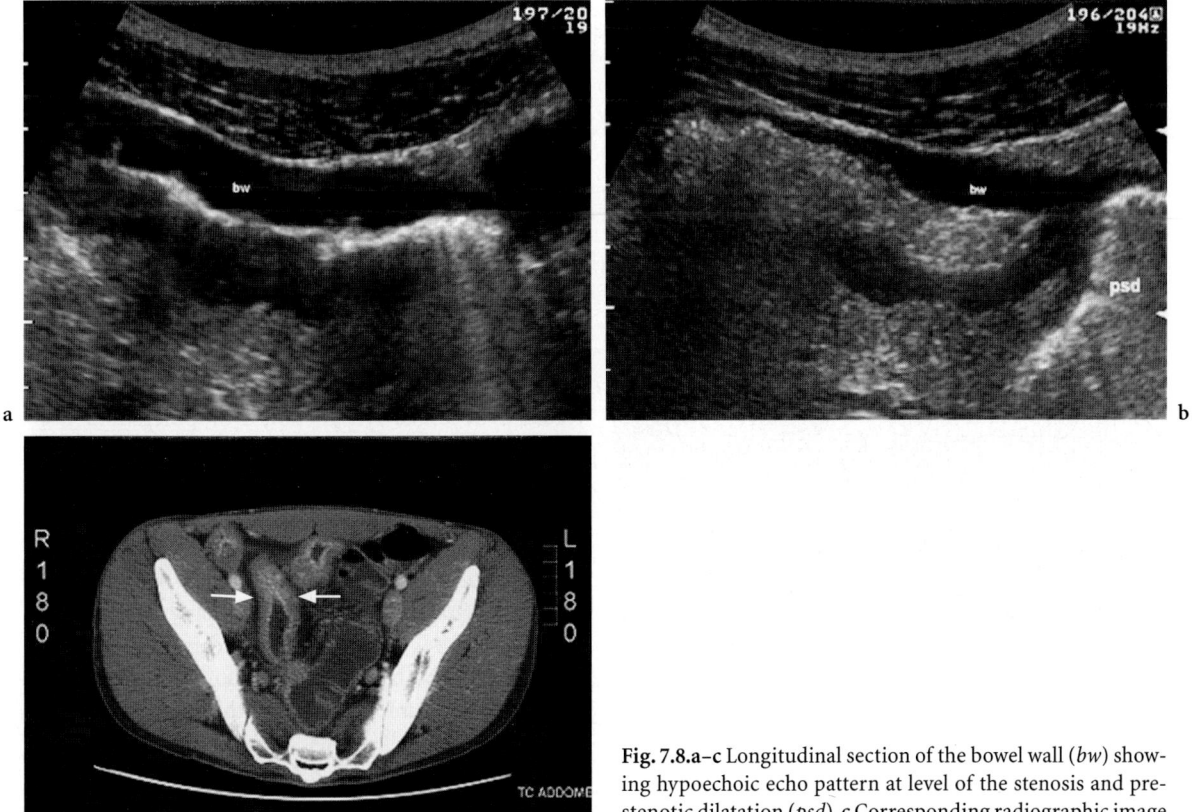

**Fig. 7.8.a–c** Longitudinal section of the bowel wall (*bw*) showing hypoechoic echo pattern at level of the stenosis and pre-stenotic dilatation (*psd*). **c** Corresponding radiographic image of the same stricture (*arrows*) at contrast CT enteroclysis

sitivity of a previous US study (GASCHE et al. 1999; MACONI et al. 2003b).

Since fistula wall is characterized by granulation tissue and neoangiogenesis, it may be easily recognized at US by detecting intramural blood flow using power Doppler or i.v. contrast enhanced US (MACONI et al. 2002).

US may also be usefully employed to define the features of external fistulae, particularly if US is combined with the injection of echoic contrast medium composed of hydrogen peroxide and povidone iodine into the fistula. This type of US fistulography defines the extension and the configuration (linear or with ramifications) of the entero-cutaneous fistulae (Fig. 7.10), is well tolerated and does not expose the patient to the risk of septic dissemination during the injection of the contrast medium (MACONI et al. 1999).

### 7.4.3
### Intra-abdominal Abscesses and Inflammatory Masses

Intra-abdominal abscesses occur in 12%–30% of CD patients, usually as a consequence of fistulising disease or as a post-surgical complication (STEINBERG et al. 1973; NAGLER et al. 1979). Although CT and magnetic resonance imaging (MRI) are considered the gold standard for the diagnosis of CD-related masses, US is usually employed as a first level procedure.

At US, abscesses appear as hypo-anechoic lesions with fluid collection and irregular thickened walls, sometimes containing internal echoes due to the presence of debris or air, and characterized by a posterior echo-enhancement (Fig. 7.11). Hypoechoic masses, especially those of small size and located close to the intestine, may be missed or mistaken for large sinus track, hypoechoic lymph nodes or phlegmon. Conventionally these lesions are diagnosed when characterised by irregular borders, non-identifiable wall or liquefaction. Inflammatory masses, phlegmon and intra-abdominal abscesses, identified or suspected at US, may be confirmed and distinguished detecting vascular signals by colour power Doppler US or, better, by i.v. contrast-enhanced US, around and/or within the lesions. Phlegmon and inflammatory masses, in fact, show increased colour signals within, whilst abscesses present fluid collections with a peripheral flow (Fig. 7.12) (TARJAN et al. 2000; MACONI et al. 2002).

US detection of intra-abdominal abscesses shows a mean sensitivity and specificity of 91.5% and 93%,

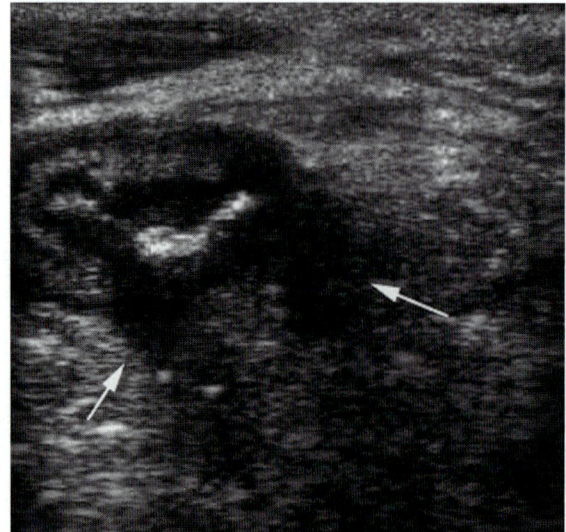
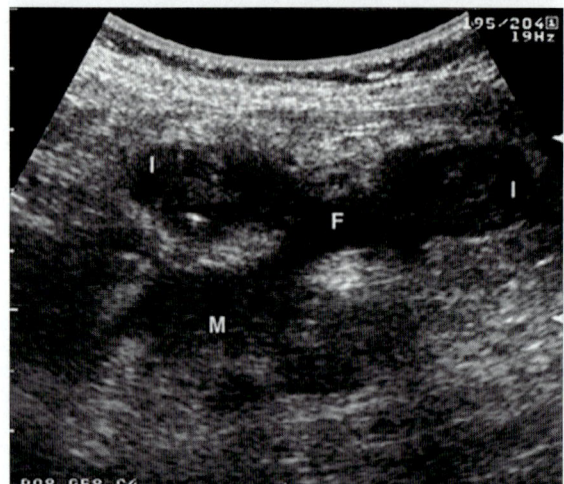
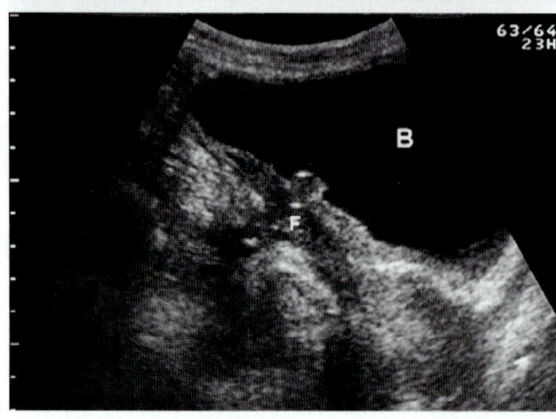

**Fig. 7.9a–c.** Ultrasonographic appearance of internal fistulae. Entero-mesenteric (**a**), entero-enteric (**b**), and entero-vesical (**c**) fistulae (*F*) revealed at US as hypoechoic area deforming the margins of bowel wall (*arrows*), as hypoechoic ducts between the intestinal loops (*l*), and as hypoechoic areas between intestinal loops and bladder (*B*), respectively. *F*, Fistula; *l*, intestinal loop; *M*, inflammatory mass; *B*, bladder

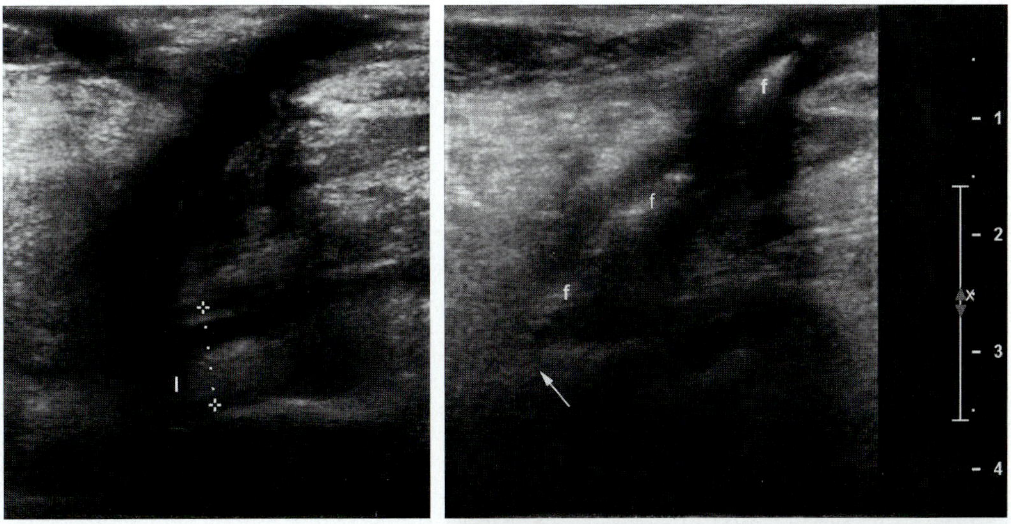

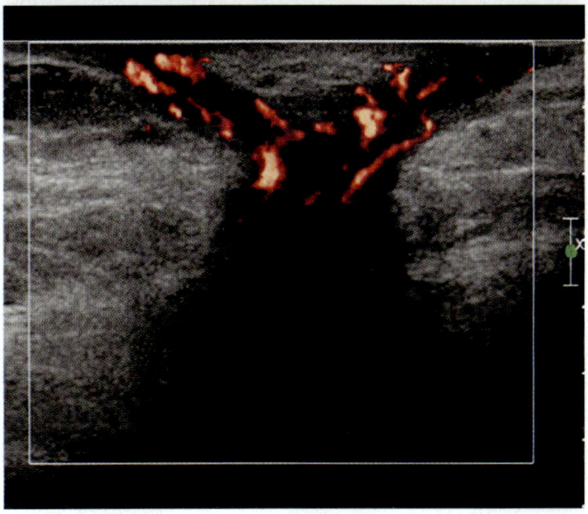

**Fig. 7.10a–c.** Assessment of enterocutaneous fistula by US fistulography. **a** US assessment of the enterocutaneous fistula and (**b**) evaluation of the same lesion following the injection of contrast agent within the fistula (*f*) revealing its openness (*arrow*), previously not clear, and defines the extension and the configuration of the lesion. **c** The presence of blood flow detected within the fistula wall can also suggest the activity of the fistula, despite the absence of conspicuous drainage. *f*, Fistula; *l*, intestinal loop

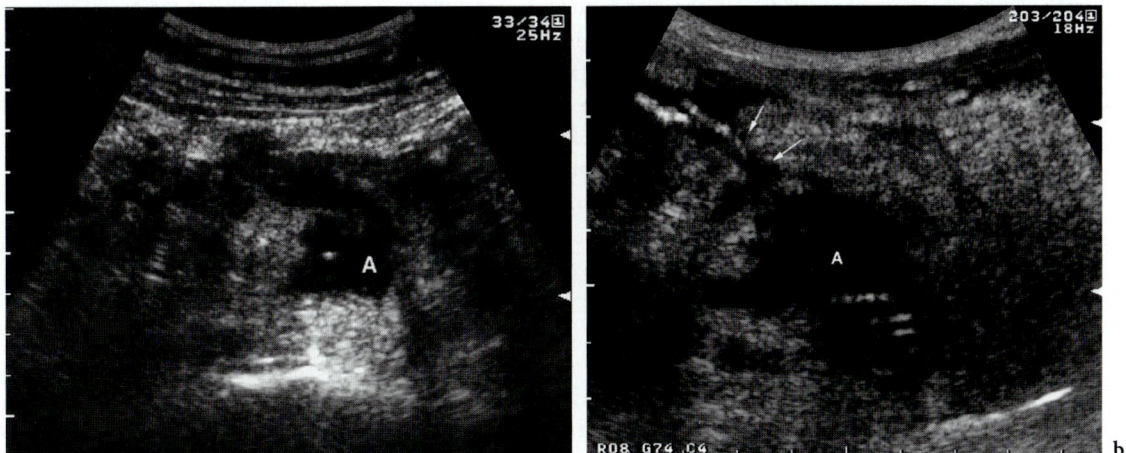

**Fig. 7.11a,b.** Intra-abdominal abscesses (*A*) appearing as hypo-anechoic lesions, often originating from a fistula (*arrows*), with irregular wall, internal echoes due to presence of debris or air, and characterised by posterior echo-enhancement

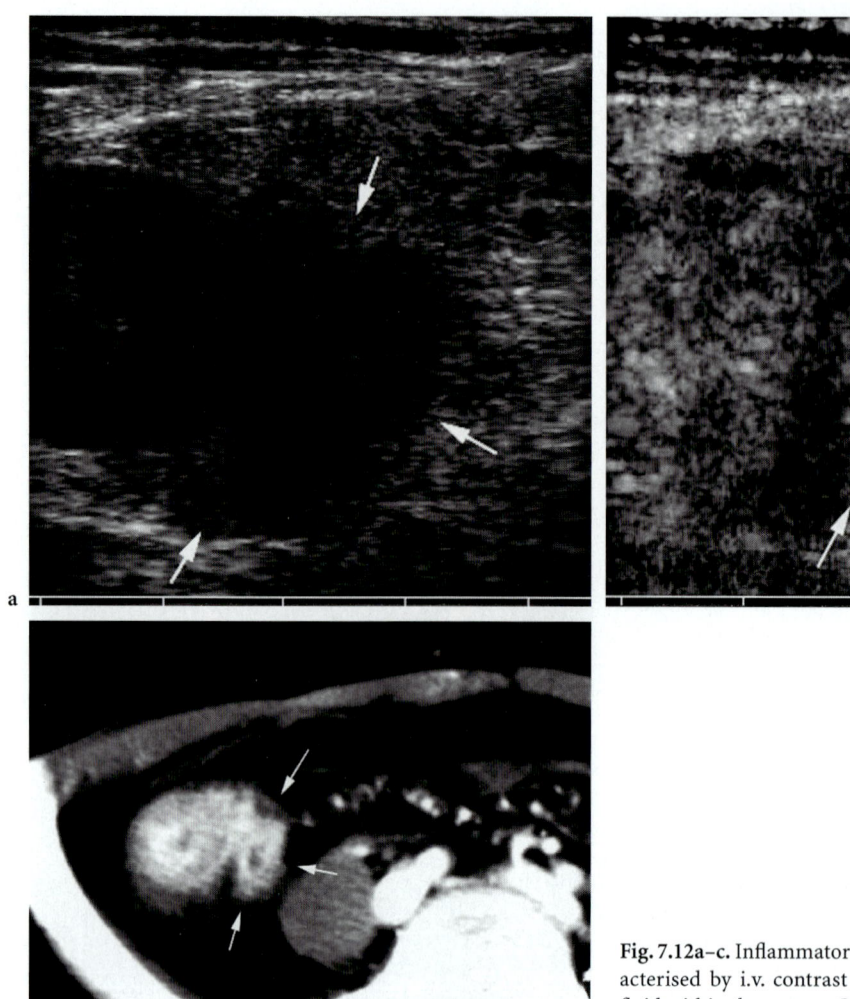

Fig. 7.12a–c. Inflammatory mass detected by US (a) and characterised by i.v. contrast agent (b) showing the absence of fluid within the mass. c Corresponding i.v. contrast CT imaging of the same lesion

respectively (SCHWERK et al. 1992; MACONI et al. 1996b, 2003b; GASCHE et al. 1999). US shows a higher sensitivity in the detection of superficial intraperitoneal abscesses, while the diagnosis of deep pelvic or retroperitoneal abscesses is more difficult due to the presence of overlying bowel gas and the difficulty in differentiating an abscess from an intestinal loop with stagnating fluid.

## 7.4.4
## Perforation

Perforation is a potentially lethal complication of CD. It occurs in 1–2% of patients as a consequence of deep fissures in the intestinal wall. Perforation should be suspected when US shows the presence of intraperitoneal liquid and air, indicative of purulent peritonitis, or the presence of free air under the diaphragm.

Focal perforations are more frequent than free perforations and may be diagnosed by US as areas of asymmetric and focal thickening of the wall associated with small periparietal collections of liquid and air.

## References

Andreoli A, Cerro P, Falasco G et al (1998) Role of ultrasonography in the diagnosis of postsurgical recurrence of Crohn's disease. Am J Gastroenterol 93:1117–1121

Brignola C, Belloli C, Iannone P et al (1993) Comparison of scintigraphy with indium-111 leukocyte scan and ultrasonography in assessment of X-ray-demonstrated lesions of Crohn's disease. Dig Dis Sci 38:433–437

Castiglione F, de Sio I, Cozzolino A et al (2004) Bowel wall thickness at abdominal ultrasound and the one-year-risk of surgery in patients with Crohn's disease. Am J Gastroenterol 99:1977–1983

Di Candio G, Mosca F, Campatelli A et al (1986) Sonographic detection of postsurgical recurrence of Crohn disease. AJR Am J Roentgenol 146:523–526

Di Mizio R, Maconi G, Romano S et al (2004) Small bowel Crohn disease: sonographic features. Abdom Imaging 29:23–35

Di Sabatino A, Ciccocioppo R, Armellini E et al (2004) Serum bFGF and VEGF correlate respectively with bowel wall thickness and intramural blood flow in Crohn's disease. Inflamm Bowel Dis 10:573–577

Esteban JM, Maldonado L, Sanchiz V et al (2001) Activity of Crohn's disease assessed by colour Doppler ultrasound analysis of the affected loops. Eur Radiol 11:1423–1428

Fenoglio-Preiser CM, Lantz PE, Listrom MB et al (1989) Gastrointestinal pathology; an atlas and text. Raven Press, New York, NY pp 427–484

Fraquelli M, Colli A, Casazza G et al (2005) Role of US in detection of Crohn's disease: meta-analysis. Radiology 236:95–101

Futagami Y, Haruma K, Hata J et al (1999) Development and validation of an US activity index of Crohn's disease. Eur J Gastroenterol Hepatol 11:1007–1012

Gasche C, Moser G, Turetschek K et al (1999) Transabdominal bowel sonography for detection of intestinal complication in Crohn's disease. Gut 44:112–117

Goldberg HI, Gore RM, Margulis AR et al (1983) Computed tomography in the evaluation of Crohn's disease. AJR Am J Roengtenol 140:277–282

Haber HP, Busch A, Ziebach R, Stern M (2000) Bowel wall thickness measured by ultrasound as a marker of Crohn's disease activity in children. Lancet 355:1239–1240

Haber HP, Busch A, Ziebach R et al (2002) US findings correspond to clinical, endoscopic, and histologic findings in inflammatory bowel disease and other enterocolitides. J Ultrasound Med 21:375–382

Hata J, Haruma K, Yamanaka H et al (1994) US evaluation of the bowel wall in inflammatory bowel disease: comparison of in vivo and in vitro studies. Abdom Imaging 19:395–399

Heyne R, Rickes S, Bock P et al (2002) Non-invasive evaluation of activity in inflammatory bowel disease by power Doppler sonography. Z Gastroenterol 40:171–175

Ko YT, Lim JH, Lee DH et al (1993) Small bowel obstruction: sonographic evaluation. Radiology 188:649–653

Kunihiro K, Hata J, Haruma K et al (2004) Sonographic detection of longitudinal ulcers in Crohn disease. Scand J Gastroenterol 39:322–326

Maconi G, Parente F, Bollani S et al (1996a) Abdominal ultrasound in the assessment of extent and activity of Crohn's disease: clinical significance and implication of bowel wall thickening. Am J Gastroenterol 91:1604–1609

Maconi G, Bollani S, Bianchi Porro G (1996b) Ultrasonographic detection of intestinal complications in Crohn's disease. Dig Dis Sci 41:1643–1648

Maconi G, Parente F, Bianchi Porro G (1999) Hydrogen peroxide enhanced ultrasound-fistulography in the assessment of enterocutaneous fistulas complicating Crohn's disease. Gut 45:874–878

Maconi G, Sampietro GM, Cristaldi M et al (2001) Preoperative characteristics and postoperative behaviour of bowel wall on risk of recurrence after conservative surgery in Crohn's disease. A prospective study. Ann Surg 233:345–352

Maconi G, Sampietro GM, Russo A et al (2002) The vascularity of internal fistulae in Crohn's disease: an in vivo power Doppler ultrasonography assessment. Gut 50:496–500

Maconi G, Carsana L, Fociani P et al (2003a) Small bowel stenosis in Crohn's disease: clinical, biochemical and US evaluation of histological features. Aliment Pharmacol Ther 18:749–756

Maconi G, Sampietro GM, Parente F et al (2003b) Contrast radiology, computed tomography and ultrasonography in detecting internal fistulas and intra-abdominal abscesses in Crohn's disease: a prospective comparative study. Am J Gastroenterol 98:1545–1555

Mayer D, Reinshagen M, Mason RA et al (2000) Sonographic measurement of thickened bowel wall segments as a quantitative parameter for activity in inflammatory bowel disease. Z Gastroenterol 38:295–300

Nagler SM, Poticha SM (1979) Intra-abdominal abscesses in regional enteritis. Am J Surg 173:350–354

Neye H, Voderholzer W, Rickes S et al (2004) Evaluation of criteria for the activity of Crohn's disease by power Doppler sonography. Dig Dis 22:67–72

Oberhuber G, Stangl PC, Vogelsang H et al (2000) Significant association of strictures and internal fistula formation in Crohn's disease. Virchows Arch 437:293–297

Parente F, Maconi G, Bollani S et al (2002) Bowel ultrasound in assessment of Crohn's disease and detection of related small bowel strictures. A prospective comparative study versus X-ray and intraoperative findings. Gut 50:490–495

Parente F, Greco S, Molteni M et al (2003) Role of early ultrasound in detecting inflammatory intestinal disorders and identifying their anatomical location within the bowel. Aliment Pharmacol Ther 18:1009–1016

Parente F, Greco S, Molteni M et al (2004a) Modern imaging of Crohn's disease using bowel ultrasound. Inflamm Bowel Dis 10:452–461

Parente F, Greco S, Molteni M et al (2004b) Oral contrast enhanced bowel ultrasonography in the assessment of small intestine Crohn's disease. A prospective comparison with conventional ultrasound, X-ray studies, and ileocolonoscopy. Gut 53:1652–1657

Sarrazin J, Wilson SR (1996) Manifestation of Crohn disease at US. Radiographics 16:499–520

Scholbach T, Herrero I, Scholbach J (2004) Dynamic color Doppler sonography of intestinal wall in patients with Crohn disease compared with healthy subjects. J Pediatr Gastroenterol Nutr 39:524–528

Schwerk WB, Beckh K, Raith M (1992) A prospective evaluation of high resolution sonography in the diagnosis of inflammatory bowel disease. Eur J Gastroenterol Hepatol 4:173–182

Simpkins KC, Gore RM (1994) Crohn's disease. In: Gore RM, Levine MS, Laufer I (eds) Textbook of gastrointestinal radiology. PA Saunders, Philadelphia, p 2660–2681

Spalinger J, Patriquin H, Miron MC et al (2000) Doppler US in patients with Crohn disease: vessel density in the diseased bowel reflects disease activity. Radiology 217:787–791

Steinberg DM, Cooke WT, Alexander Williams J (1973) Abscesses and fistulae in Crohn's disease. Gut 14:865–869

Tarjan Z, Toth G, Gyorke T et al (2000) Ultrasound in Crohn's disease of the small bowel. Eur J Radiol 35:176–182

Truong M, Atri M, Bret PM et al (1998) Sonographic appearance of benign and malignant conditions of the colon. Am J Roentgenol 170:1451–1455

Yekeler E, Danalioglu A, Movasseghi B et al (2005) Crohn disease activity evaluated by Doppler ultrasonography of the superior mesenteric artery and the affected small-bowel segments. J Ultrasound Med 24:59–65

# Ulcerative Colitis

Giovanni Maconi, Salvatore Greco, and Gabriele Bianchi Porro

## CONTENTS

8.1 Introduction 73
8.2 Clinical and Pathological Features 73
8.3 Ultrasonographic Features of Bowel Walls 75
8.4 Detection and Determination of Extension 78
8.5 Assessment of Disease Activity 78
8.6 Toxic Megacolon 79
8.7 Differential Diagnosis Between Ulcerative Colitis, Crohn's Disease and Other Inflammatory Diseases 79
References 80

However, transabdominal US has been demonstrated to be a reliable diagnostic tool both for diagnostic purposes and to detect disease extension and activity in UC, thus providing important information if endoscopy is incomplete (due to tight strictures) or contraindicated (severe active disease) (Table 8.1).

Table 8.1. Potential indications for bowel ultrasound in ulcerative colitis

- Early evaluation of patients with suspected UC
- Evaluation of extension of UC
- Differential diagnosis in chronic inflammatory colitis
- Diagnosis of CD abdominal complications
  - Toxic megacolon
  - Massive pseudopolyposis
- Assessment of UC activity
- Prediction of UC recurrence

## 8.1 Introduction

The role of abdominal ultrasound (US) has been less extensively investigated in ulcerative colitis (UC) than in Crohn's disease (CD). This is due to the different features between these two intestinal diseases. In fact, in UC, unlike in CD, inflammatory lesions are confined to the colon, have a predictable spread involving mainly the rectum, which is considered difficult to image by transabdominal US, and affects only the inner wall layer of the colon. Therefore, endoscopy is considered the method of choice in the diagnosis and in assessing extent and severity of the disease.

## 8.2 Clinical and Pathological Features

Ulcerative colitis is a chronic idiopathic inflammatory disease of unknown origin. Depending on extension and activity, the presence and severity of leading symptoms of the disease such as diarrhoea, rectal blood loss, abdominal pain and fever can vary and laboratory parameters of the acute phase response (e.g., C-reactive protein, erythrocyte sedimentation rate) may be normal or abnormal. These findings usually depend on the severity and extent of colonic involvement.

Ulcerative colitis involves the rectum and extends proximally to all or different portions of the colon (ulcerative proctitis, sigmoiditis, left-sided colitis or pancolitis). Rectosigmoid involvement is present in almost all patients at endoscopy, with approximately 40–50% of patients having disease limited to the rectum

---

G. Maconi, MD
S. Greco, MD; G. Bianchi Porro, MD, PhD
Chair of Gastroenterology, Department of Clinical Science, "L. Sacco" University Hospital, Via G.B. Grassi 74, 20157 Milan, Italy

and rectosigmoid, 30–40% disease extending beyond the sigmoid colon but not involving the entire colon, and 20% total colitis. Mucosal inflammation of the terminal ileum, the so-called backwash ileitis, is rare. Proximal spread of the disease occurs in continuity, without areas of uninvolved mucosa, and although macroscopic activity may suggest skip areas, endoscopic biopsies from mucosa with a normal appearance are usually abnormal.

Indeed, the mucosa may appear normal when disease is in remission, whereas with mild and moderate inflammation it is erythematous and of granular appearance. In more severe cases, the mucosa is ulcerated and haemorrhagic (Fig. 8.1). In long-standing disease, the mucosa may appear atrophic and inflammatory polyps, or pseudopolyps, may be present as a result of epithelial regeneration.

In UC, histological changes are limited to the mucosa and superficial submucosa with deeper layers being unaffected, except in fulminant colitis. The major changes are distortion of crypt architecture and basal plasma cells and basal lymphoid cell infiltrate. Mucosal vascular congestion with oedema, focal haemorrhage and inflammatory cell infiltration may also be present (Fig. 8.2).

These histological changes, as well as endoscopic features, correlate well with sonographic images. However, since the disease is confined to the inner layers of the colon, endoscopy alone may be sufficient to detect and assess the extent and activity of the disease in UC, unlike in CD. In this context the role of cross sectional imaging, US included, may be marginal although useful, in some instances, since it can be repeated and is non-invasive.

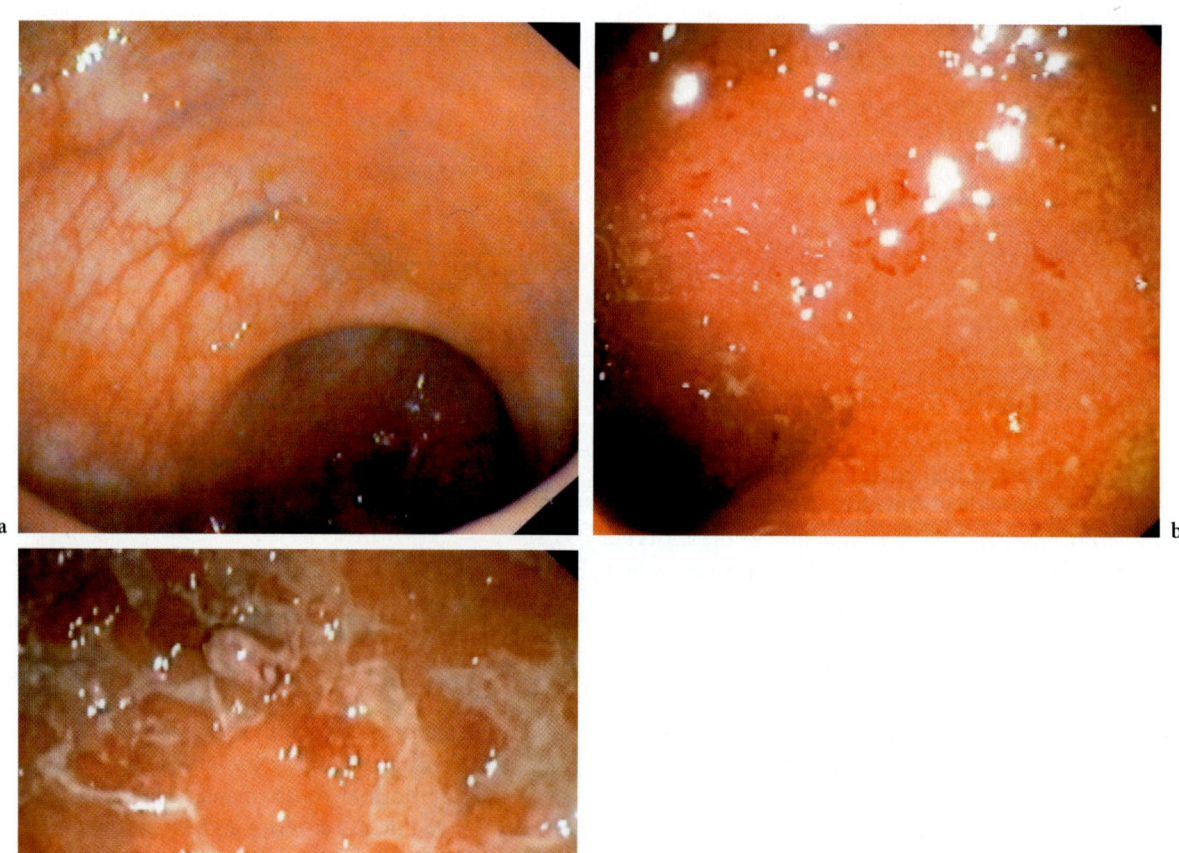

**Fig. 8.1a–c.** Different endoscopic aspects of colon in ulcerative colitis. **a** Inactive disease: presence of distorted mucosal vascular pattern without ulcerations, friability or spontaneous bleeding. **b** Moderate disease: marked erythema, absent vascular pattern, friability, coarse granularity with small erosions. **c** Severe disease: gross ulceration and spontaneous bleeding

# Ulcerative Colitis

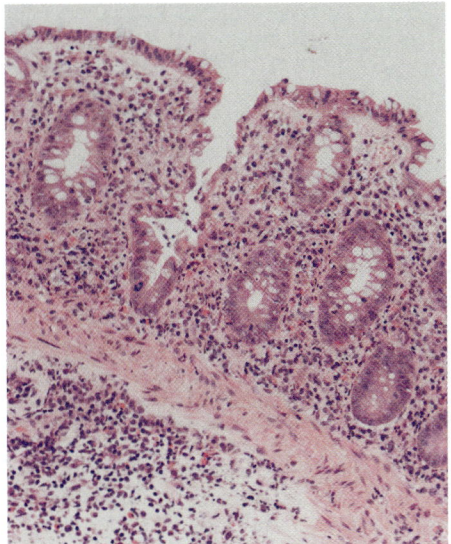

**Fig. 8.2.** Histological feature of ulcerative colitis. Changes are limited to mucosa (*muscularis mucosae* is normal) and consist in distortion of crypt architecture, vascular congestion of mucosa, oedema, and basal inflammatory cell infiltrate

## 8.3
## Ultrasonographic Features of Bowel Walls

The US features of UC reflect the pathological aspects of the bowel wall. The main abnormalities of the bowel wall include thickening, alterations of bowel wall echo pattern, hyperaemia and loss of haustra coli. Occasionally mesenteric hypertrophy and mesenteric nodes, or complications such as stenosis or toxic megacolon, can be found.

US features of bowel wall, and particularly bowel wall thickening, largely depend on the activity of the disease. In active UC patients, US frequently reveals thickened bowel walls, usually >4 mm (which is considered the limit of normal bowel wall in the ileum and colon), frequently ranging from 5 to 7 mm, and only rarely reaching 10 mm, in the most severe disease (WORLICEK et al. 1987; VALLETTE et al. 2001) (Fig. 8.3).

However, as mentioned elsewhere in this volume, the abnormal thickening of bowel walls at US (bowel

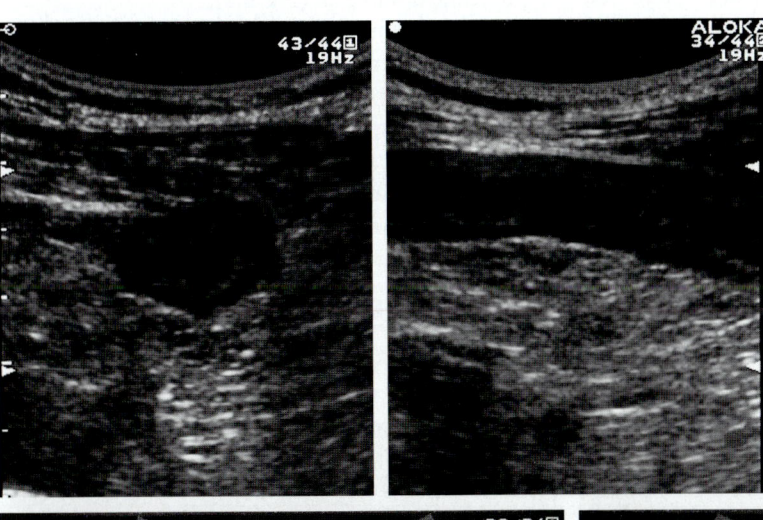

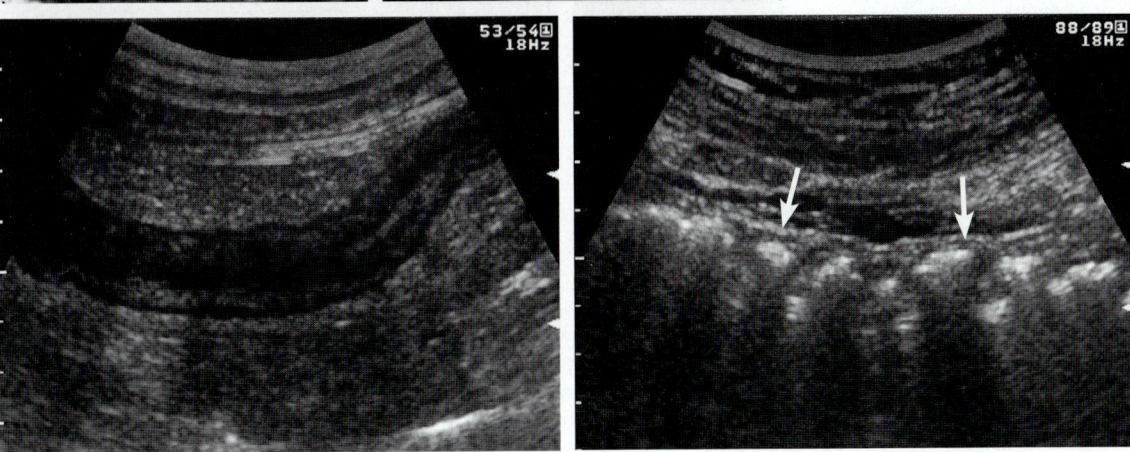

**Fig. 8.3a–d.** Ultrasonographic features of bowel wall in a patient with ulcerative colitis. Transverse (**a**) and longitudinal (**b**) sections of descending colon in patient with left-sided active ulcerative colitis. Thickened bowel walls characterised by stratified echo pattern and absence of haustra coli (**c**) in the left colon. The presence of haustra coli (*arrows*) in the transverse colon (**d**) clearly define the extension of the disease

wall thickness >4 mm) is not specific since several intestinal disorders, including UC, are characterised by US thickening of bowel walls. The degree of thickness depends on disease activity, being greater in active disease, and normal in the quiescent phases (Fig. 8.4).

For this reason, sonographic diagnosis of UC relies on different features of the bowel wall. In UC, the thickness of the bowel wall is continuous, predominates in the left colon and is, therefore, usually found in left iliaca fossa and in hypogastric regions and extends throughout the entire colon in pancolitis (Fig. 8.5). Loss of haustration is a frequent finding in active and extensive disease. The thickness of the bowel wall is circumferential and symmetrical.

Since inflammation involves the mucosa and the superficial submucosa, the stratified echo pattern of the bowel wall is usually preserved (Fig. 8.5). However, in cases of acute inflammation, the thickening involves the submucosa which may appear slightly hypoechoic and dyshomogeneous, sometimes giving the bowel wall the US appearance of pathological wall thickening with loss of stratification and increased bowel wall vascularity (Fig. 8.6).

The muscularis propria, which is imaged at US as an external hypoechoic line is preserved; therefore, external profiles of the bowel walls, in UC, are usually linear and regular (Figs. 8.4 and 8.5).

Unlike Crohn's disease, ulcerations are superficial and, therefore, not usually revealed by US. No deep or penetrating ulcers are present, except in severe UC in which a pre-perforative laceration of the submucosa is found. Therefore, in mild to moderate active UC, the inner layers of the colonic wall are usually

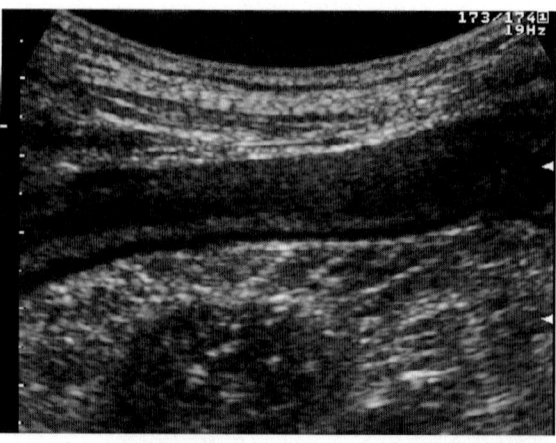

**Fig. 8.5.** Frequent US feature of ulcerative colitis. Thickness of bowel wall is continuous, symmetrical, regular and usually found in the left iliaca fossa when it affects the left colon

regular. On the contrary, in severe active disease, the inner layer may be regular or even irregular with fine multiple hyperechoic spots, representing deep penetrating ulcers, but within a severely thickened and hypoechoic bowel wall (Fig. 8.7).

Since the colon returns, at endoscopy, to a normal appearance after resolution of inflammation, also US reveals a normal colonic wall. Indeed, after several recurrences, in quiescent disease, as well as in some cases with mild inflammation, the colonic wall shows normal or only slight thickening with a predominant echogenic submucosa contrasting with the hypoechoic inner mucosa and outer muscularis propria (Fig. 8.8).

Particular US findings may be observed in UC patients with extensive pseudopolyposis (Fig. 8.9).

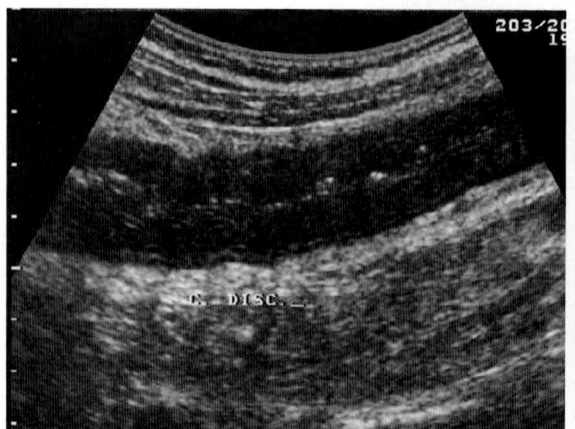 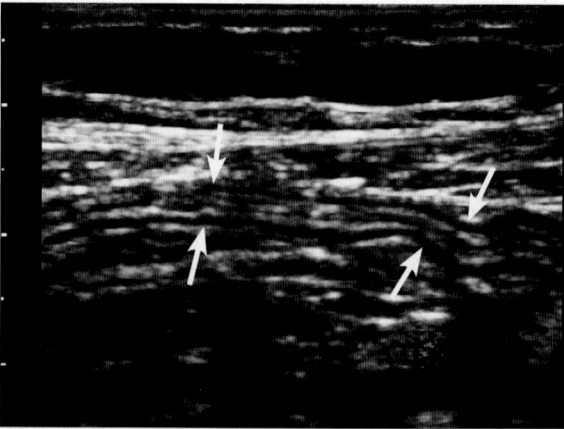

**Fig. 8.4a,b.** Longitudinal ultrasonographic sections of descending colon in patients with active (**a**) and non-active (**b**) ulcerative colitis. Note increased wall thickness and hypoechoic echo pattern in a patient with active disease and normal aspect of bowel wall (*arrows*) in a patient with quiescent disease

Pseudopolyps have been described as small echogenic nodules visible at the surface of the mucosa or echogenic indentations into the fluid-filled intestinal lumen. However, while a few isolated inflammatory polyps can be imaged only by hydrocolonic sonography, extensive pseudopolyposis appears as an increased and dyshomogeneous thickness of the bowel wall (up to 15 mm) without the typical wall stratification (at least in inactive UC), markedly irregular internal margins and/or as dilated incompressible bowel with echogenic dyshomogeneous content

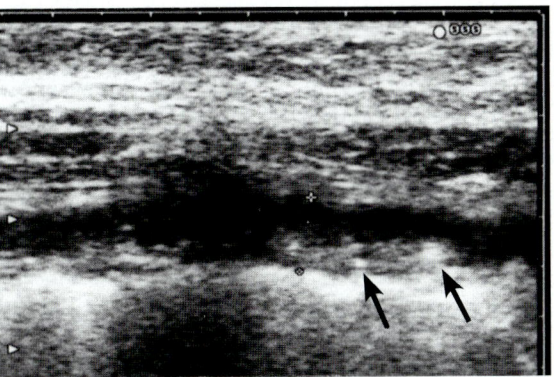

**Fig. 8.7.** Severe active ulcerative colitis showing severely thickened and hypoechoic bowel walls, with irregular inner layer due to fine multiple hyperechoic spots, representing deep penetrating ulcers (*arrows*)

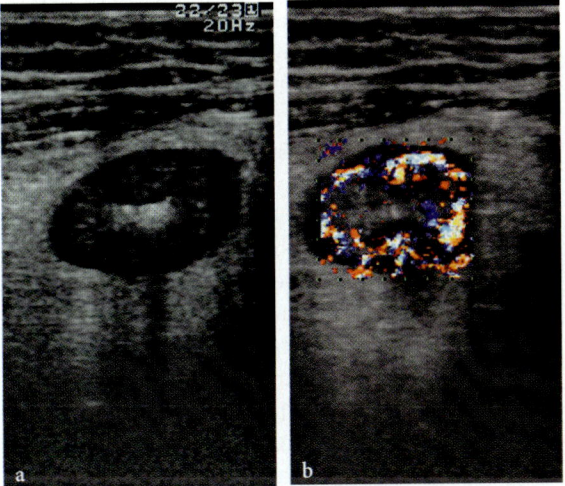

**Fig. 8.6a,b.** Ultrasonographic aspect of bowel wall in patient with active ulcerative colitis. The thickening involves submucosa which may appear slightly hypoechoic (**a**), with increased bowel wall vascularity (**b**)

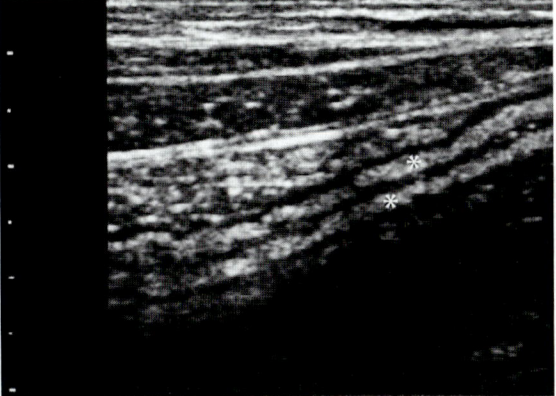

**Fig. 8.8.** Quiescent ulcerative colitis, showing colonic wall presenting normal or slight thickening, with a predominant echogenic submucosa (*asterisks*) contrasting with the hypoechoic inner mucosa and outer muscularis propria

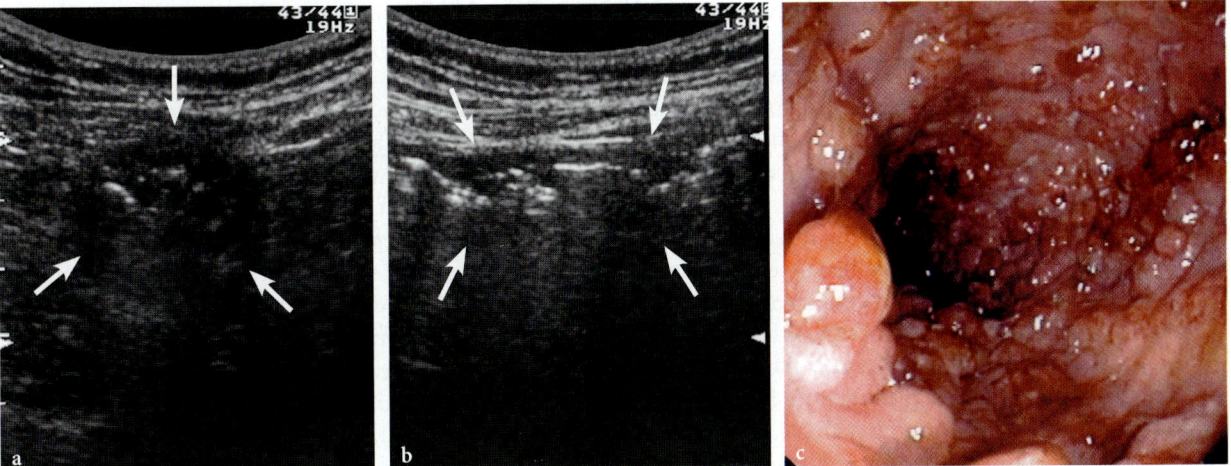

**Fig. 8.9a–c.** Ultrasonographic (**a,b**) and endoscopic (**c**) findings in an ulcerative colitis patient with extensive pseudopolyposis. Note dyshomogeneous thickness of distal descending colon at US without typical wall stratification. Bowel was also incompressible with echogenic dyshomogeneous content (**a**)

(Fig. 8.9). To obtain confirmation of the pseudopolypoid nature of the intestinal content, colour-power Doppler can be used to assess the blood flow within the echogenic material.

## 8.4
## Detection and Determination of Extension

The US diagnosis of UC relies upon the above-mentioned findings, but mainly upon visualisation of bowel wall thickening greater than 4 mm.

So far, few studies have focused on the accuracy of bowel US in diagnosing UC and in assessing the extent of inflammation (ARIENTI et al. 1996; MACONI et al. 1999). When bowel wall thickness >4 mm was used for abnormality in adults, the sensitivity of conventional transabdominal US in detecting bowel inflammation in UC showed a mean of 74% and a median of 76% (range: 53–89%) (LIMBERG 1989; PASCU et al. 2004; HOLLERBACH et al. 1998; SCHWERK et al. 1992; WORLICEK et al. 1987; HATA et al. 1994; PARENTE et al. 2003; ASTEGIANO et al. 2001; SONNENBERG et al. 1982). As demonstrated by these authors, these results are inferior to those observed in Crohn's disease. The lower accuracy of US in detecting UC may be explained by the superficial mucosal involvement of the disease, the less marked bowel wall thickening in UC and, in particular, by the distal localisation of the disease. In fact, inactive disease or UC characterised by mild inflammation have, or may have, a normal bowel wall thickening (<4 mm) and, therefore, can be missed by US. However, the main problem in detecting UC is that distal localisation of the disease is difficult to reveal by US and, therefore, proctitis or diseases confined to the rectum and distal part of the sigmoid colon cannot usually be identified with this technique.

In fact, studies assessing the accuracy of bowel US in evaluating the anatomical extension of the inflammatory process, during disease flare-up, have shown that the technique has a very high sensitivity in detecting left-sided colitis and a very low sensitivity in identifying proctitis. In particular, in our experience, the involvement of the rectum was the most difficult location to identify by US, sensitivity being only 15% (PARENTE et al. 2003). In contrast, UC involvement of other colonic diseased segments can be correctly detected in >70% of patients.

These findings suggest that bowel US may be a valid alternative to invasive procedures in assessing the extension of UC, provided that the disease is active (e.g. bowel examination should be performed only during flare-up of the disease) and not limited to the rectum (e.g. bowel examination may be negative in patients presenting without diarrhoea and only with rectal bleeding).

## 8.5
## Assessment of Disease Activity

Assessment of bowel wall features, namely the degree of wall thickening in diseased segments and their echo pattern, together with bowel wall and mesenteric vascularity, can provide useful information to evaluate the activity in UC. Unlike Crohn's disease, where the role of these US features in assessing disease activity are still controversial, in UC, most studies have demonstrated a significant correlation between the degree of bowel wall thickening, hypoechoic echo pattern and increased mesenteric and bowel wall vascularity, and active disease.

Indeed, several studies have shown that the degree of bowel wall thickening correlates well with clinical activity (WORLICEK et al. 1987; SCHWERK et al. 1992; ARIENTI et al. 1996; MACONI et al. 1999; RUESS et al. 2000; BRU et al. 2001; HABER et al. 2002), biochemical (namely C-reactive protein and erythrocyte sedimentation rate values) (MACONI et al. 1999; RUESS et al. 2000), endoscopic (MACONI et al. 1999; BRU et al. 2001) and scintigraphic (ARIENTI et al. 1996) activity of UC. Indeed, other studies have shown that the loss of bowel wall stratification (hypoechoic echo pattern) (HATA et al. 1994) and increased bowel wall vascularity (HEYNE et al. 2002) strongly suggest the presence of active UC. On the contrary, very few studies fail to show any correlation between US features of bowel wall (e.g. bowel wall thickening) and disease activity in UC (MAYER et al. 2000).

Following these results, bowel US has been proved useful to evaluate the response to medical treatment in active UC (MACONI et al. 1999; ARIENTI et al. 1996) and, in particular, to depict the absence of response and predict the failure of treatment and future relapses of the disease.

In this regard, mesenteric vascularity, unlike CD, has been shown to be well correlated with disease activity. Doppler sonography of the inferior mesenteric artery and superior mesenteric artery are closely related to clinical and endoscopic activity in patients with UC. Indeed, several studies have shown that mean velocity is significantly reduced, and pulsatility and resistance indexes of these arteries are increased compared to those in control subjects (Pascu et al. 2004; Kalantzis et al. 2002; Sigirci et al. 2001; Ludwig et al. 1999; Mirk et al. 1999; Maconi et al. 1996; Bolondi et al. 1992), thus suggesting their potential usefulness in the evaluation of inflammation of the colon and to document response to therapy.

## 8.6
## Toxic Megacolon

The presence of toxic megacolon should be suspected when, at US, marked decrease in thickness (< 2 mm) of the colonic wall is found associated with dilatation (> 6 cm) of the trasverse colon and presence of increased fluid and dilatation of the ileal loops (Fig. 8.10) (Maconi et al. 2004). US plays a supportive role in the event of clinical suspicion of this type of complication. Despite the advantage of rapid diagnostic and therapeutic interventions, its role is marginal in comparison to the reference investigation of plain abdominal radiography.

## 8.7
## Differential Diagnosis Between Ulcerative Colitis, Crohn's Disease and Other Inflammatory Diseases

Unfortunately, there are no specific US features of the intestinal walls that can be usefully employed in the differential diagnosis between UC and Crohn's disease or other inflammatory bowel diseases. However, the site and degree of bowel wall thickness and other features of the bowel wall may be helpful in differentiating between UC and CD (Table 8.2). Indeed, the diagnosis of Crohn's disease seems to be easier than

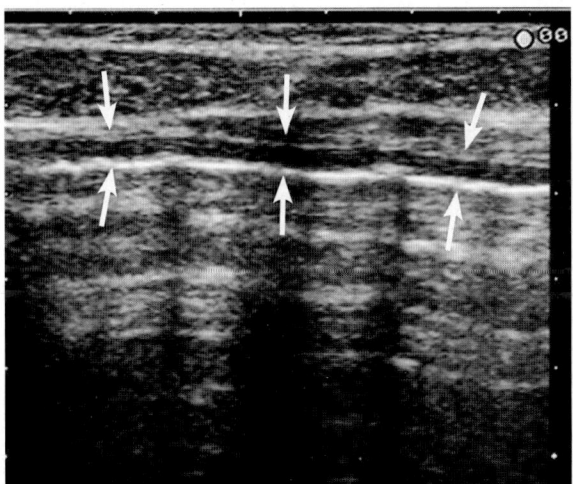
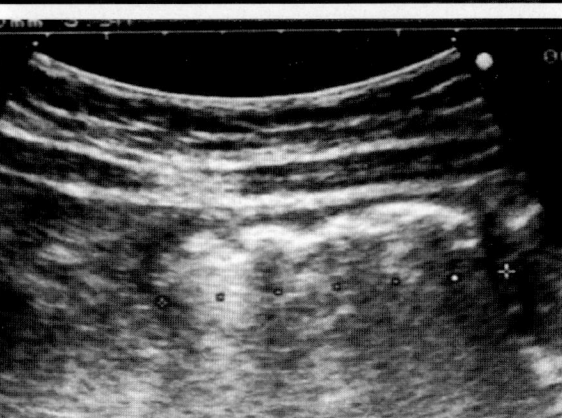
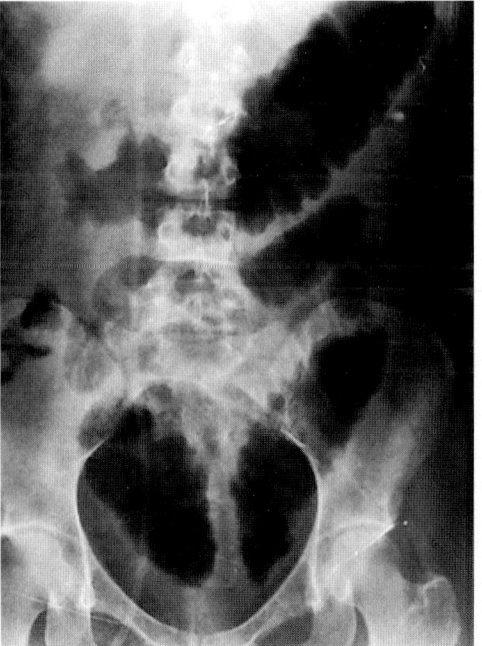

**Fig. 8.10a–c.** Ultrasonographic (a,b) and radiographic (c) findings in an ulcerative colitis patient with toxic megacolon. Note the thin bowel wall (*arrows*) without haustration (a) and dilated transverse colon (b). Plain X-ray of the abdomen shows the typical dilated transverse colon (c)

Table 8.2. Main ultrasonographic features in differential diagnosis between ulcerative colitis and Crohn's disease

|  | Ulcerative colitis | Crohn's disease |
|---|---|---|
| **Bowel wall** | | |
| • Thickness | 5–7 mm | 5–14 mm |
| • Echo pattern | Variable | Variable |
| • Vascularity | Variable | Variable |
| • Contour | Well defined | Variable |
| • Stiffness | Absent | Often present |
| • Haustra coli | Absent | Absent |
| • Peristalsis |  | Often weak or absent |
| **Location and extension** | | |
| • Site | Recto-sigmoid and colon | Ileum (70%), colon (60%) |
| • Bowel involvement | Continuous | Often divided in segments |
| **Extra-intestinal alterations** | | |
| • Mesenteric hypertrophy | Rare | Common |
| • Enlarged lymph nodes | Uncommon | Common |
| • Fistulae and abscesses | Rare | Common |

that of UC due to specific features that are not usually present in this disease: namely, abdominal complications (e.g. strictures and fistulae), skip areas, ileal localisation, and deep ulcerations with transmural involvement. The assessment of these signs may be useful to differentiate chronic inflammatory bowel diseases, in particular in patients who, for various reasons (e.g. colonic stricture, lack of tolerance to radiographic examinations, pregnancy) are not amenable to adequate endoscopic or radiological evaluation of the bowel. The US features of the colonic wall may discriminate between UC and Crohn's disease in approximately 80% of cases, relying only on features of the bowel walls (PERA et al. 1988; LIMBERG 1989; LIMBERG and OSSWALD 1994).

The differential diagnosis is more difficult between UC and acute inflammatory conditions such as infectious colitis, diverticular sigmoiditis and ischaemic lesions. Infectious colitis shows a similar echo pattern to that of UC, although the more frequent right localisation of infectious colitis may help in differentiating these entities.

Diverticular sigmoiditis is different from UC since the thickening is classically segmental and eccentric, the bowel wall echo pattern is different and frequently diverticula can be observed on the outer border of the colon. The differential diagnosis between UC and ischaemic colitis may be very difficult. Bowel wall thickening and echo pattern may vary depending on the extent of devascularisation and type of vascular obstruction, and, in this context, study of mesenteric circulation may be significant.

## References

Arienti V, Campieri M, Boriani L et al (1996) Management of severe ulcerative colitis with the help of high resolution ultrasonography. Am J Gastroenterol 91:2163–2169

Astegiano M, Bresso F, Cammarota T et al (2001) Abdominal pain and bowel dysfunction: diagnostic role of intestinal ultrasound. Eur J Gastroenterol Hepatol 13:927–931

Bolondi L, Gaiani S, Brignola C et al (1992) Changes in splanchnic hemodynamics in inflammatory bowel disease. Non-invasive assessment by Doppler ultrasound flowmetry. Scand J Gastroenterol 27:501–507

Bru C, Sans M, Defelitto MM et al (2001). Hydrocolonic sonography for evaluating inflammatory bowel disease. AJR Am J Roentgenol 177:99–105

Haber HP, Busch A, Ziebach R, Dette S, Ruck P, Stern M (2002) Ultrasonographic findings correspond to clinical, endoscopic, and histologic findings in inflammatory bowel disease and other enterocolitides. J Ultrasound Med 21:375–382

Hata J, Haruma K, Yamanaka H et al (1994) Ultrasonographic evaluation of the bowel wall in inflammatory bowel disease: comparison of in vivo and in vitro studies. Abdom Imaging 19:395–399

Heyne R, Rickes S, Bock P, Schreiber S, Wermke W, Lochs H (2002) Non-invasive evaluation of activity in inflammatory bowel disease by power Doppler sonography. Z Gastroenterol 40:171–175

Hollerbach S, Geissler A, Schiegl H et al (1998) The accuracy of abdominal ultrasound in the assessment of bowel disorders. Scand J Gastroenterol 33:1201–1208

Kalantzis N, Rouvella P, Tarazis S et al (2002) Doppler US of superior mesenteric artery in the assessment of ulcerative colitis. A prospective study. Hepatogastroenterology 49:168–171

Limberg B (1989) Diagnosis of acute ulcerative colitis and colonic Crohn's disease by colonic sonography. J Clin Ultrasound 17:25–31

Limberg B, Osswald B (1994) Diagnosis and differential diagnosis of ulcerative colitis and Crohn's disease by hydrocolonic sonography. Am J Gastroenterol 89:1051–1057

Ludwig D, Wiener S, Bruning A et al (1999) Mesenteric blood flow is related to disease activity and risk of relapse in ulcerative colitis: a prospective follow-up study. Gut 45:546–552

Maconi G, Imbesi V, Bianchi Porro G (1996) Doppler ultrasound measurement of intestinal blood flow in inflammatory bowel disease. Scand J Gastroenterol 31:590–593

Maconi G, Ardizzone S, Parente F, Bianchi Porro G (1999) Ultrasonography in the evaluation of extension, activity, and follow-up of ulcerative colitis. Scand J Gastroenterol 34:1103–1107

Maconi G, Sampietro GM, Ardizzone S et al (2004) US detection of toxic megacolon in inflammatory bowel diseases. Dig Dis Sci 49:138–142

Mayer D, Reinshagen M, Mason RA et al (2000) Sonographic measurement of thickened bowel wall segments as a quantitative parameter for activity in inflammatory bowel disease. Z Gastroenterol 38:295–300

Mirk P, Palazzoni G, Gimondo P (1999) Doppler sonography of hemodynamic changes of the inferior mesenteric artery in inflammatory bowel disease: preliminary data. AJR Am J Roentgenol 173:381–387

Parente F, Greco S, Molteni M et al (2003) Role of early ultrasound in detecting inflammatory intestinal disorders and identifying their anatomical location within the bowel. Aliment Pharmacol Ther 18:1009–1016

Pascu M, Roznowski AB, Muller HP, Adler A, Wiedenmann B, Dignass AU (2004) Clinical relevance of transabdominal ultrasonography and magnetic resonance imaging in patients with inflammatory bowel disease of the terminal ileum and large bowel. Inflamm Bowel Dis 10:373–382

Pera A, Cammarota T, Comino E et al (1988) Ultrasonography in the detection of Crohn's disease and in the differential diagnosis of inflammatory bowel disease. Digestion 41:180–184

Ruess L, Blask AR, Bulas DI (2000) Inflammatory bowel disease in children and young adults: correlation of sonographic and clinical parameters during treatment. AJR Am J Roentgenol 175:79–84

Schwerk WB, Beckh K, Raith M (1992) A prospective evaluation of high resolution sonography in the diagnosis of inflammatory bowel disease. Eur J Gastroenterol Hepatol 4:173–182

Sigirci A, Baysal T, Kutlu R, Aladag M, Sarac K, Harputluoglu H (2001) Doppler sonography of the inferior and superior mesenteric arteries in ulcerative colitis. J Clin Ultrasound 29:130–139

Sonnenberg A, Erckenbrecht J, Peter P, Niederau C (1982) Detection of Crohn's disease by ultrasound. Gastroenterology 83:430–434

Vallette PJ, Rioux M, Pilleul F, Saurin JC, Fouque P, Henry L (2001) Ultrasonography of chronic inflammatory bowel diseases. Eur Radiol 11:1859–1866

Worlicek H, Lutz H, Heyder N, Matek W (1987) Ultrasound findings in Crohn's disease and ulcerative colitis: a prospective study. J Clin Ultrasound 15:153–163

# Malabsorption

# Coeliac Disease

Mirella Fraquelli

CONTENTS

9.1 Introduction 85
9.2 Abdominal Ultrasound in the Diagnosis of Coeliac Disease 85
9.2.1 Rare Manifestations of Coeliac Disease 88
9.3 Splanchnic Circulation in Coeliac Disease 89
9.4 Role of Ultrasonography in Diagnosing the Complications of Coeliac Disease 89
9.4.1 Intestinal Lymphoma and Small Bowel Adenocarcinoma 89
9.5 Gallbladder Motility and Gastric Emptying in Coeliac Disease: Ultrasonographic Studies 90

References 91

## 9.1 Introduction

Coeliac disease (CD) is a chronic disorder in which the small bowel mucosa of susceptible subjects is damaged by dietary gluten. The aetiology of the disease is unknown, but enviromental, genetic and immunological factors all seem to contribute to its development. Its prevalence is now known to be far greater than previously reported, with an increasing number of silent cases being diagnosed: according to population-based studies of Caucasians using serological screening, it ranges from 0.2 to about 1%. The incidence pattern of the disease is also changing, and a larger number of cases are now diagnosed during adulthood (Farrell and Kelly 2002; Rewers 2005).

Absorption is impaired to varying degrees, and patients can experience gastrointestinal symptoms and malabsorption leading to the development of diarrhoea, anaemia, osteoporosis or other complications; however, the clinical picture is highly variable, and can range from pauci-symptomatic to severe forms. The diagnosis is supported by the determination of endomysial (EmA) and transglutaminase (tTG) antibodies, which is characterised by >85% sensitivity and nearly 100% specificity, and confirmed by consistent histological duodenal findings (Rostom et al. 2005). Overt disease is pathologically characterised by a flattened small intestine mucosa, with lymphocytic infiltrate, crypt hyperplasia and villous atrophy (Farrell and Kelly 2002).

Untreated CD is associated with significant morbidity and increased mortality, largely related to the development of enteropathy-associated T-cell lymphomas (EATL). Other less common complications include refractory sprue, carcinomas of the oropharynx, oesophagus and small bowel, and ulcerative jejuno-ileitis and its collagenous variant (Logan et al. 1989; Holmes et al. 1976; Catassi et al. 2005).

Patients with gastrointestinal symptoms normally first undergo abdominal ultrasonography (US), the accuracy of which has been markedly improved by the widespread availability of high-resolution transducers, and a number of US signs have proved to be valuable in supporting or ruling out a diagnosis of CD. In addition, several US studies have reported impaired gallbladder and gastric motility in association with gastrointestinal hormone abnormalities in patients with untreated CD.

## 9.2 Abdominal Ultrasound in the Diagnosis of Coeliac Disease

Different US signs have been reported in association with CD in scattered case reports, a paediatric series, and a retrospective case-control study of adults (Peck et al. 1997; Riccabona and Rossipal

M. Fraquelli, MD, PhD
Department of Gastroenterology and Endocrinology, IRCCS Fondazione Ospedale Maggiore, Mangiagalli e Regina Elena, Pad. Granelli 3 piano, Via F Sforza 35, 20122 Milan, Italy

1993; RETTENBACHER et al. 1999; FRAQUELLI et al. 2004).

In a case series of 39 children with overt malabsorption and a definite, histology-based CD diagnosis (Table 9.1), RICCABONA and ROSSIPAL (1993) found that 36 (92%) had an "abnormal-looking" small intestine, 32 (82%) showed increased peristalsis, and 30 (76%) the presence of free abdominal fluid. Interestingly, half of the cases also presented pericardial effusion. On the basis of these findings, the authors concluded that, although intestinal biopsy remains the reference standard for diagnosing CD, an awareness of CD-associated US abnormalities can accelerate the diagnostic work-up and allow the earlier introduction of a gluten-free diet (GFD) (RICCABONA and ROSSIPAL 1993).

In a case-control study of 11 adults with histologically proven CD and 20 healthy subjects (Table 9.2), RETTENBACHER et al. (1999) found that the controls were negative, whereas the cases showed an increase in intraluminal fluid content, the presence of moderate small bowel dilatation, increased peristalsis and moderate bowel wall thickness. Further extra-intestinal signs, such as mesenteric lymph node enlargement, free abdominal fluid, a dilated superior mesenteric artery or portal vein, and hepatic steatosis, were also identified with overall frequencies of 52–84% (RETTENBACHER et al. 1999).

A recent prospective study (FRAQUELLI et al. 2004) evaluated the diagnostic accuracy of various US signs in predicting CD in a cohort of 162 consecutive patients examined because of chronic diarrhoea, iron-deficiency anaemia and dyspepsia (all frequent manifestations of CD): a population with a pre-test CD probability of about 10%, as estimated from previous series (HIN et al. 1999). All of the patients underwent anti-endomysial IgA antibody determinations and a duodenal biopsy. Two operators unaware of the clinical, serological and histological findings evaluated six US signs: the increased transverse diameter of small bowel loops containing increased fluid (Fig. 9.1a,b), increased small bowel wall thickness with hypertrophic valvulae conniventes (Fig. 9.1c), the pattern of peristalsis, the presence of free abdominal fluid within the abdominal cavity (Fig. 9.2a,b), and the enlarged mesenteric lymph nodes (Fig. 9.3) as well as the enlarged fasting gallbladder volume (Fig. 9.4).

Twelve patients (7%) were diagnosed as having CD on the basis of EmA positivity and histological duodenal findings consistent with Marsh grade-III (11 cases) or IV (1 case). Of the 150 EmA-negative cases, all of whom had normal duodenal histology,

Table 9.1. Ultrasound findings in a series of 39 paediatric patients with histologically proven coeliac disease (From RICCABONA and ROSSIPAL 1993)

| Ultrasonographic findings | No. of patients with a positive sign |
|---|---|
| Abnormal aspect of the small intestine | 36 |
| Increased peristalsis | 32 |
| Abdominal fluid | 30 |
| Pericardial effusion | 18 |

Table 9.2. Ultrasound findings in a series of 11 adult patients with histologically proven coeliac disease (From RETTENBACHER et al. 1999)

| Ultrasonographic findings | No. of patients with a positive sign |
|---|---|
| Moderate small bowel dilatation | 8 |
| Increased intraluminal fluid content | 11 |
| Small bowel wall thickness | 7 |
| Increased peristalsis | 8 |
| Mesenteric lymph node hypertrophy | 9 |
| Free abdominal fluid | 5 |
| Dilated superior mesenteric artery or portal vein | 7 |
| Hepatic stenosis | 6 |

72 (48%) were eventually diagnosed as having functional disease, and 78 (52%) as having organic disease, including nine showing ileal involvement (six with Crohn's disease and three with final diagnoses of giardiasis and common variable immunodeficiency, primary lymphangiectasia, and ileal carcinoid). Interestingly, the US pattern in the patients with ileal Crohn's disease, showing a localised and marked bowel wall thickening, was completely different from that observed in CD patients. The details concerning the diagnostic accuracy of the six US signs are shown in Table 9.3.

Interestingly, the positive likelihood ratios (LR+) of >10 observed for increased gallbladder volume, free abdominal fluid and enlarged mesenteric lymph nodes allowed a confirmatory strategy, whereas the negative likelihood ratios (LR-) of 0.1 observed for dilated small bowel loops and increased peristalsis supported an exclusion strategy (SACKETT and HAYNES 2002).

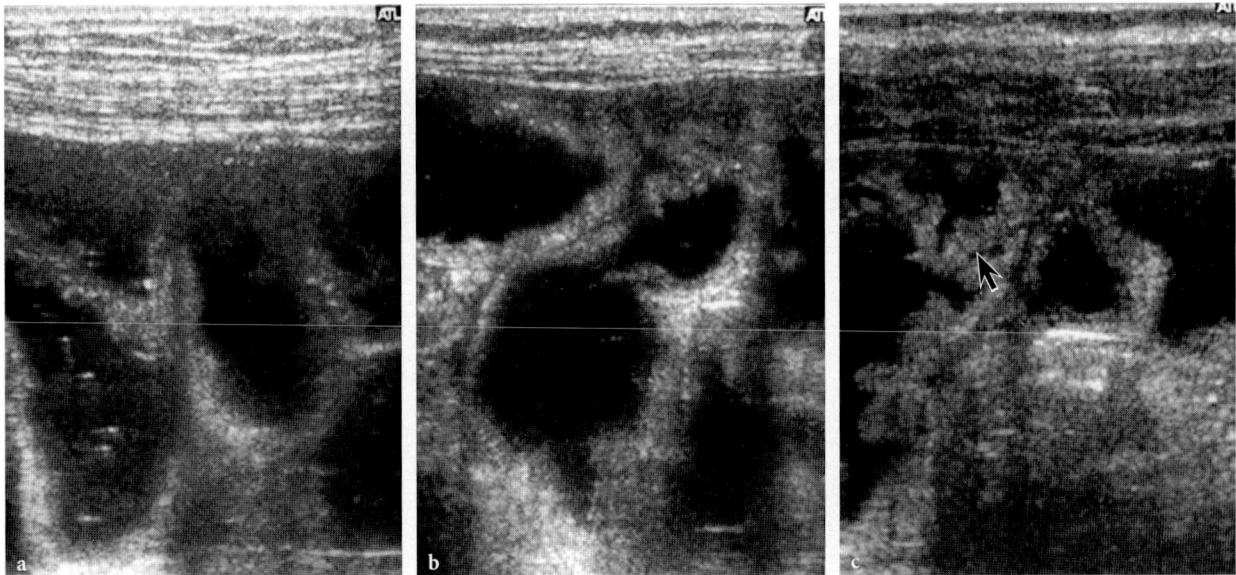

**Fig. 9.1. a,b** Dilated small bowel loops with anechoic liquid content in coeliac disease. **c** Moderately dilated small bowel loops with hypertrophic valvulae conniventes (*arrow*) in coeliac disease

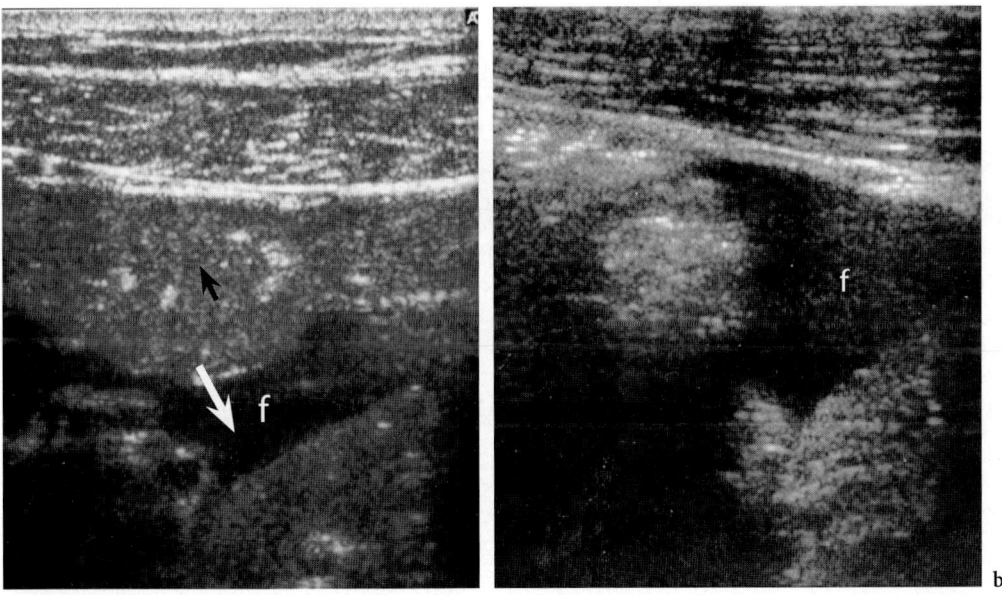

**Fig. 9.2a,b.** Ultrasound images show a small amount of anechoic free fluid (*f*) within the abdominal cavity in coeliac disease. Free fluid (*white arrow*), bowel loop (*black arrow*)

The κ values (i.e. the percentage agreement between US sign and duodenal histologic findings) ranged from 0.76 for increased peristalsis to 0.95 for dilated small bowel loops, and were consistent with the good inter-observer agreement in evaluating the US signs. It is interesting to note that a strict GFD led to EmA negativity and the complete reversal of the US abnormalities after 1 year.

Overall, increased gallbladder volume, abdominal free fluid and mesenteric lymph node enlargement reliably and accurately predict CD, whereas the lack of intestinal dilatation and increased peristalsis makes it possible to rule out the diagnosis. The specificity of US was 99% in the presence of all six signs, with an obvious decrease in sensitivity (33%); moreover, an LR+ value of 50 allowed a confirmatory strategy and

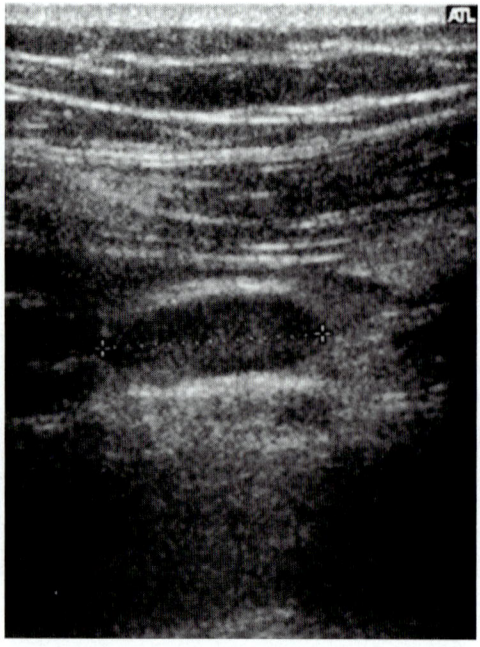

**Fig. 9.3.** Enlarged mesenteric lymph node in coeliac disease

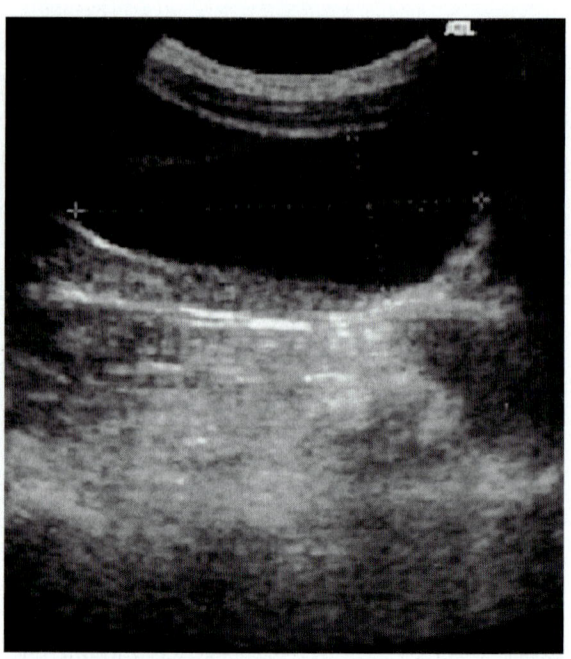

**Fig. 9.4.** Enlarged gallbladder in coeliac disease

**Table 9.3.** Sensitivity, specificity, positive and negative likelihood ratio (LR+ and LR-), and positive and negative predictive value (PPV, NPV) of six ultrasound signs in predicting coeliac disease. The corresponding 95% confidence intervals are given in parentheses

| Ultrasound parameters | Sensitivity (%) | Specificity (%) | LR+ | LR- | PPV (%) | NPV (%) |
|---|---|---|---|---|---|---|
| Increased gallbladder volume (reference value: ≤20 ml) | 73 (46–99) | 96 (92–99) | 17.0 (7.3–41.0) | 0.28 (0.1–0.7) | 57 (31–83) | 98 (95–100) |
| Dilated small bowel loops + increased fluid content (reference value: ≤2.5 cm) | 92 (76–100) | 77 (70–84) | 4.0 (2.8–5.5) | 0.10 (0.1–0.7) | 24 (11–36) | 99 (97–100) |
| Thickened small bowel wall (reference value: ≤3mm) | 75 (50–99) | 91 (86–95) | 8.0 (4.4–14.5) | 0.27 (0.1–0.7) | 39 (19–59) | 98 (95–100) |
| Increased peristalsis | 83 (62–100) | 87 (82–92) | 6.6 (4.0–10.7) | 0.10 (0.05–0.7) | 34 (17–51) | 98 (96–100) |
| Free abdominal fluid | 50 (22–78) | 96 (93–99) | 12.5 (4.7–33) | 0.52 (0.3–0.9) | 50 (22–78) | 96 (92–99) |
| Enlarged mesenteric lymph nodes (reference value: ≤5 mm) | 42 (14–69) | 97 (95–99) | 15.6 (6.8–50.6) | 0.59 (0.4–0.9) | 55 (23–88) | 95 (92–99) |

a predictive positive value (PPV) of 80%. Conversely, in the presence of at least one US sign, sensitivity was 92% with an LR- value of 0.10 and an NPV of 99%, a diagnostic performance that was comparable to that of dilated small bowel loops.

The above findings support the role of US in predicting CD; however, its role in a diagnostic algorithm should be varied on the basis of the probability of the disease in a given population.

### 9.2.1
### Rare Manifestations of Coeliac Disease

Other less common manifestations of CD that can be revealed by abdominal US are the presence of mesenteric lymph node cavitation and transient small bowel intussusception.

The cavitation of mesenteric lymph nodes is a rare complication of CD the pathogenesis which is remains to be clarified. It has been described as being revealed by US or computed tomography (CT) in a few cases, and was sometimes associated with hyposplenism (BURRELL et al. 1994; BAHLOULI et al. 1998; BARDELLA et al. 1999; REDDY et al. 2002).

Transient small bowel intussusception is a rare event that has been described in case reports of both paediatric and adult patients, in some of whom it was demonstrated by US (COHEN and LINTOTT 1978; GONZALES et al. 1998; MUSHRAQ et al. 1999).

## 9.3
## Splanchnic Circulation in Coeliac Disease

Basal and post-prandial splanchnic blood flow (i.e., in the superior mesenteric artery and portal vein) has been evaluated in CD patients by means of Doppler US. Under fasting conditions, increased superior mesenteric artery velocity and flow with a lower resistance index, and greater portal vein velocity and flow have been uniformly observed in comparison with controls (ARIENTI et al. 1996; ALIOTTA et al. 1997; GIOVAGNORIO et al. 1998; MAGALOTTI et al. 2003).

Interestingly, in addition, in the post-prandial phase all of these parameters vary significantly less than in healthy subjects.

Once again, the use of a long-term GFD reverses all of these abnormalities.

## 9.4
## Role of Ultrasonography in Diagnosing the Complications of Coeliac Disease

### 9.4.1
### Intestinal Lymphoma and Small Bowel Adenocarcinoma

Enteropathy-associated, T-cell non-Hodgkin's lymphoma (EATL-NHL), the annual incidence of which is 0.5–1 per million people, is confined to patients with previously or concomitantly diagnosed CD and also complicates the refractory form of the enteropathy (SWINSON et al. 1983). An increased risk of small bowel adenocarcinoma (an exceedingly rare malignancy with an annual incidence of 0.6–0.7 per 100,000 of the general population) has also been reported.

The typical US pattern is similar in the presence of both of these neoplasms, with evidence of the "bull's eye", "target" or "pseudokidney" sign related to eccentric and localised bowel wall thickening (Fig. 9.5).

Under the above-mentioned conditions, US is useful in locating and staging the disease, and also allows the detailed characterisation of adjacent or

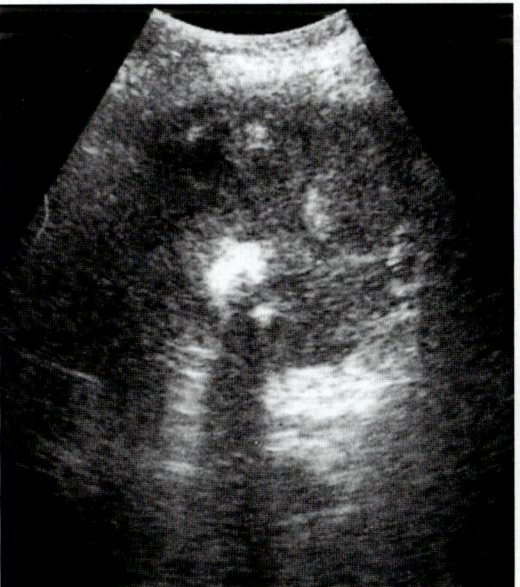
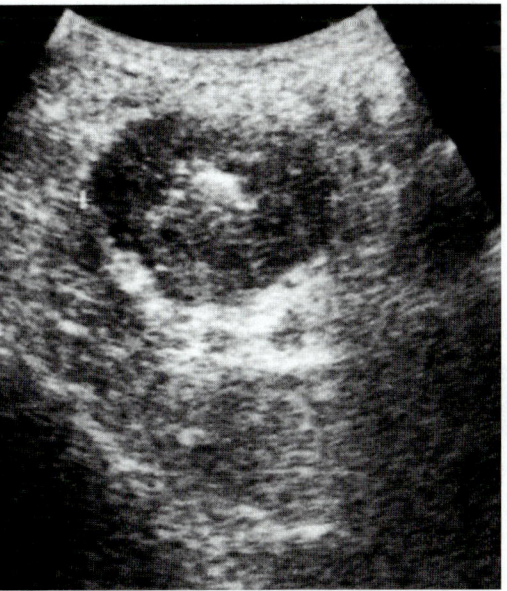

**Fig. 9.5a,b.** Ultrasound images show a target lesion in the small bowel due to the presence enteropathy-associated, T-cell non-Hodgkin's lymphoma

distant lymph nodes and, when indicated, their sampling for histological purposes; however, US should not generally be considered the reference technique in diagnosing an intestinal lymphoma superimposed on CD because of its poor sensitivity even when performed by well-trained operators. It should therefore be considered an ancillary technique to endoscopy in identifying and staging EATL in CD patients.

## 9.5
## Gallbladder Motility and Gastric Emptying in Coeliac Disease: Ultrasonographic Studies

Impaired gallbladder (GB), stomach and small bowel motility have been reported in patients with untreated CD, and attributed to the impaired secretion of enteric hormones or decreased sensitivity to them (BROWN et al. 1987; BARDELLA et al. 2000; FRAQUELLI et al. 1999; TURSI 2004).

As shown in Table 9.4, a number of studies of untreated CD patients have reported a reduction in absolute and net GB emptying in response to various stimuli, which could be attributed mainly to reduced cholecystokinin (CCK) secretion by the specialised cells located in the upper tract of the duodenum (LOW-BEER et al. 1975; DELAMARRE et al. 1984; MATON et al. 1985; MASCLEE et al. 1991; BROWN et al. 1987; FRAQUELLI et al. 1999).

Some authors have reported decreased post-prandial CCK levels in untreated CD patients despite a concomitant increase in the number of CCK-secreting duodenal cells, which are not adequately stimulated to release the hormone because of the impaired lipolysis of exogenous fat (LOW-BEER et al. 1975; MATON et al. 1985; MASCLEE et al. 1991; HOPMAN et al. 1995; FRAQUELLI et al. 2003). The resulting gallbladder inertia also contributes to impairing small bowel transit time and the enterohepatic circulation of bile salts.

In addition, somatostatin (SS) secretion is also altered in CD patients at diagnosis, and fasting SS levels are significantly higher than in controls. This could be due to an increased number of SS-secreting cells accounting for increased basal gallbladder volume, as a correlation between SS levels and gallbladder size under fasting conditions has been clearly confirmed in patients with somatostatinomas and those treated with SS or SS analogues.

Gallbladder ultrasonography is reliable to estimate volume in fasting state and in response to test meal or exogenous stimulus. Figure 9.6 shows a simple and reliable method, the ellipsoid one (DODDS et al. 1985), to determine GB volume by measuring the longitudinal (a), transverse (b) and anteroposterior (c) GB diameters, applying the following formula:

GB volume = 1/6 π (a × b × c).

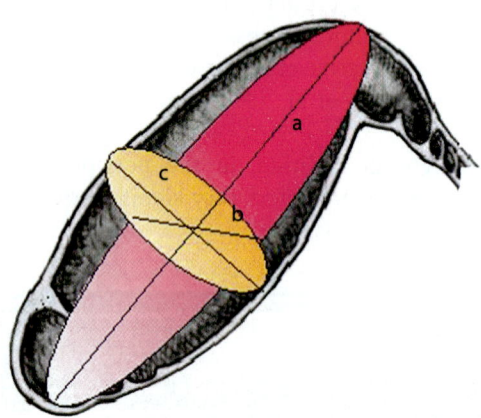

Fig. 9.6. The gallbladder (GB). The lines represent the longitudinal, transverse and anteroposterior GB diameters which are used to calculate GB volume using the ellipsoid formula

Table 9.4. Main data from studies evaluating gallbladder (GB) motility in coeliac disease patients

| Reference | No. of patients | Technique | Type of stimulus | Post-prandial GB motility |
|---|---|---|---|---|
| LOW-BEER et al. (1975) | 18 | Scintigraphy | CCK analogue | ↓ |
| BROWN et al. (1987) | 8 | Scintigraphy | CCK analogue | ↓ |
| FRAQUELLI et al. (1999) | 10 | US | Liquid | ↓ |
| MATON et al. (1985) | 8 | US | Liquid | ↓ |
| DELAMARRE et al. (1984) | 4 | US | Solid | ↓ |

*CCK* cholecystokinin

Untreated CD patients also have increased serum levels of neurotensin (NT), a hormone, the physiological post-prandial increase of which, is a reliable index of nutrient delivery to the ileum, and which may impair GB motility directly and indirectly by delaying gastric emptying. Interestingly, the abnormalities in GI hormone release and their effects on GB, gastric and small bowel motility completely revert after successful treatment with a GFD.

Various scintigraphic and US studies have assessed gastric emptying in patients with untreated CD, and the results of most of them are consistent with a marked delay in gastric emptying that returned to normal after gluten withdrawal (BENINI et al. 2001; BARDELLA et al. 2000).

## References

Aliotta A, Pompili M, Rapaccini GL et al (1997) Doppler ultrasonographic evaluation of blood flow in the superior mesenteric artery in celiac patients and in healthy controls in fasting conditions and after saccharose. J Ultrasound Med 16:85–91

Arienti V, Califano C, Brusco G et al (1996) Doppler ultrasonographic evaluation of splanchnic blood flow in coeliac disease. Gut 39:369–373

Bahlouli F, Seror O, Mathieu E et al (1998) Mesenteric lymph node cavitation disclosing celiac disease in adults. J Radiol 79:431–433

Bardella MT, Trovato C, Quatrini M, Conte D (1999) Mesenteric lymph node cavitation: a rare hallmark of celiac disease. Scand J Gastroenterol 34:1257–1259

Bardella MT, Fraquelli M, Peracchi M et al (2000) Gastric emptying and plasma neurotensin levels in untreated celiac patients. Scand J Gastroenterol 35:269–273

Benini L, Sembenini C, Salandini L et al (2001) Gastric emptying of realistic meals with and without gluten in patients with coeliac disease. Effect of jejunal mucosal recovery. Scand J Gastroenterol 36:1044–1048

Brown AM, Bradshaw MJ, Richardson R et al (1987) Pathogenesis of the impaired gall bladder contraction of coeliac disease. Gut 28:1426–1432

Burrell HC, Trescoli C, Chow K, Ward MJ (1994) Case report: mesenteric lymph node cavitation, an unusual complication of coeliac disease. Br J Radiol 67:1139–1140

Catassi C, Bearzi I, Holmes GK (2005) Association of celiac disease and intestinal lymphomas and other cancers. Gastroenterology 128:S79–S86

Cohen MD, Lintott DJ (1978) Transient small bowel intussusception in adult coeliac disease. Clin Radiol 29:529–534

Delamarre J, Capron JP, Joly JP et al (1984) Gallbladder inertia in celiac disease: ultrasonographic demonstration. Dig Dis Sci 29:876–877

Dodds WJ, Groh WJ, Darweesh RMA et al (1985) Sonographic measurement of gallbladder volume. Am J Roentgenol 145:1009–1011

Farrell LJ, Kelly CP (2002) Celiac sprue. N Engl J Med 346:180–188

Fraquelli M, Bardella MT, Peracchi M et al (1999) Gallbladder emptying and somatostatin and cholecystokinin plasma levels in celiac disease. Am J Gastroenterol 94:1866–1870

Fraquelli M, Pagliarulo M, Colucci A et al (2003) Gallbladder motility in obesity, diabetes mellitus and coeliac disease. Digest Liver Dis 35:S12–S16

Fraquelli M, Colli A, Colucci A et al (2004) Accuracy of ultrasonography in predicting celiac disease. Arch Intern Med 164:169–174

Giovagnorio F, Picarelli A, Di Giovanbattista F, Mastracchio A (1998) Evaluation with Doppler sonography of mesenteric blood flow in celiac disease. Am J Roentgenol 171:629–632

Gonzalez JA, Gonzalez JB, Crespo MJ, Sancho CI (1998) Acute gallbladder distension and recurrent small bowel intussusception in a child with celiac disease. J Pediatr Gastroenterol Nutr 27:444–445

Hin H, Bird G, Fisher P et al (1999) Coeliac disease in primary care: case finding study. Br Med J 318:164–167

Holmes GK, Stokes PL, Sorahan TM et al (1976) Coeliac disease, gluten-free diet, and malignancy. Gut 17:612–619

Hopman WP, Rosenbusch G, Hectors MP, Jansen JB (1995) Effect of predigested fat on intestinal stimulation of plasma cholecystokinin and gall bladder motility in coeliac disease. Gut 36:17–21

Logan RF, Rifkind EA, Turner ID, Ferguson A (1989) Mortality in celiac disease. Gastroenterology 97:265–271

Low-Beer TS, Harvey RF, Davies ER, Read AF (1975) Abnormalities of serum cholecystokinin and gallbladder emptying in celiac disease. N Engl J Med 292:961–963

Magalotti D, Volta U, Bonfiglioli A et al (2003) Splanchnic haemodynamics in patients with coeliac disease: effects of a gluten-free diet. Digest Liver Dis 35:262–268

Masclee AA, Jansen JB, Driessen WM et al (1991) Gallbladder sensitivity to cholecystokinin in coeliac disease. Correlation of gallbladder contraction with plasma cholecystokinin-like immunoreactivity during infusion of cerulein. Scand J Gastroenterol 26:1279–1284

Maton PN, Selden AC, Fitzpatrick ML, Chadwick VS (1985) Defective gallbladder emptying and cholecystokinin release in celiac disease. Reversal by gluten-free diet. Gastroenterology 88:391–396

Mushraq N, Marven S, Walker J et al (1999) Small bowel intussusception in celiac disease. J Pediatr Surg 3:1833–1835

Peck RJ, Jackson A, Gleeson D (1997) Case report: ultrasound of coeliac disease with demonstration of response to treatment. Clin Radiol 52:244–245

Reddy D, Salomon C, Demos TC (2002) Mesenteric lymph node cavitation in celiac disease. Am J Roentgenol 178:247

Rettenbacher T, Hollerweger A, Macheiner P et al (1999) Adult celiac disease: US signs. Radiology 211:389–394

Rewers M (2005) Epidemiology of celiac disease: What are the prevalence, incidence, and progression of celiac disease? Gastroenterology 128:S47–S51

Riccabona M, Rossipal E (1993) Sonographic findings in celiac disease. J Pediatr Gastroenterol Nutr 17:198–200

Rostom A, Dube C, Cranney A et al (2005) The diagnostic accuracy of serologic tests for celiac disease: a systematic review. Gastroenterology 128:S38–S46

Sackett DL, Haynes RB (2002) The architecture of diagnostic research. Br Med J 324:539–541

Swinson CM, Slavin G, Coles EC, Booth CC (1983) Coeliac disease and malignancy. Lancet 8316:111–115

Tursi A (2004) Gastrointestinal motility disturbances in celiac disease. J Clin Gastroenterol. 38:642–645

# Lymphangiectasia, Whipple's Disease and Eosinophilic Enteritis

Mirella Fraquelli

CONTENTS

10.1 Primary Intestinal Lymphangiectasia 93
10.2 Whipple's Disease 94
10.3 Ultrasonography in the Diagnosis and Follow-Up of Eosinophilic Enteritis 95

References 96

## 10.1
## Primary Intestinal Lymphangiectasia

Primary intestinal lymphangiectasia is a rare disorder characterised by a protein-losing gastroenteropathy leading to secondary hypoproteinaemia due to lymphatic vessel obstruction and the loss of lymphatic fluid in the gastrointestinal tract. It is believed to be a congenital disorder, although the time of its clinical onset can vary widely.

Clinically, the most relevant symptoms are oedema, diarrhoea and lymphocytopenia due to both lymphatic leakage and rupture. The small bowel biopsy finding of numerous dilated lymphatic vessels consistent with diffuse or focal lymphangiectasia definitely support the diagnosis.

M. Fraquelli, MD, PhD
Department of Gastroenterology and Endocrinology, IRCCS Fondazione Ospedale Maggiore, Mangiagalli e Regina Elena, Pad. Granelli 3 piano, Via F. Sforza 35, 20122 Milano, Italy

A strict dietary regimen including only medium-chain triglycerides (MCT) is recommended as the initial treatment. It has been reported that tissue fibrinolytic activity in the mucosa of intestinal lymphangiectasia is increased, and there are some reports indicating that antiplasmin therapy can dramatically reduce protein loss by inhibiting lymphatic permeability; some authors have recently observed that octreotide, a somatostatin analogue, may play a therapeutic role.

There are only a few published case reports concerning the ultrasonography (US) findings observed in association with primary intestinal lymphangiectasia. Although diagnosis still relies on intestinal histology, the US picture is fairly indicative of the disease, especially in patients with protein-losing enteropathy. In the first study of three paediatric patients, Dorne and Jequier (1986) most frequently observed ascites, diffuse bowel wall thickening, mesenteric oedema, dilated mesenteric lymphatic vessels, and thickening of the gallbladder and urine bladder wall.

In 1998, Maconi et al. described the case of a 20-year-old female patient with histologically proven primary intestinal lymphangiectasia presenting with protein-losing enteropathy and right leg lymphoedema. The US findings showed dilatation of the intestinal loops with regular and diffuse thickening of the bowel wall, plical hypertrophy and considerable mesenteric oedema (Maconi et al. 1998). Similar findings were also reported by Loreti et al. (2003) in a 26-year-old female presenting with protein-losing enteropathy, lymphedema, severe steatorrhoea and malabsorption.

Frequent US findings of primary intestinal lymphangiectasia are a markedly dilated small intestinal loop with increased (mixed but mainly echogenic) fluid content (Fig. 10.1), and small bowel tract with regular and diffuse bowel wall thickening and mesenteric oedema (Fig. 10.2).

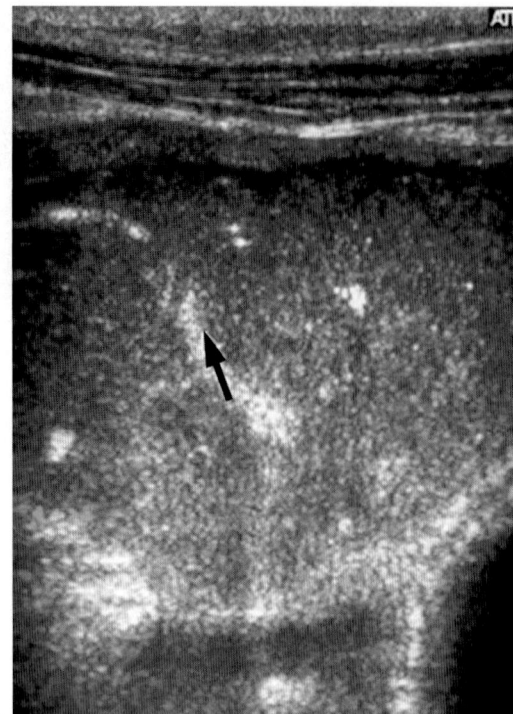

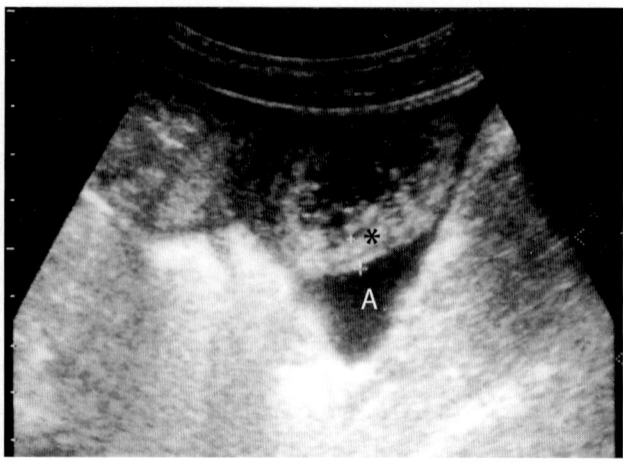

**Fig. 10.1a,b.** US images showing dilated small bowel loops (**a**) with increased mixed, mainly echogenic intraluminal fluid content and (**b**) diffuse bowel wall thickening (*asterisk*) with ascites (*A*)

## 10.2 Whipple's Disease

Whipple's disease is a chronic disorder characterised by diarrhea, weight loss, arthralgias, and cardiac and neurological involvement. It is caused by a small gram-positive bacillus, *Tropheryma whippelii*, a low-virulence but highly infectious actinobacterium. The onset can be very insidious and is characterised by GI symptoms such as diarrhoea, steatorrhoea and abdominal pain, associated with migratory large joint arthropathy, fever, and ophthalmological and neurological manifestations (Bai et al. 2004).

Whipple's disease occurs most frequently in middle-aged Caucasian men. Its diagnosis is suggested by the clinical findings, and confirmed by tissue sampling from the small intestine and/or other involved organs (lymph nodes, liver, central nervous system, etc.). The presence of PAS-positive (periodic acid Schiff stain) macrophages containing small bacilli definitely support the diagnosis. The treatment is based on a prolonged antibiotic course, with the first-choice regimen being 1 year of trimethoprim/sulphamethoxazole, and the second choice chloramphenicol. PAS-positive bacilli can persist after successful treatment, and their presence outside macrophages is indicative of persistent infection. The

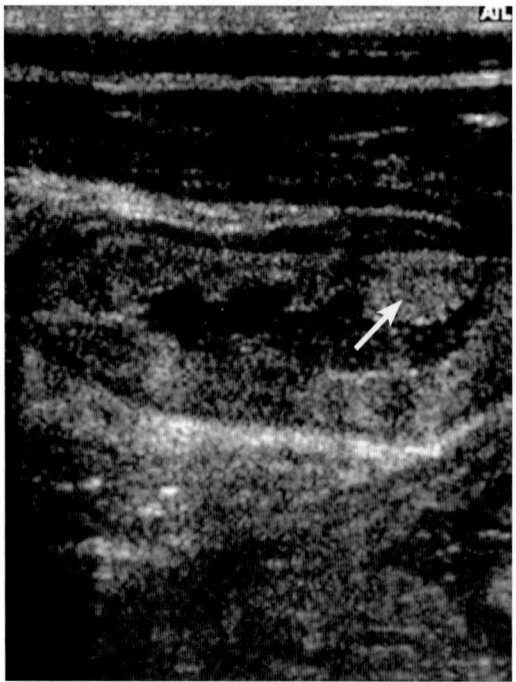

**Fig. 10.2.** US image showing a dilated small bowel loop with a thickened bowel wall with plical hypertrophy (*arrow*), and mesenteric oedema

recurrence of the disease, especially with dementia, carries an extremely poor prognosis and, in this case, the use of antibiotics crossing the blood-brain barrier can be very useful.

A number of reports of individual cases and a few case series have described the US abdominal findings, which can suggest the presence of the disease even if they are not very specific (ALBANO et al. 1984; BRUGGEMANN et al. 1992; CARROCCIO et al. 1996; CASTAGNONE et al. 1991). In particular, most of these studies have identified a moderately dilated and thickened small bowel wall, with the disappearance of normal bowel wall stratification and brilliant, hyperechoic luminal contents mixed with a few hypoechogenic parts (Fig. 10.3), as well as an unusual, distinctive and diffusely echogenic retroperitoneal lymphadenopathy (DAVIS and PATEL 1990), sometimes with concomitant free abdominal fluid. It is interesting to note that the US abnormalities revert with appropriate long-term antibiotic therapy.

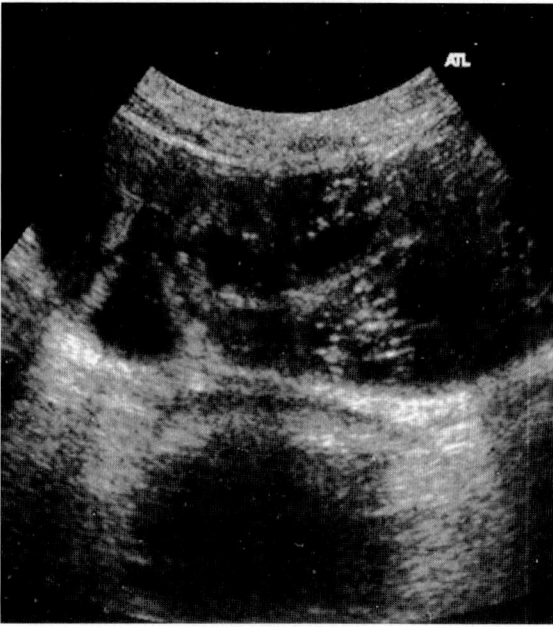

**Fig. 10.3.** US image showing dilated and thickened small bowel loops with the disappearance of normal bowel wall stratification and brilliant, hyperechoic luminal contents

## 10.3 Ultrasonography in the Diagnosis and Follow-Up of Eosinophilic Enteritis

Eosinophilic gastroenteritis is an uncommon condition of unknown aetiology, although it is generally believed to be due to intestinal allergy. Its clinical manifestations can be very heterogeneous, and the disease may mimic peptic ulcer, subacute (or chronic) intestinal obstruction, gastroenteritis, irritable bowel syndrome, or inflammatory bowel disease.

It is characterised by a selective eosinophilic infiltration of the stomach and/or small intestine. Primary eosinophilic gastroenteritis includes multiple disease entities depending on the level of histological involvement, and may be mucosal, muscular or serosal (LEE et al. 1993).

The *mucosal* form (the most common variant) is characterised by vomiting, abdominal pain, diarrhoea, blood loss, iron deficiency anaemia, malabsorption, and protein-losing enteropathy. The *muscular* form is characterised by eosinophilic infiltration in the muscular layer leading to a thickening of the bowel wall that may cause bowel obstruction. The *serological* form occurs in only a minority of cases, and is characterised by exudative ascites and a higher peripheral eosinophil count than that associated with the other forms (TALLEY et al. 1990; LEE et al. 1993; ROTHENBERG 2004).

Diagnosis is often difficult, and most cases are only diagnosed after a surgical procedure and histological sampling. The withdrawal of the food the involvement of which is suggested by means of skin prick testing (or RASTs: radio-allergo sorbent test) has variable effects. The treatment of choice is the administration of anti-inflammatory drugs, such as systemic or topical steroids. In severe cases, when dietary restriction fails, intravenous feeding or immunosuppressive antimetabolite therapy (azathioprine or 6-mercaptopurine) should be considered (TALLEY et al. 1990).

The most frequently reported US finding is a moderate thickening of the part of the gastrointestinal wall running from the stomach to the terminal ileum. Normal bowel wall stratification is lost, and the wall is hyperechoic with hypertrophic *valvulae conniventes*; the contents of the lumen may be anechoic (completely liquid) or slightly brilliant (in the case of a corpusculate content) (Fig. 10.4). (BULJEVAC et al. 2005). Abundant ascitic fluid is sometimes present, and should be sampled as it may reveal a diagnostic increase in the proportion of eosinophilic cells.

The pancreas is sometimes swollen, and the mesenteric lymph nodes (Fig. 10.5) may be enlarged.

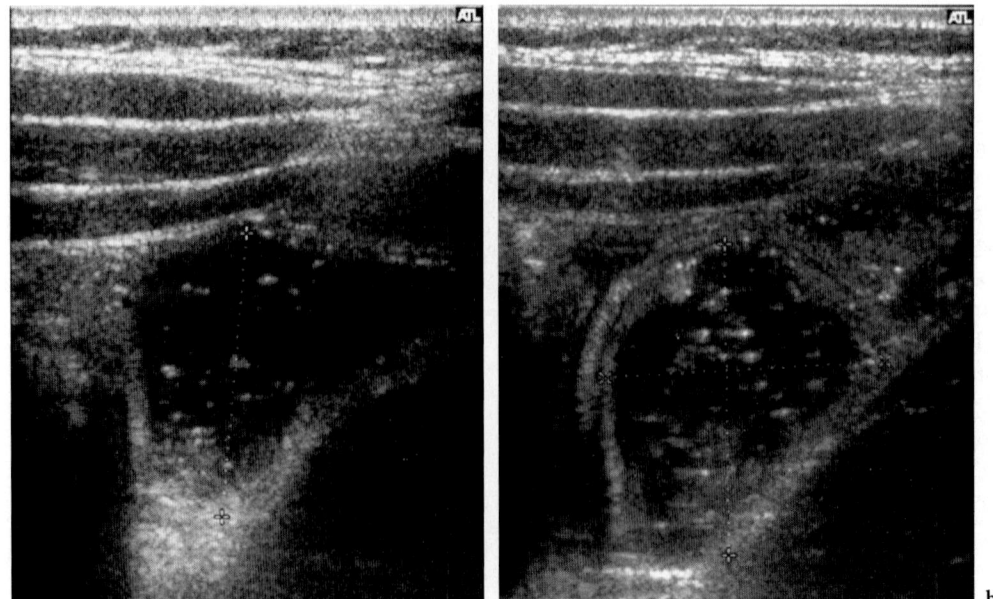

**Fig. 10.4a,b.** US images showing moderately dilated small bowel loops with a slightly thickened bowel wall and increased, prevalently anechoic intraluminal contents

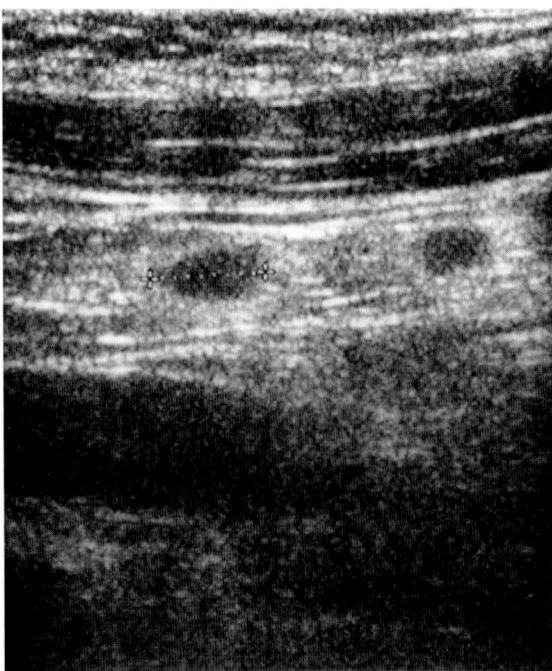

**Fig. 10.5.** US image showing some mesenteric lymph nodes slightly enlarged

Similar US findings have been reported also in a case of eosinophilic enteritis presenting as acute abdomen (SEELEN et al. 1992).

BULJEVAC et al. (2005) have recently published a case report concerning an 18-year-old patient with the serosal form of the disease. Basal US visualised nodular peritoneal deposits associated with ascites, whose cytological sampling revealed the presence of numerous eosinophils. After 2 weeks of corticosteroid treatment, the clinical, laboratory and US findings normalised (BULJEVAC et al. 2005).

## References

Albano O, Carrieri V, Vinciguerra V et al (1984) Ultrasonic findings in Whipple's disease. J Clin Ultrasound 12:286–288

Bai JC, Mazure RM, Vazquez H et al (2004) Whipple's disease. Clin Gastroenterol Hepatol 2:849–860

Bruggemann A, Burchardt H, Lepsien G (1992) Sonographical findings in Whipple's disease. A case report with regard to the literature. Surg Endosc 6:138–140

Buljevac M, Urek MC, Stoos-Veic T (2005) Sonography in the diagnosis and follow up of serosal gastroenteritis treated with corticosteroid. J Clin Ultrasound 33:43–46

Carroccio A, Soresi M, Montalto G et al (1996) Whipple's disease: a non-invasive approach for suspected diagnosis. Case report. Ital J Gastroenterol 28:229–231

Castagnone D, Mandelli C, Rivolta R et al (1991) Echography and computerized tomography of the abdomen in Whipple's disease. Radiol Med 82:540–542

Davis SJ, Patel A (1990) Distinctive echogenic lymphadenopathy in Whipple's disease. Clin Radiol 42:60–62

Dorne HL, Jequier S (1986) Sonography of intestinal lymphangiectasia. J Ultrasound Med 5:13–16

Lee CM, Changchien CS, Chen PC et al (1993) Eosinophilic gastroenteritis: 10 years experience. Am J Gastroenterol 88:70–74

Loreti L, Masselli G, Melisi MT et al (2003) Intestinal lymphangiectasia. Rays 28:409–416

Maconi G, Molteni P, Manzionna G et al (1998) Ultrasonographic features of long-standing primary intestinal lymphangiectasia. Eur J Ultrasound 7:195–198

Rothenberg ME (2004) Eosinophilic gastrointestinal disorders (EGID). J Allergy Clin Immunol 113:11–28

Seelen JL, You PH, de Vries AC, Puylaert JB (1992) Eosinophilic enteritis presenting as acute abdomen: US features of two cases. Gastrointest Radiol 17:19–20

Talley NJ, Shorter RG, Phillips SF, Zinsmeister AR (1990) Eosinophilic gastroenteritis: a clinicopathological study of patients with disease of the mucosa, muscle layer, and subserosal tissue Gut 31:54–58

# Infections

# Infectious Enteritis

Giovanni Maconi, Luciano Tarantino, and Gabriele Bianchi Porro

CONTENTS

11.1 Clinical Features 101

11.2 Infectious Enteritis and Colitis 102
11.2.1 Salmonellosis 102
11.2.2 Shigellosis 104

11.3 Infectious Bacterial Ileocecitis 104

11.4 Neutropenic Enterocolitis 106

References 107

## 11.1
## Clinical Features

Bacterial infectious enteritis is one of the most frequent causes of morbidity worldwide. Major causes are Salmonellosis, Shigellosis and infections due to *Yersina enterocolitis*, *Yersinia paratuberculosis* and *Campylobacter jejuni*. In otherwise healthy adults, infections due to these agents are frequently of short course and self-limiting. However, morbidity and

G. Maconi, MD
Chair of Gastroenterology, Department of Clinical Sciences, "L. Sacco" University Hospital, Via G.B. Grassi 74, 20157 Milan, Italy
L. Tarantino, MD
Interventional Ultrasound Unit, Department of Medicine, S. Giovanni di Dio Hospital, Via Mario Vergara Padre 187, 80027 Frattamaggiore, Naples, Italy
G. Bianchi Porro, MD, PhD
Chair of Gastroenterology, Department of Clinical Sciences, "L. Sacco" University Hospital, Via G.B. Grassi 74, 20157 Milan, Italy

mortality due to these infections are highest among the elderly, infants and children, as well as immunocompromised individuals.

Enteric infections result in gastroenteritis occurring 6–48 h after ingestion of contaminated food or water. The most common symptoms are diarrhoea, fever, nausea and vomiting, as well as abdominal pain. Abdominal pain usually consists of cramping and may be, in most cases, the most prominent symptom. It may be generalised but, in some instances, may be localised and cause a syndrome or disorder that mimics appendicitis or inflammatory bowel disease.

Indeed, symptoms of pathogen-specific enteritis are not sufficiently unusual to distinguish a disorder form those due to Salmonella, Shigella, Campylobacter or Yersinia or other pathogens. The combination of fever and faecal leukocytes or erythrocytes is indicative of inflammatory diarrhoea, but the definite diagnosis is based on culture or demonstration of specific organisms on stained faecal smears.

For this reason, the importance of radiographic and sonographic imaging in the diagnosis of infectious enteritis is limited. However, since ultrasound is a rapid, simple, cheap and non-invasive diagnostic tool, it may be usefully employed, in some instances, to discriminate between self-limiting infectious conditions and severe enterocolitic syndromes, such as inflammatory bowel diseases or appendicitis and their complications, or other conditions requiring surgery or specific medical treatment. Therefore, in individuals presenting with abdominal pain, diarrhoea and fever, or patients with acute or atypical symptoms and infants, as well as immunocompromised and elderly patients where a differential diagnosis between bacterial infectious enteritis and other acute abdominal conditions is mandatory, ultrasound can be usefully employed to avoid unnecessary laparotomy or, on the other hand, to avoid delay of surgery or specific therapy (Fig. 11.1) (Puylaert 1994; Tarantino et al. 2003).

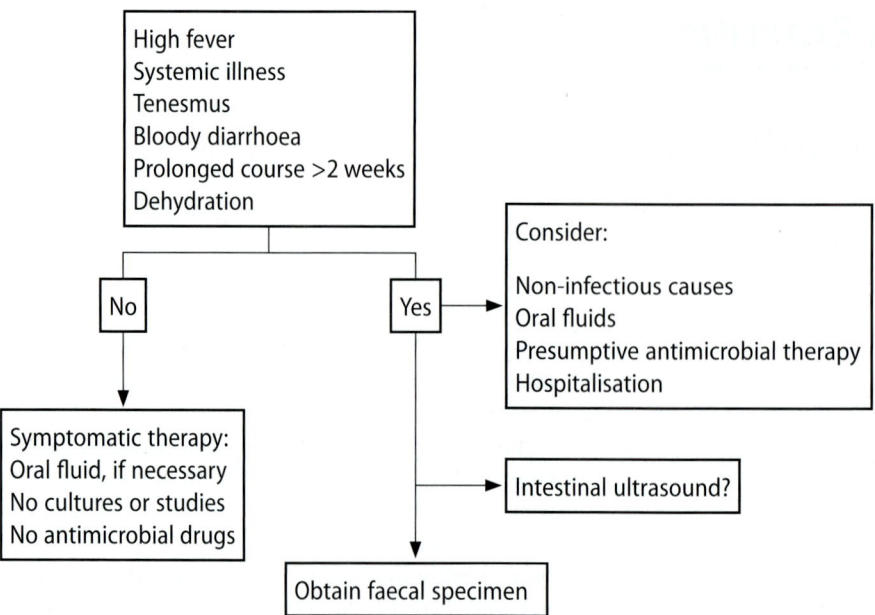

Fig. 11.1. Algorithm in patients presenting with suspicious infectious gastroenteritis

## 11.2 Infectious Enteritis and Colitis

### 11.2.1 Salmonellosis

Gastroenteritis infection with non-typhoidal salmonella often results in gastroenteritis indistinguishable from that caused by other bacterial or viral pathogens. It is usually self-limited, and fever and diarrhoea resolve within 3 and 7 days, respectively. In a minority of patients (<5%), particularly neonates, infants, elderly and immunocompromised patients, carriage of the pathogen and/or a bacteraemia is prolonged with endovascular or localised (intra-abdominal, central nervous system, pulmonary) infections.

Sonographic features of Salmonella enterocolitis have been described both in children and in adults. The first report described ileocaecal wall thickening and lymph node enlargement in a single case report of a patient with typhoid fever (PUYLAERT 1989). In a series of 27 patients, a concentric thickening (up to 7 mm; range 5–11 mm) of the left side of the colonic wall was observed in 81% of cases and in individual cases enlarged mesenteric lymph nodes and ascites were seen (MATHIS and METZLER 1992). In a large series of adult patients with typhoid fever, wall thickening of the ileum (Fig. 11.2a) and/or ascending colon was reported in 36% and mesenteric lymph node enlargement (Fig. 11.2 b) in 56% of patients (TARANTINO et al. 1997).

In a more recent study carried out in children, increased colonic wall thickening has been observed in up to 40% of cases. The mean thickness was 6.2 mm, resulting predominantly from a gross submucosa oedema. Peristalsis has been described as either increased or attenuated. Ascites has been observed in 60% of patients and enlarged mesenteric lymph nodes in less than 10% of patients (UEDA et al. 1999). In children, the sonographic detection of ascites and the increased colonic wall thickening correlated well with serum levels of C-reactive protein and stool occult blood and, therefore, these may be useful signs by which to determine the severity of Salmonella enterocolitis. However, whether they also represent a significant prognostic factor is still unknown. In this regard, the persistence of positive stool culture 3 months after infection may result in the persistence of slight bowel wall thickening and in enlarged intra-abdominal lymph nodes (Fig. 11.3). Sonographic detection of ascites or intra-abdominal fluid in children with infectious enteritis can distinguish Salmonella enteritis from colitis due to Rotavirus. In fact, ascites is usually absent in Rotavirus colitis (UEDA et al. 1999; BASS et al. 2004).

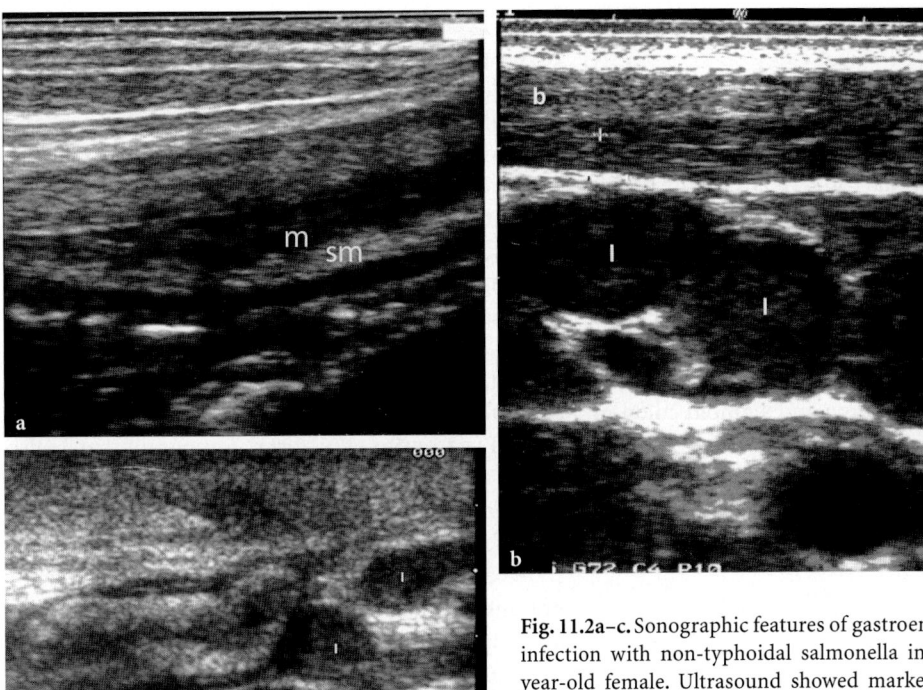

**Fig. 11.2a–c.** Sonographic features of gastroenteritis infection with non-typhoidal salmonella in a 16-year-old female. Ultrasound showed marked wall thickening of ileum (**a,c**) and caecum, confined to mucosa (*m*) and submucosa (*sm*) and multiple enlarged mesenteric lymph nodes (*l*) distributed in "rosary-like" appearance (**b**). Ascites was also present

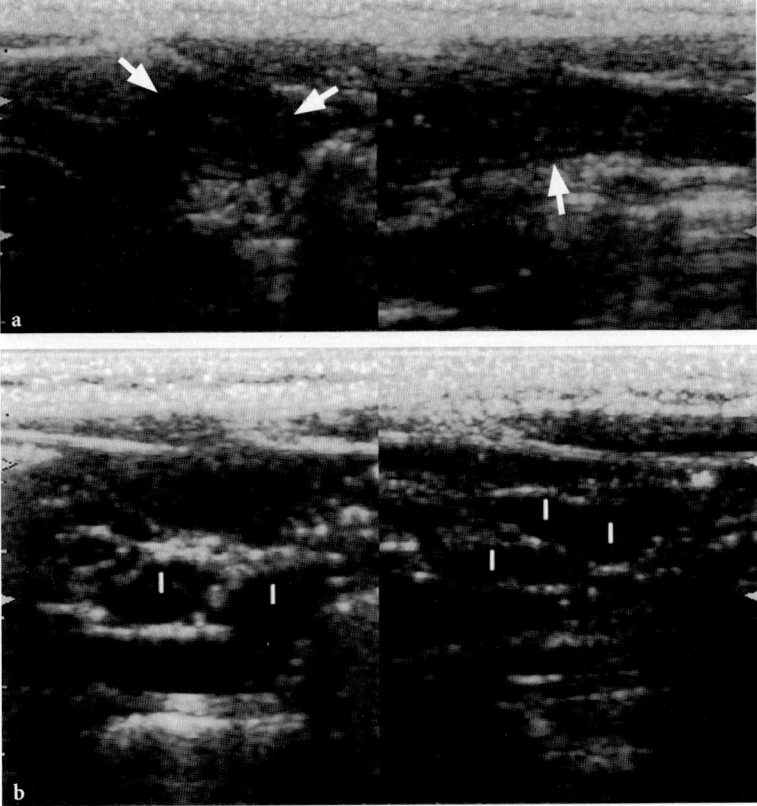

**Fig. 11.3a,b.** Presence of (**a**) slight bowel wall thickening (*arrows*) and (**b**) enlarged intra-abdominal lymph nodes (*l*) in a 10-year-old patient with persistence of positive stool culture 3 months after infection with Salmonella

## 11.2.2
## Shigellosis

Shigellosis is the main bacterial cause of dysentery and should be taken into consideration in patients presenting with bloody diarrhoea. It is an acute bacterial infection caused by Shigella species (*S. dysenterie, S. flexneri, S. sonnei*) usually involving the distal colon and progressively decreasing in the more proximal segments of the large bowel. Sporadic case reports have depicted the sonographic features of Shigellosis. A diffuse wall thickening (8 mm) with distinct layer stratification in the descending and sigmoid colon in an 81-year-old female was observed, ruling out the presence of ischaemic colitis on the basis of clinical history and sonographic findings (FUJII et al. 2001).

## 11.3
## Infectious Bacterial Ileocecitis

Infectious ileocecitis is an infection of the terminal ileum and caecum that is caused by *Yersinia enterocolitica, Campylobacter jejuni* or *Salmonella enteritidis*. The clinical features of infectious ileocecitis are very similar to those commonly found in acute appendicitis, with localized pain in the right lower quadrant being the main symptom, whereas diarrhoea is absent or mild. Local tenderness may be less prominent and acute phase reactants more elevated than in appendicitis. Due to these symptoms, infectious ileocecitis may lead to unnecessary laparotomy for suspected appendicitis.

At laparotomy, the appendix is normal, whereas the wall of the ileum and caecum is thickened and surrounded by enlarged mesenteric lymph nodes. However, these findings may be subtle and underestimated at laparotomy. Stool cultures are rarely requested since diarrhoea is absent and, therefore, the diagnosis is rarely made.

It has been widely shown that ultrasound may reveal a high incidence of infectious ileocecitis in patients with acute right lower quadrant pain suspicious for appendicitis (PUYLAERT et al. 1988, 1989, 1997; TARANTINO et al. 2003). Sonography may also reveal the features of the bowel wall useful in the differential diagnosis between infectious ileocolitis, Crohn's disease and appendicitis (Table 11.1).

According to PUYLAERT et al. (1997) the sonographic involvement of the terminal ileum, caecum, ascending colon and mesenteric lymph nodes in infectious ileocecitis caused by different microorganisms may be different, thus suggesting a possible aetiological diagnosis.

The sonographic features of infectious enterocolitis are characteristic, consisting of thickening of the mucosa and (less frequently) submucosa of the ileum, caecum and ascending colon together with enlarged regional mesenteric lymph nodes (Fig. 11.4). Usually, the thickened ileo-caecal valve can be seen in these cases (Fig. 11.5). The appendix is normal.

In the differential diagnosis between infectious ileocecitis and Crohn's disease, the latter is characterized by transmural inflammation and intestinal com-

Table 11.1. Main differences in sonographic features of infectious ileocecitis caused by Yersinia, Campylobacter or Salmonella, Crohn's disease and appendicitis

|  | Infectious ileocecitis | Crohn's disease | Appendicitis |
|---|---|---|---|
| Bowel Wall Thickening | Mild and confined to superficial layers | Moderate and involving all layers | Absent or Mild (ileum) |
| Echo Pattern | Preserved | Preserved, altered or loss | Preserved (ileum) |
| Compressibility of ileum | Preserved | Usually not preserved | Preserved |
| Mesenteric hypertrophy | Sometimes present | Often present | Often present |
| Haustration of right colon | Preserved | Often lost (in diseased tract) | Preserved |
| Appendix | Normal | Normal or enlarged | Enlarged |
| Regional lymph nodes | Moderately to grossly enlarged | Often present | Often present |
| Abscess | Absent | Often present | Sometimes present |
| Fistula | Absent | Often present | Absent |
| Pre-stenotic dilatation | Absent | Often present | Absent |

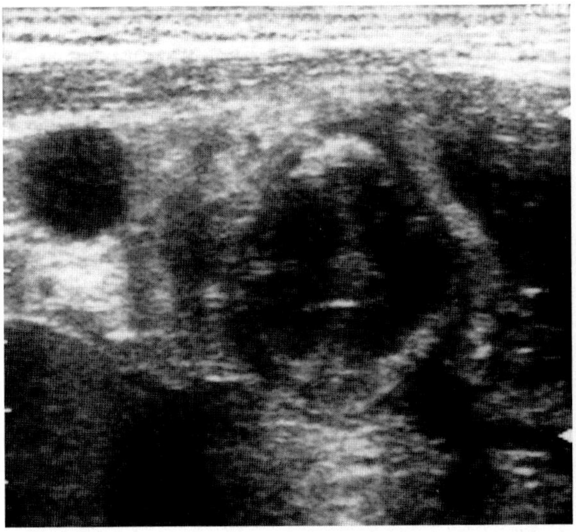

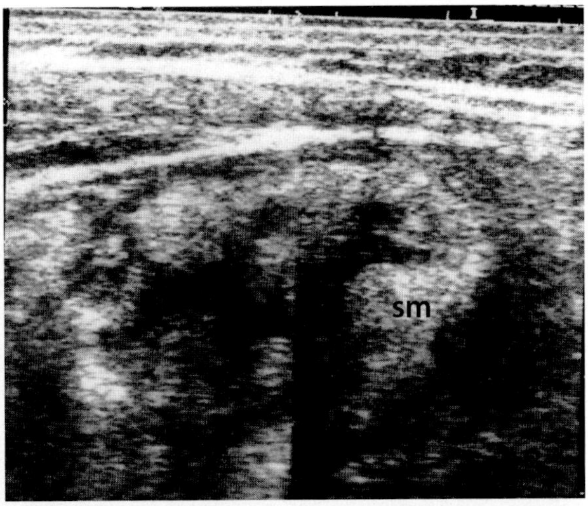

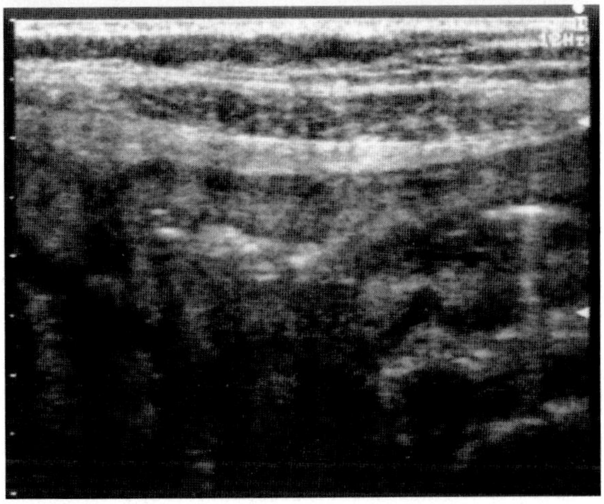

**Fig. 11.4a–c.** Infectious ileocecitis in a 20-year-old male with clinical signs of appendicitis. **a** Ultrasound showed marked wall thickening of ileum confined to mucosa and submucosa. **b** Marked thickening of the caecal wall mainly confined to submucosa (*sm*). **c** Wall thickening of the ascending colon

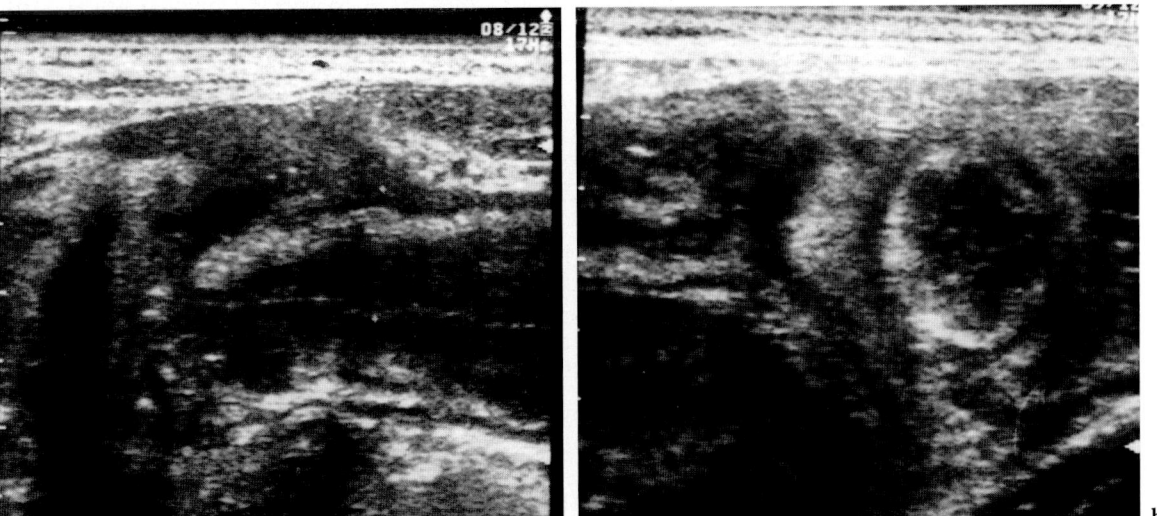

**Fig. 11.5a,b.** Sagittal view of caecum, ileocaecal valve and ascending colon (**a**), and axial view of the ileum ileocaecal valve and caecum (**b**) are the most typical US features of infectious ileocecitis

plications. Therefore, the bowel wall is usually thicker than in infectious ileocecitis, and may be non-compressible with transmural inflammation involving the muscularis layer and resulting in disappearance of the normal stratified echo pattern. The thickened bowel wall may be surrounded by mesenteric hypertrophy and complications such as abscess or fistula and prestenotic dilatation can be found. None of these features are present in infectious ileocecitis. Nevertheless, when sonographic features suggest the presence of an inflammatory/infectious ileocecitis, bacteriological tests are mandatory to differentiate between Crohn's disease and infectious ileocecitis.

## 11.4
## Neutropenic Enterocolitis

Neutropenic enterocolitis is a life-threatening complication in neutropenic patients with acute leukaemia undergoing aggressive myelosuppressive chemotherapy (GORSCHLÜTER et al. 2001), the incidence varying between 1.8% and 32.5% (highest frequency in children) with a mortality of at least 50% (WADE et al. 1992; GORSCHLÜTER et al. 2001).

It is difficult to differentiate between infectious and non-infectious causes of abdominal symptoms in these patients. In fact, symptoms suggesting an abdominal infection, such as diarrhoea, abdominal pain, nausea and vomiting may also be caused by intestinal mucositis or other toxic effects of chemotherapy. The diagnosis of abdominal infections is usually based on a combination of clinical findings (fever, abdominal pain, diarrhoea) and abnormalities in imaging studies. Bowel wall thickening reflects the pathology of neutropenic enterocolitis characterized by marked mucosal and submucosal oedema and occasionally haemorrhage (Fig. 11.6) (CARTONI et al. 2001; GORSCHLÜTER et al. 2002). Therefore, it has been proposed as the main criterion to establish the diagnosis of neutropenic enterocolitis (PICARDI et al. 1999) and it has been demonstrated that the degree of thickening is a valuable prognostic factor that adversely affects the outcome (CARTONI et al. 2001).

The sonographic detection of increased colonic wall thickening (>4 mm) 2–4 days after the end of intensive chemotherapy, in neutropenic (neutrophils below $0.5 \times 10^9/l$) patients with a clinical syndrome characterized by fever, diarrhoea and abdominal pain confirms the clinical diagnosis of infectious neutropenic enterocolitis and should not be considered as a sign of chemotherapy-induced mucositis. These patients have a higher mortality rate than patients not presenting colonic wall thickening and require, particularly those with a thicker bowel wall (>10 mm), intensive supportive treatment consisting of bowel rest with total parenteral nutrition and antibiotic and antimycotic therapy, as they have a very poor prognosis.

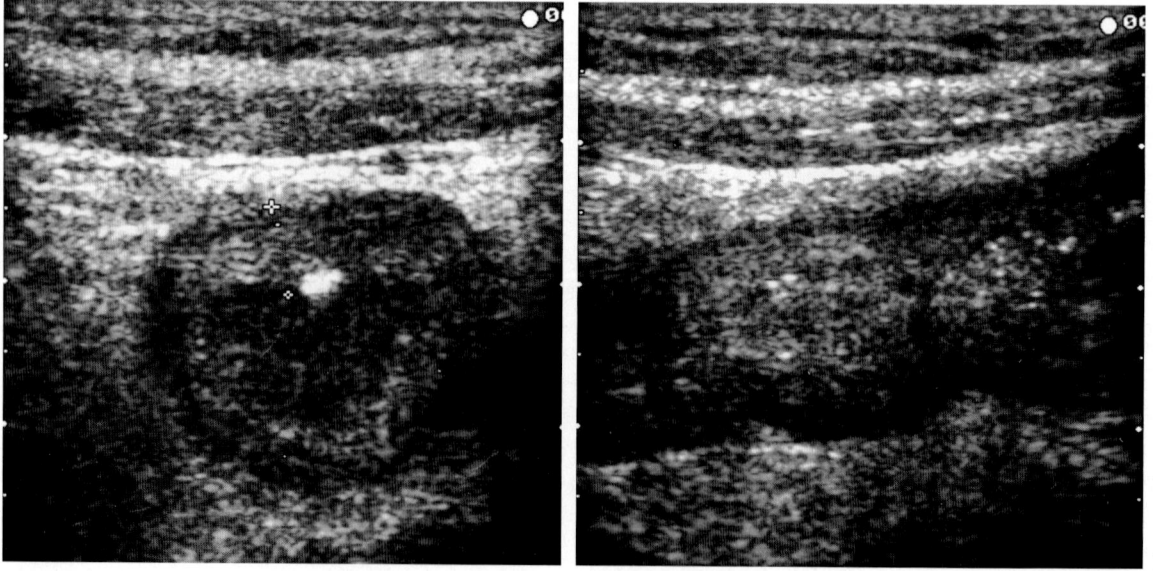

**Fig. 11.6a,b.** Transverse (a) and axial (b) views of ascending colon wall thickening, reflecting neutropenic enterocolitis characterized by marked mucosal and submucosal oedema and occasional haemorrhage

# References

Bass D, Cordoba E, Dekker C, Schuind A, Cassady C (2004) Intestinal imaging of children with acute rotavirus gastroenteritis. J Pediatr Gastroenterol Nutr 39:270–274

Cartoni C, Dragoni F, Micozzi A et al (2001) Neutropenic enterocolitis in patients with acute leukemia: prognostic significance of bowel wall thickening detected by ultrasonography. J Clin Oncol 19:756–761

Fujii Y, Taniguchi N, Itoh K (2001) Sonographic findings in Shigella colitis. J Clin Ultrasound 29:48–55

Gorschlüter M, Glasmacher A, Hahn C et al (2001) Severe abdominal infections in neutropenic patients. Cancer Invest 19:669–677

Gorschlüter M, Marklein G, Höfling K et al (2002) Abdominal infections in patients with acute leukaemia: a prospective study applying ultrasonography and microbiology. Br J Haematol 117:351–358

Mathis G, Metzler J (1992) Sonography in salmonella enterocolitis. Ultraschall Med 13:106–109

Picardi M, Selleri C, Camera A, Catalano L, Rotoli B (1999) Early detection by ultrasound scan of severe post-chemotherapy gut complications in patients with acute leukemia. Haematologica 84:222–225

Puylaert JMBC (1989) Typhoid fever: diagnosis by ultrasonography. Am J Roentgenol 153:745–746

Puylaert JBCM (1994) When in doubt, sound it out. Radiology 191:320–321

Puylaert JB, Lalisang RI, van der Werf SD, Doornbos L (1988) Campylobacter ileocolitis mimicking acute appendicitis: differentiation with graded-compression US. Radiology 166:737–740

Puylaert JB, Vermeijden RJ, van der Werf SD, Doornbos L, Koumans RK (1989) Incidence and sonographic diagnosis of bacterial ileocaecitis masquerading as appendicitis. Lancet 2:84–86

Puylaert JB, Van der Zant FM, Mutsaers JA (1997) Infectious ileocecitis caused by Yersinia, Campylobacter, and Salmonella: clinical, radiological and US findings. Eur Radiol 7:3–9

Tarantino L, Giorgio A, de Stefano G et al (1997) Value of bowel ultrasonography in the diagnosis of typhoid fever. Eur J Ultrasound 5:77–83

Tarantino L, Giorgio A, de Stefano G et al (2003) Acute appendicitis mimicking infectious enteritis: diagnostic value of sonography. J Ultrasound Med 22:945–950

Ueda D, Sato T, Yoshida M (1999) Ultrasonographic assessment of Salmonella enterocolitis in children. Pediatr Radiol 29:469–471

Wade DS, Nava HR, Douglass-Ho J (1992) Neutropenic enterocolitis. Clinical diagnosis and treatment. Cancer 69:17–23

# Intestinal Tuberculosis

Dong Ho Lee and Jae Hoon Lim

CONTENTS

12.1 Introduction  109
12.2 Pathology  109
12.3 Sonographic Findings of Intestinal Tuberculosis  109
12.3.1 Bowel Wall Thickening  109
12.3.2 Hyperemia  110
12.3.3 Stricture  111
12.3.4 Mesenteric Lymphadenitis  111
12.4 Sonographic Findings of Tuberculous Peritonitis  112
12.4.1 Ascites  112
12.4.2 Omental Cake  113
12.4.3 Thickened Mesentery with Matted Small Bowel Loops  113
12.5 Differential Diagnosis  113
References  114

## 12.1
## Introduction

Sonography may be used in patients with intestinal tuberculosis to document its classic features, i.e., bowel wall thickening, hyperemia, stricture, and mesenteric lymphadenopathy. When tuberculous peritonitis coexists, sonography shows ascites, omental cake, and thickened mesentery with an adherent small bowel loop; thus, ultrasonography may be used as a primary investigative tool in patients with suspected or recurrent tuberculosis.

D. H. Lee, MD
Professor of Radiology, Department of Radiology and Center for Imaging Science, Kyung Hee University Hospital, 1, Hoeki-dong, Dongdaemun-gu, Seoul, Korea
J. H. Lim, MD
Professor of Radiology, Department of Radiology, Samsung Medical Center, Sungkyunkwan University School of Medicine, 50, Ilwon-dong, Kangnam-ku, Seoul, Korea

## 12.2
## Pathology

Intestinal tuberculosis is a chronic inflammation of the bowel caused by *Mycobacterium tuberculosis*. The ileocecal area is the most common site. The classic radiographic appearance of ileocecal tuberculosis on barium enema has been described as a conical, shrunken, retracted cecum associated with a narrow ulcerated terminal ileum (Reeder and Palmer 1989). This cecal deformity is the result of spasm early in the disease and transmural infiltration with fibrosis in advanced phases. Narrowing of the terminal ileum may be caused by persistent irritability with rapid emptying of the narrowed segment, corresponding to the acute inflammatory phase, or it may be the result of stricture with thickening and ulceration.

Grossly, there is ulceration with diffuse fibrosis extending through the bowel wall, causing stenosis and obstruction (Rosai 2004). Coexisting tuberculous peritonitis is observed in relatively few cases. Microscopically, typical granulomas are usually present accompanied by ulceration and extensive desmoplasia. These granulomas can be caseating or non-caseating, suppurative, or fibrous. Features favoring tuberculosis are caseation and granuloma coalescence.

## 12.3
## Sonographic Findings of Intestinal Tuberculosis

### 12.3.1
### Bowel Wall Thickening

The normal bowel wall is visualized as a single, circular, hypoechoic layer surrounding hyperechoic bowel contents, such as gas, foodstuffs, or feces. The hypoechoic layer is considered to be the muscle layer (LIM 2000). The normal bowel wall is uniform with an average thickness of 2–3 mm if distended and 3–5 mm if not (WILSON 1998). When the wall thickness in the transverse section is more than 5 mm, the bowel wall is regarded as being pathologically thickened (MALIK and SAXENA 2003).

The ileocecal region is most commonly involved in tuberculosis. The principal sonographic features of intestinal tuberculosis are diffuse, uniform, concentric, and circumferential wall thickenings of the terminal ileum, cecum, and ascending colon (Figs. 12.1–12.3; LEE et al 1993; KEDAR et al 1994). These wall thickenings are continuous without skip lesions. Concentric involvement is more common than eccentric involvement (Fig. 12.4; LEE et al 1993). The detection of bowel wall thickening is important when making a diagnosis of intestinal tuberculosis and the detection rates range from 86% to 96% (MALIK and SAXENA 2003; LEE et al 1993; LIM et al 1994). Mild wall thickening of small bowel may be overlooked (Fig. 12.5), and it is difficult to distinguish individual loops when they adhere to each other (LEE et al 1991).

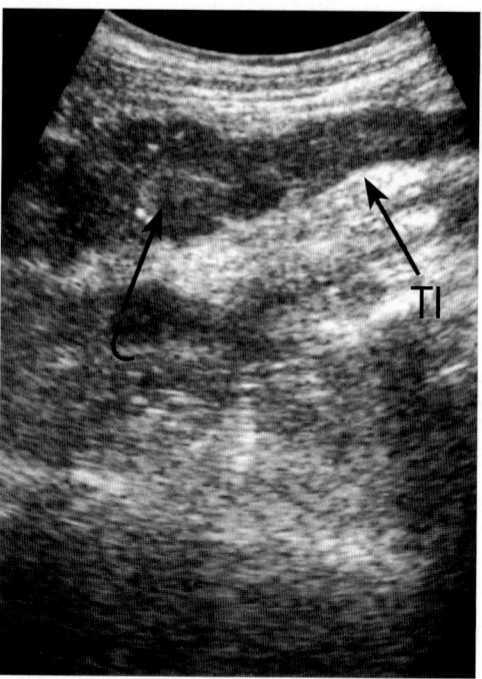

Fig. 12.1. Ileocecal tuberculosis. Transverse sonogram of the right lower abdomen shows diffuse thickening of the terminal ileum (*TI*) and cecum (*C*)

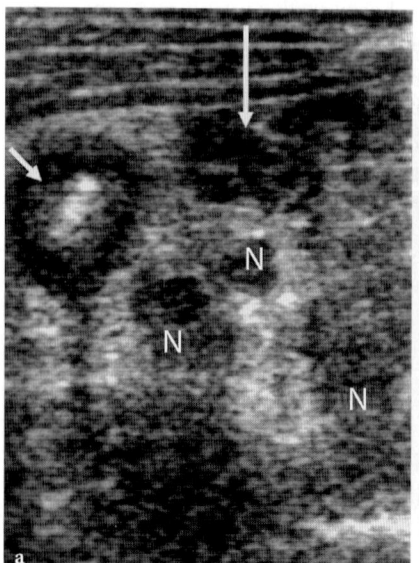 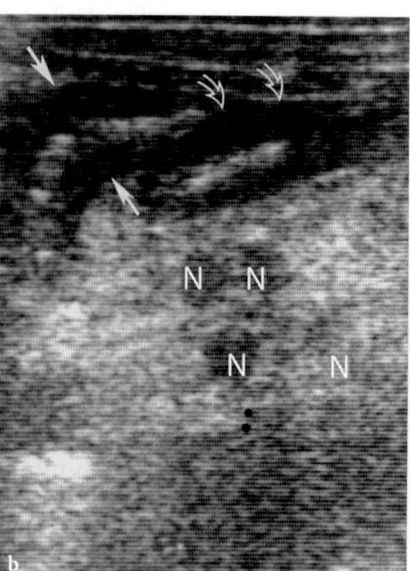 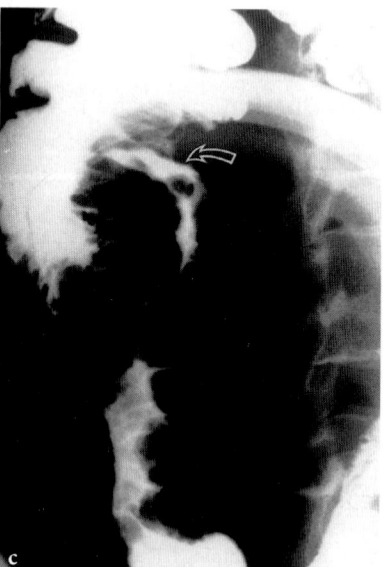

Fig. 12.2a–c. Ileocecal tuberculosis and associated mesenteric lymphadenitis. a Transverse sonogram of ileocecal region shows thickening of the wall of the cecum (*short arrow*) and terminal part of the ileum (*long arrow*). Note enlarged mesenteric lymph nodes (*N*) and thickened mesentery around lymph nodes. b Longitudinal sonogram shows thickening of the cecum (*solid arrows*) and terminal part of the ileum (*open arrows*) and enlarged lymph nodes (*N*). c Barium examination shows irregular narrowing of the terminal part of the ileum and cecum. Note longitudinal ulcer (*arrow*) at the terminal part of the ileum. Mucosal folds are markedly thickened and irregular

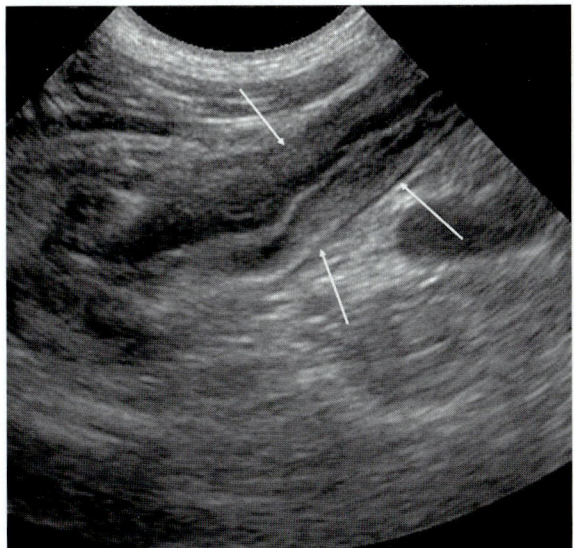

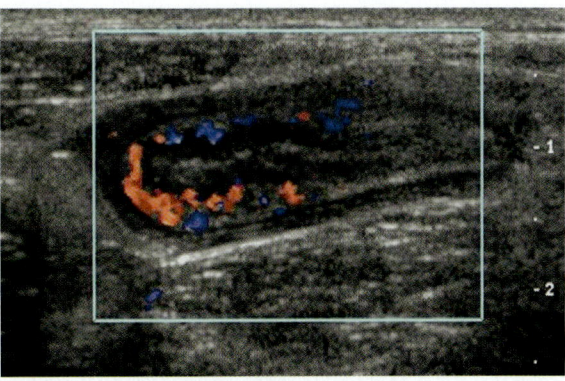

Fig. 12.3a,b. Ileal tuberculosis. a Transverse sonogram of right lower quadrant abdomen shows diffuse mural thickening of the terminal ileum. The terminal ileum shows concentric thickening (*arrows*). The thickness of the anterior and posterior walls is the same. b Transverse color Doppler sonogram of the terminal ileum shows numerous color signals

### 12.3.2
### Hyperemia

Although subjective, color Doppler imaging is helpful in distinguishing active inflammatory changes in the thickened bowel wall from other disorders (Fig. 12.3; WILSON 1998; TEEFEY et al 1996). Power Doppler imaging may improve the visualization of intramural gastrointestinal vascularity (CLAUTICE-ENGLE et al 1996); thus, recent advances in color Doppler and power Doppler imaging improve the accuracy of sonography by allowing the detection of hyperemia of the inflamed bowel wall and of adjacent inflamed fat.

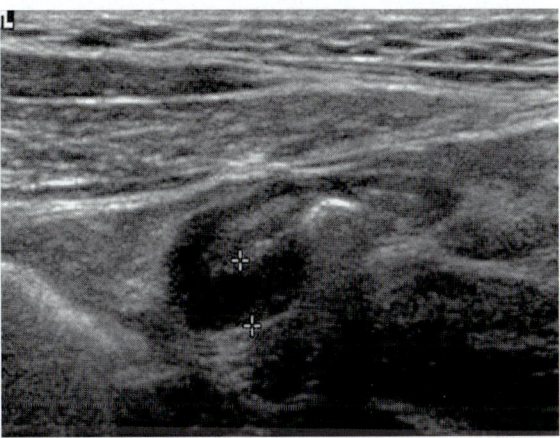

Fig. 12.4. Ileal tuberculosis. Transverse sonogram of the right lower quadrant abdomen discloses eccentric thickening of the posterior wall of the terminal ileum

### 12.3.3
### Stricture

In the active stage of intestinal tuberculosis, bowel wall thickening is usually accompanied by luminal narrowing, which results from spasm and edema. Later, fibrosis and scarring lead to permanent stricture (Fig. 12.5); however, it is difficult to detect stricture during sonographic examinations (KEDAR et al 1994).

Ultrasonography detects ulceration within the thickened wall in only a few cases, whereas it is seen frequently during small bowel follow through examination or barium enema studies. This low sensitivity for the detection of ulcers on sonography may be due to the associated spasm (KEDAR 1994). Lymphoid tissue involvement in the ileal wall with ulceration, necrosis, fibrosis, and often with extensive granulomatous infiltrate can be observed (KHAW 1991). In a few cases of intestinal tuberculosis, a spasm of the cecum is identified by a collapsed lumen and irritability of the thickened wall (LEE et al. 1993).

### 12.3.4
### Mesenteric Lymphadenitis

In active tuberculosis, enlarged mesenteric nodes are frequent. Lymphadenopathy is located mainly at the mesentery around the ileum (Fig. 12.2; LEE 1993), but is sometimes found at the periportal (Fig. 12.6), peri-

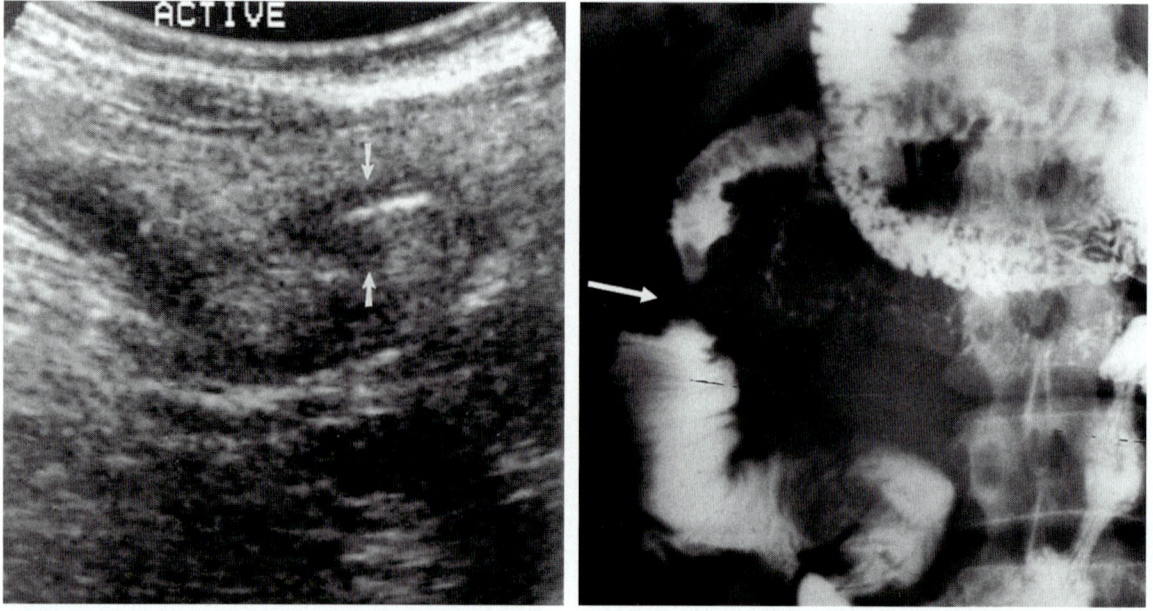

**Fig. 12.5a,b.** Jejunal tuberculosis. **a** Transverse sonogram of the right upper abdomen shows a short segmental wall thickening of the jejunum (*arrows*). **b** Small bowel follow-through examination shows a segmental stricture of the jejunum (*arrow*). Note thickening of the mucosal folds at the proximal loop

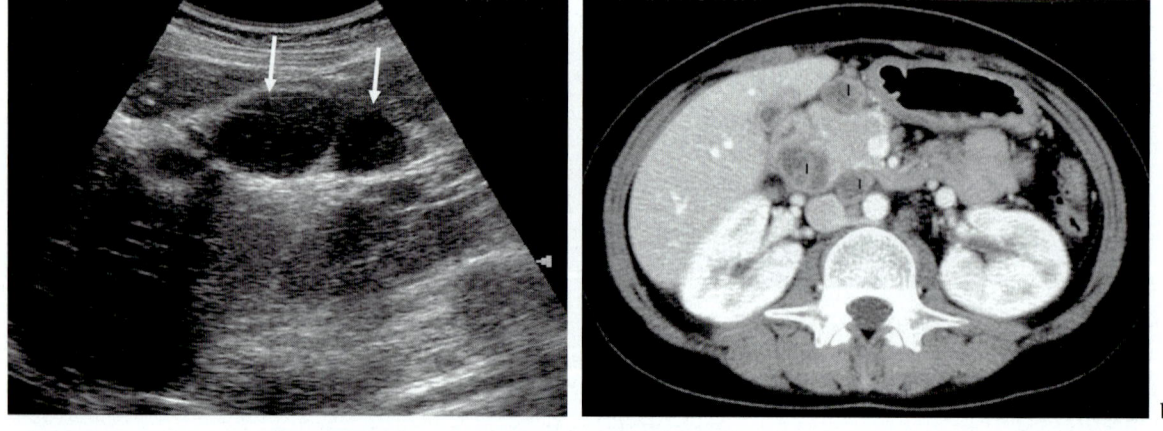

**Fig. 12.6a,b.** Tuberculous lymphadenitis. **a** Transverse sonogram of the right upper quadrant abdomen shows hypoechoic lymph node enlargement at porta hepatis (*arrows*). **b** Abdominal CT shows multiple peripancreatic lymph nodes (*l*) enlargement. The enlarged lymph nodes show central low attenuation with marginal rim enhancement due to central caseous necrosis

pancreatic, mesenteric, and upper periaortic regions (MALIK and SAXENA 2003); however, the retroperitoneal lymph node is rarely involved, which can be explained by the fact that mesenteric lymph nodes drain directly into the thoracic duct via the cisterna chyli (JAIN et al. 1995). Enlarged lymph nodes are hypoechoic, round to ovoid, and variable in size. Sometimes the nodes may be calcified (MALIK and SAXENA 2003; KEDAR et al. 1994). Calcification in healing tuberculosis is seen as a discrete reflective arc with posterior shadowing.

## 12.4
## Sonographic Findings of Tuberculous Peritonitis

### 12.4.1
### Ascites

Three types of tuberculous peritonitis are generally recognized: the wet-ascitic type; the dry-plastic type; and the fibrotic-fixed type (MALIK and SAXENA 2003;

LEE et al. 1991). The wet-ascitic type is characterized by ascites that may be free or loculated, whereas the dry-plastic type presents with enlarged lymph nodes with central caseation necrosis and adhesion, and the fibrotic-fixed type is observed as an omental mass and matted loops of bowel and mesentery. Combinations of these three forms are also found (KEDAR et al. 1994). The characteristic sonographic finding of tuberculous peritonitis of the wet-ascitic type is ascites. The most common pattern of ascites is clear fluid, though sometimes ascites is associated with membranes, septa, fine mobile strands, or floating debris (Fig. 12.7).

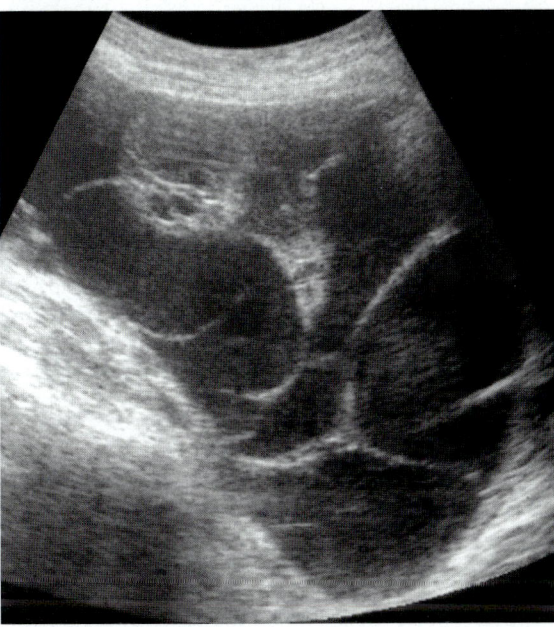

**Fig. 12.7.** Tuberculous peritonitis. Longitudinal sonogram of low abdomen shows a large amount of ascites with multiple, interlacing, thin septae

## 12.4.2
## Omental Cake

About 20–30% of patients with tuberculous peritonitis have omental cake (LEE et al. 1991). Omental cake is defined as a pancake-like diffuse thickening of the greater omentum, stretching from the greater curvature of the stomach down to the lower abdomen. Omental cakes are depicted as diffuse, hyperechoic, or heterogeneously echogenic thickening on sonographic examination (LEE et al. 1991). They may be seen in cancer peritonitis, and thus, it is impossible to differentiate by means of sonography.

## 12.4.3
## Thickened Mesentery with Matted Small Bowel Loops

The important sonographic features of early abdominal tuberculosis are a mesenteric thickness of 15 mm or more, and an increase in mesenteric echogenicity (JAIN et al. 1995), which increases markedly, presumably because of fat deposition due to lymphatic obstruction. Pathologically, this mesenteric thickening results from edema, lymphadenopathy, and fat deposition. Another sonographic finding is matted, fixed small bowel loops and mesenteric strands, resembling spokes radiating from the mesenteric root, i.e., the sonographic "stellate" sign (KEDAR et al. 1994).

## 12.5
## Differential Diagnosis

The principal sonographic features of intestinal tuberculosis are diffuse wall thickening of the terminal ileum and ascending colon with mesenteric lymphadenopathy. Other diseases that show wall thickening of the terminal ileum and colon are Crohn's disease, bacterial ileocolitis, and lymphoma (LEE et al. 1993). In Crohn's disease, bowel wall thickening is more severe and lymphadenopathy is rare (LIMBERG 1990; WORLICEK et al. 1987). Frequently, the normal stratification of the bowel wall is no longer evident in involved areas due to transmural inflammation (LIMBERG 1990). Abscess, fistula, and skip lesions are often seen in Crohn's disease, but they are rare in tuberculosis (SARRAZIN and WILSON 1996). In *Yersinia* ileitis, thickening of the ileal wall and mesenteric lymphadenopathy are the main findings, but the cecum and the ascending colon are usually spared (MATSUMOTO et al. 1991). In neutropenic typhlitis, wall thickening is confined to the right colonic wall and patients are usually in an immunosuppressed state (TEEFEY et al. 1987). In typhoid fever, there may be mural thickening of the terminal ileum and cecum and enlarged mesenteric lymph nodes (PUYLAERT et al. 1989). Clinical symptoms and course are usually different in *Campylobacter* ileocolitis from those in tuberculosis (PUYLAERT et al. 1988). In lymphoma, bowel wall thickening is severe. However, the sonographic findings of all these diseases are sometimes similar; therefore, it is necessary to confirm the nature of bowel pathology by barium studies, CT, or colonoscopic biopsy.

## References

Clautice-Engle T, Jeffrey RB Jr, Li KC, Barth RA (1996) Power Doppler imaging of focal lesions of the gastrointestinal tract: comparison with conventional color Doppler imaging. J Ultrasound Med 15:63–66

Jain R, Sawhney S, Bhargava DK, Berry M (1995) Diagnosis of abdominal tuberculosis: sonographic findings in patients with early disease. Am J Roentgenol 165:1391–1395

Kedar RP, Shah PP, Shivde RS, Malde HM (1994) Sonographic findings in gastrointestinal and peritoneal tuberculosis. Clin Radiol 49:24–29

Khaw KT, Yeoman LJ, Saverymuttu SH, Cook MG, Joseph AEA (1991) Ultrasonic patterns in inflammatory bowel disease. Clin Radiol 43:171–175

Lee DH, Lim JH, Ko YT, Yoon Y (1991) Sonographic findings in tuberculous peritonitis of wet-ascitic type. Clin Radiol 44:306–310

Lee DH, Ko YT, Yoon Y, Lim JH (1993) Sonographic findings of intestinal tuberculosis. J Ultrasound Med 12:537–540

Lim JH (2000) Ultrasound examination of gastrointestinal tract diseases. J Korean Med Sci 15:371–379

Lim JH, Ko YT, Lee DH, Lim JW, Kim TH (1994) Sonography of inflammatory bowel disease: findings and value in differential diagnosis. Am J Roentgenol 163:343–347

Limberg B (1990) Sonographic features of colonic Crohn's disease: comparison of in vivo and in vitro studies. J Clin Ultrasound 18:161–166

Malik A, Saxena NC (2003) Ultrasound in abdominal tuberculosis. Abdom Imaging 28:574–579

Matsumoto T, Iida M, Sakai T, Kimura Y, Fujishima M (1991) Yersinia terminal ileitis: sonographic findings in eight patients. Am J Roentgenol 156:965–967

Puylaert JBCM, Lalisang RI, van der Werf SDJ, Doornbos L (1988) *Campylobacter* ileocolitis mimicking acute appendicitis: differentiation with graded-compression US. Radiology 166:737–740

Puylaert JBCM, Kristjansdottir S, Golterman KL, de Jong GM, Knecht NM (1989) Typhoid fever: diagnosis by using sonography. Am J Roentgenol 153:745–746

Reeder MM, Palmer PES (1989) Infections and infestations. In: Freeny PC, Stevenson GW, Margulis AR (eds) Burhenne's alimentary tract radiology, 4th edn. St. Louis, Mosby, pp 1479–1481

Rosai J (2004) Rosai and Ackerman's surgical pathology, 9th edn. Mosby, Edinburgh, pp 793–794

Sarrazin J, Wilson SR (1996) Manifestations of Crohn disease at US. RadioGraphics 16:499–520

Teefey SA, Montana MA, Goldfogel GA, Shuman WP (1987) Sonographic diagnosis of neutropenic typhlitis. Am J Roentgenol 149:731–733

Teefey SA, Roarke MC, Brink JA et al (1996) Bowel wall thickening: differentiation of inflammation from ischemia with color Doppler and duplex US. Radiology 198:547–551

Wilson SR (1998) The gastrointestinal tract. In: Rumack CM, Wilson SR, Charboneau JW (eds) Diagnostic ultrasound, 2nd edn. Mosby, St. Louis, 279–327

Worlicek H, Lutz H, Heyer N, Matek W (1987) Ultrasound findings in Crohn's disease and ulcerative colitis: a prospective study. J Clin Ultrasound 15:153–163

# Pseudomembranous Colitis

Etienne Danse and Daphne Geukens

CONTENTS

13.1 Introduction 115
13.2 Microbiology 116
13.3 Clinical Manifestations 116
13.4 Endoscopy 116
13.5 Imaging Study 116
13.5.1 Plain Films 116
13.5.2 Sonography 116
13.5.3 Computed Tomography 118

References 119

## 13.1
## Introduction

Pseudomembranous colitis (PMC) is a severe form of colitis characterized by a wide spectrum of clinical manifestations, observed in poorly symptomatic or critically ill patients. The PMC is included in the group of pseudomembranous enterocolites (PMEC). This condition is defined as an affection of the intestine related to the presence of pseudomembranes covering the colic or the small bowel mucosal surface. The colon is the most frequent affected site, but small bowel involvement is described, alone or in association with the colon (Ros et al. 1996). The PMC is most frequently due to the mucosal effect of the toxins produced by *Clostridium difficile*. Other unusual infectious agents have been considered as cause for a similar condition (*Staphylococcus aureus*). The proliferation of *Clostridium* is due to antibiotic therapy, most frequently ampicillins, clindamycin, and cephalosporins. Erythromycin and tetracyclines have also been reported as causes of PMC. Diarrhoea appears between 2 and 10 weeks after the beginning of the antibiotic treatment (Megibow et al. 1984). The PMC is so-called antibiotic-associated diarrhoea. The PMC can also develop without *Clostridium difficile* infection. In this setting, similar macroscopic colic wall changes are due to mucosal ischaemia related to ischemic colitis, mechanical bowel obstruction, intestinal surgery, or chemotherapy (Ros et al. 1996).

Risk factors contributing to the development of PMC are: age (>60 years); previous surgical intervention; non-surgical gastrointestinal procedures; presence of a nasogastric tube and enteral feeding; anti-ulcer medication, hospitalisation in an intensive care unit; malignancies (lymphoma, leukaemia); immunosuppression; transplantation; irradiation; pulmonary disease; severe cardiac disease; and heavy-metal exposure (Ros et al. 1996; Cleary 1998; Dallal et al. 2002).

The mortality rate in patients with *Clostridium difficile* colitis is reported to be 1.6–3.2%, but these percentages can increase to 13.5% when we take into account all causes of death for patients with the diagnosis of *Clostridium difficile* colitis (Dallal et al. 2002).

The role of radiology in the management of PMC has to be considered in two fields. Firstly, acute abdominal pain, fever, and leucocytosis are initial symptoms in patients with pseudomembranous colitis. These clinical data may require imaging studies, usually including sonography and/or computed tomography (CT). These imaging procedures are mandatory to rule out acute abdominal diseases needing prompt therapy. Acute intestinal disorders are on the list of the diagnostic conditions that the radiologist has to look for during these imaging procedures performed

E. Danse, MD, PhD
Dept. of Radiology, St. Luc University Hospital, Université Catholique de Louvain, 10, Av Hippocrate, 1200 Brussels, Belgium
D. Geukens, MD
Dept. of Radiology, University Hospital Center, 6000 Charleroi, Belgium

in emergency situations (Ros et al. 1996); therefore, the radiologist has to be prepared to detect suggestive radiological signs of PMC. Secondly, in patients with a confirmed diagnosis of PMC, cross-sectional imaging studies can contribute to the evaluation of the extension of the disease initially demonstrated with rectosigmoidoscopy. Sonography and/or CT can also be helpful for the recognition of complications including toxic megacolon, ischaemia, abscesses, and perforation (Merine et al. 1987; Ros et al. 1996).

## 13.2
## Microbiology

*Clostridium difficile* is a Gram-positive bacteria, spore-forming, responsible for 15–20% of the antibiotic-associated diarrhoeas (Hamrick et al. 1989; Eckel et al. 2002). The gold-standard technique for the detection of *Clostridium difficile* is the stool cytotoxin assay. The microbiological mechanism is related to the production of two toxins (toxins A and B) by *Clostridium difficile* (Kyne et al. 2000). Disturbance of the normal bacterial flora in the colonic lumen is an important factor for the development of PMC (Ros et al. 1996). Children younger than 1 year develop symptomatic disease probably because of immature enterocytic membrane receptors for the toxin (Ros et al. 1996).

## 13.3
## Clinical Manifestations

Clinical manifestations of PMC classically include watery or bloody diarrhoea (Ros et al. 1996). The patients have moderate fever, abdominal cramps, leukocytosis, and hypoalbuminaemia. Severe forms can cause electrolyte disturbances, dehydratation, hypoalbuminaemia (with anasarca), and even life-threatening conditions such as toxic megacolon and perforation of the colon. Hypoalbuminaemia is due to the rapid loss of protein in the gastrointestinal tract (Merine et al. 1987).

The diagnosis of PMC is based on endoscopy and stool assays. When the endoscopic findings are non-specific, sonography or CT can show signs suggesting PMC.

## 13.4
## Endoscopy

Endoscopy is helpful for the diagnosis of PMC by showing typical raised yellowish-white plaques separated by areas of normal mucosa, oedema or erythema (Megibow et al. 1984). The plaques usually have a thickness of 2–10 mm. These plaques can be larger, extended, and are adherent to the mucosa (Ros et al. 1996). Epithelial necrosis, infiltration of the lamina propria with polymorphonuclear cells, and eosinophilic exudates are histologically demonstrated. The "pseudomembrane" is composed of cellular debris, fibrin, mucous, and polymorphonuclear cells (Hamrick et al. 1989).

## 13.5
## Imaging Study

### 13.5.1
### Plain Films

Non-specific abnormalities can be seen on plain films in patients with PMC. These findings include bowel dilatation, haustral fold thickening, thumbprinting, small bowel and colonic ileus. Rare complications of the disease can be seen and include toxic megacolon and perforation (Merine et al. 1987; Ros et al. 1996).

### 13.5.2
### Sonography

Finding suggesting of acute colitis can be detected during this examination by showing modification of colic wall thickness, which is considered as thickened when the colic wall is thicker than 5 mm. Other colonic wall changes due to acute colitis and detected with sonography include disappearance of the wall stratification (related to the severity of the disease regardless off the type of colitis, whether infectious, ischaemic or inflammatory), increasing or absence of mural flow (in relation to colonic wall vascularisation and oedema) and mural gas indicating pneumatosis (Fig. 13.1; Danse et al. 2004; Danse et al. 2005). Ascites is also visible with sonography.

Specific sonographic findings related to PMC include pronounced colic wall thickening related to oedema of the haustral folds and giving the "accor-

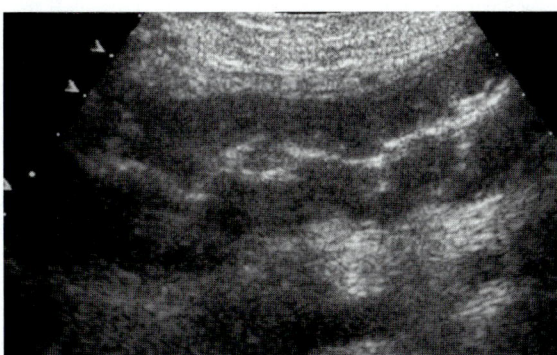

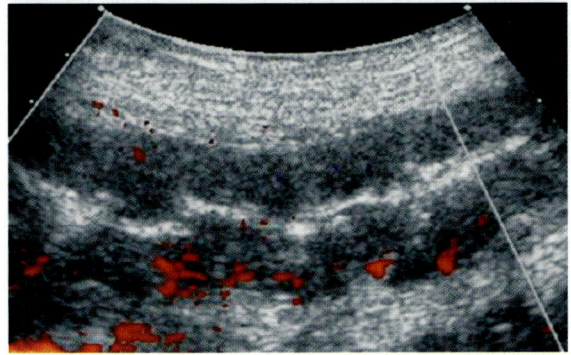

**Fig. 13.1a,b.** Sagittal views of the left colon in a severe form of pseudomembranous colitis. **a** B-mode sonogram shows hypoechoic, nodular, and diffuse thickening of the haustral relief of the colonic wall. **b** Discrete mural flow of the thickened colonic wall is observed in the same patient when colour Doppler evaluation is performed. On both images, there is a mild hyperechogenicity of the pericolic fat tissue

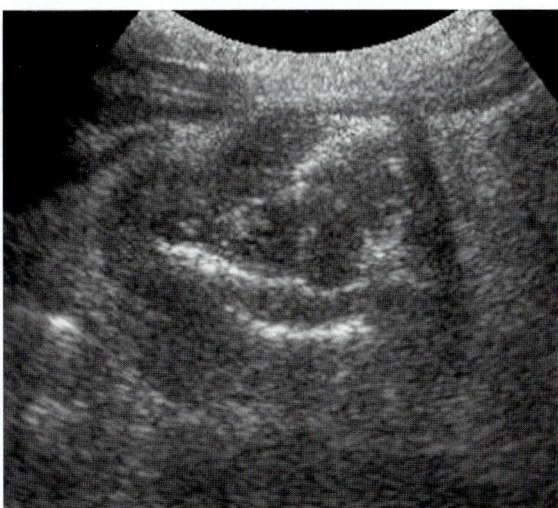

**Fig. 13.2.** Pseudomembranous colitis affecting the right colon. Transverse view on B-mode imaging shows the "accordion sign" related to oedema of the haustral folds

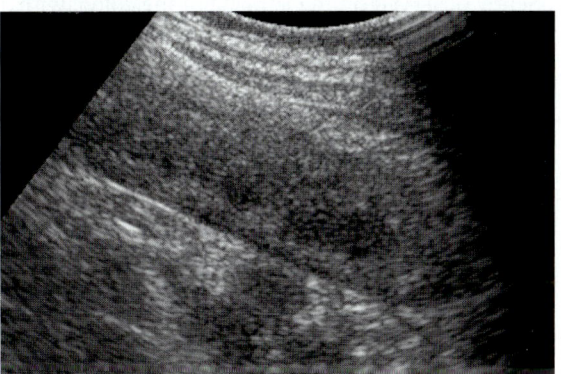

**Fig. 13.3.** Pseudomembranous colitis of the right colon. Thickening of the colonic wall with preserved wall stratification

dion sign" or a "gyral" pattern (Fig. 13.2; O'MALLEY and WILSON 2003). The lumen of the colon is narrowed and the submucosa appears as congestive due to the acute inflammation of the colonic wall (FRISOLI et al. 2000; O'MALLEY and WILSON 2003). The wall thickness ranges from 10 to 30 mm (mean 11 mm; DOWNEY and WILSON 1991; TRUONG et al. 1998). Despite the increased wall thickness, the colonic wall stratification is usually preserved (Fig. 13.3; TRUONG et al. 1998). Reduced or absent mural flow is noted and ascitis is present in 30–77% of the cases (DOWNEY and WILSON 1991; TRUONG et al. 1998; LEDERMANN et al. 2000). Infiltration of the pericolic fatty tissue is noted in 50% of the cases (TRUONG et al. 1998).

A prospective study evaluating sonography as a first-line method for the detection of PMC has shown a sensitivity of this technique of 78% for the diagnosis of PMC and a specificity of 94% (GALLIX et al. 1997). In this setting, relevant sonographic signs were the increased wall thickness, the hyperechoic thickening of the submucosa and the presence of the "accordion sign". On the other hand, mural vascularisation, pericolic wall changes and presence of ascites were not demonstrated to significantly contribute to the positive sonographic diagnosis of PMC.

The PMC can be differentiated from other colitides (ischaemic colitis and inflammatory colitis) when colonic wall changes are evaluated. These sonographic colonic wall changes include the wall thickness, the presence of wall stratification, detection of mural flow, the visualisation of the haustration and the localisation of the disease along the colon (Table 13.1; TRUONG et al. 1998; DANSE et al. 2004; DANSE et al. 2005).

In comparison with PMC, which is more frequently seen on the left colon, acute forms of Crohn's disease have a predisposition for the right colon, are associated with a wall thickness less than 13 mm,

Table 13.1. Synoptic view of the main sonographic findings used for the differential diagnosis of acute diseases of the colon (*PMC*, pseudomembranous colitis)

|  | Localisation | Thickness (mm) | Stratification | Mural flow (%) |
|---|---|---|---|---|
| Crohn's colitis | Right colon | <13 | Preserved | 100 |
| Ulcerative colitis | Left colon | < 9 | Preserved | 100 |
| PMC | Left colon | 11 | Preserved or Absent | – |
| Infection | Right colon | 9 | Preserved (apart from neutropaenic colitis) | 90 |
| Ischaemic colitis | Left colon >right colon | 9 | 50% | 60 |
| Malignancy | Anywhere | 12 | 20% | 80 |

have a preserved stratification with visualisation of the haustral folds and present an increased mural flow when colour Doppler study of the colonic wall is performed.

Acute forms of ulcerative colitis are more frequently observed on the left side of the colon, with a mild wall thickness (<9 mm), a preserved stratification and an increased mural flow. Infectious colitis is more frequently detected in the right colon together with limited or extended involvement of the distal small bowel. The colonic thickness is usually <9 mm. Preserved stratification is noted as well as the persistence of the haustral relief. Mural flow is present in 90% of the cases. Ischaemic colitis is most frequently detected on the left colon but can affect any part of the colon. Wall thickness of ischaemic colitis is in the same range as in PMC (11–12 mm; TRUONG et al. 1998; DANSE et al. 2000; DANSE et al. 2004). Stratification is present in 50% of patients; disappearance of haustral folds is the rule. Absence of mural flow is noted in 60% of cases. Disappearance of the stratification and absence of flow in the colonic wall are related to the severity of the disease (DANSE et al. 2000; DANSE et al. 2004). Malignancy of the colon are related to pronounced colonic wall thickening (>12 mm; TRUONG et al. 1998; DANSE et al. 2004). The wall thickening has a limited extension (length <10 cm). Preservation of the stratification is noted in only 20% of cases and mural flow is visible in 80% of cases (DANSE et al. 2004).

### 13.5.3
### Computed Tomography

The diagnosis of PMC can be suggested with CT. As with sonography, there is a need for further examinations to confirm the diagnosis (MEGIBOW et al. 1984; MERINE et al. 1987; HAMRICK et al. 1989; BLICKMAN et al. 1995; WILCOX et al. 1995). The CT signs of PMC include pronounced hypodense or heterogeneous colic wall thickening (ranging from 3 to 32 mm; Ros et al. 1996). Wall nodularity combined with the entrapment of contrast medium within the thickened haustra leads to the "accordion sign" (Fig. 13.4; Ros et al. 1996). This latter CT sign was presented as specific for PMC, but it has been described as a non-specific colonic wall oedema, observed in severe Crohn's disease, infectious or ischaemic colitis, or in

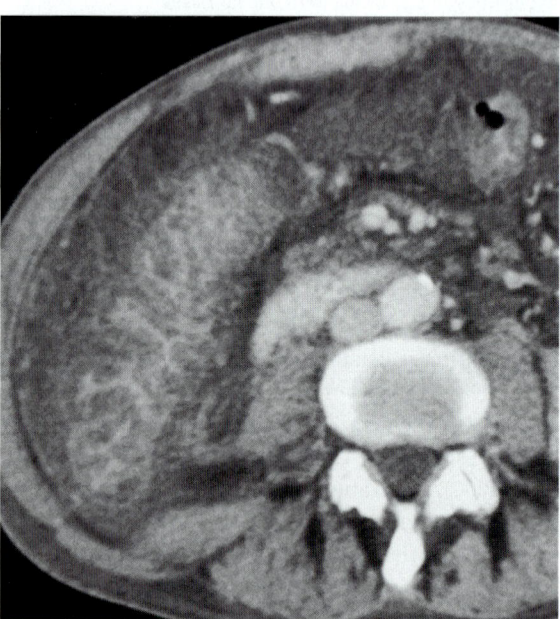

Fig. 13.4. A CT scan of the abdomen in a case of pseudomembranous colitis shows the "accordion sign", due to contrast trapping between thickened haustral folds. In this case, pericolic fat stranding and ascites are also visible

colic wall congestion related to cirrhosis (Macari et al. 1999; Mountanos and Manolakakis 2001). Ascites is noted in 20–57% of the patients, as well as pericolic stranding.

## References

Blickman JG, Boland GWL, Cleveland RH, Bramson RT, Lee MJ (1995) Pseudomembranous colitis: CT findings in children. Pediatr Radiol 25:S157–S159

Cleary RK (1998) *Clostridium difficile*-associated diarrhea and colitis. Dis Colon Rectum 41:1435–1449

Dallal RM, Harbrecht BG, Boujoukas AJ et al (2002) Fulminant *Clostridium difficile*: an underappreciated and increasing cause of death and complications. Ann Surg 235:363–372

Danse E, Van Beers BE, Jamart J et al (2000) Prognosis of ischemic colitis: comparison of color Doppler sonography with early clinical and laboratory findings. AJR Am J Roentgenol 175:1151–1154

Danse E, Jamart J, Hoang P, Laterre PF, Kartheuser A, Van Beers BE (2004) Focal bowel wall changes detected with colour Doppler ultrasound: diagnostic value in acute non-diverticular diseases of the colon. Br J Radiol 77:917–921

Danse E, Dewit O, Goncette L, Sempoux C, Kartheuser A, Van Beers B (2005) Que faire en cas d'affection aiguë du colon? Une échographie, un scanner, des clichés conventionnels ou une endoscopie? SFR Paris Octobre, Formation Médicale Continue 23:241–253

Downey DB, Wilson SR (1991) Pseudomembranous colitis: sonographic features. Radiology 180:61–64

Eckel F, Huber W, Weiss W, Lersch C (2002) Recurrent pseudomembranous colitis as a couse of recurrent severe sepsis. Z Gastroenterol 40:255–258

Frisoli JK, Desser TS, Jeffrey RB (2000) Thickened submucosal layer: a sonographic sign of acute gastrointestinal abnormality representing submucosal edema or hemorrhage. 2000 ARRS Executive Council Award II. American Roentgen Ray Society. AJR Am J Roentgenol 175:1595–1599

Gallix B, Atri M, Bret P (1997) Evaluation prospective de l'échographie haute résolution pour le diagnostic des colites pseudomembraneuses (CPM). J Radiol 78:S877

Hamrick KM, Tishler JM, Schwartz ML, Koslin DB, Han SY (1989) The CT findings in pseudomembranous colitis. Comput Med Imaging Graph 13:343–346

Kyne L, Warny M, Qamar A, Kelly CP (2000) Asymptomatic carriage of *Clostridium difficile* and serum levels of IgG antibody against toxin. N Engl J Med 342:390–397

Ledermann HP, Börner N, Strunk H et al (2000) Bowel wall thickening on transabdominal sonography. AJR Am J Roentgenol 174:107–117

Macari M, Balthazar EJ, Megibow AJ (1999) The accordion sign at CT: non-specific finding in patients with colonic edema. Radiology 211:743–746

Megibow AJ, Streiter ML, Balthazar EJ, Bosniak MA (1984) Pseudomembranous colitis: diagnosis by computed tomography. J Computed Assist Tomogr 8:281–283

Merine D, Fishman EK, Jones B (1987) Pseudomembranous colitis: CT evaluation. J Comput Assist Tomogr 11:1017–1020

Mountanos GI, Manolakakis IS (2001) The accordion sign at CT: report of a case of Crohn's disease with diffuse colonic involvement. Eur Radiol 11:1433–1434

O'Malley ME, Wilson SR (2003) US of gastrointestinal tract abnormalities with CT correlation. Radiographics 23:59–72

Ros PR, Buetow PC, Pantograg-Brown L, Forsmark CE, Sobin LH (1996) Pseudomembranous colitis. Radiology 198:1–9

Truong M, Atri P, Bret P et al (1998) Sonographic appearance of benign and malignant conditions of the colon. AJR Am J Roentgenol 170:1451–1455

Wilcox MC, Gryboski D, Fernandez M, Stahl W (1995) Computed tomographic findings in pseudomembranous colitis: an important clue to the diagnosis. South Med J 88:929–933

# Amoebic, Ascariasis and Other Parasitic and Infectious Enteritis

S. Boopathy Vijayaraghavan

CONTENTS

14.1 Amoebiasis  121
14.2 Ascariasis  122
14.3 Trichuriasis  124
14.4 Oesophagostomiasis  124
References  125

## 14.1 Amoebiasis

Amoebiasis is a disease caused by infection with a unicellular parasite *Entamoeba histolytica*. It is most common in people living in developing counties of tropical and subtropical regions in areas with poor sanitary conditions. The main source of infection is the cyst-passing chronic patient or asymptomatic carrier. The cyst reaches humans through contaminated water and vegetables. The cyst, which is resistant to the acidic digestive juices of the stomach, passes to the lower part of the small intestine. There, under the influence of the neutral or alkaline juices, the cyst wall disintegrates, releasing a metacystic amoeba, which moves downwards to the large intestine. The lesions produced are primary intestinal and secondary extraintestinal. The most frequent primary sites are the caecal and sigmoidorectal regions (Neva and Brown 1994). As the infection progresses, additional colonic sites of invasion develop. The severity of the disease depends on (a) the resistance of the host, (b) the virulence and invasiveness of the amoebic strain and (c) the condition of the intestinal tract. The early lesion is a tiny area of necrosis in the superficial mucosa or a small nodular elevation with a minute opening that leads to a flask-shaped cavity containing cytolysed cells, mucus and amoebas. There is rapid lateral and downward extension of the ulcerative process to both superficial and deep layers of the intestine. Eventually, the mucosa may slough off, exposing large necrotic areas (Neva and Brown 1994). The complications of intestinal amoebiasis include granuloma, appendicitis, perforation, haemorrhage and stricture. Amoebic granulomas (amoeboma) are firm, painful, nodular, inflammatory thickening of the intestinal wall around ulcers. It occurs most commonly in the caecum and rarely in the sigmoid colon. Perforation occurs most frequently in the caecum. Erosion of a large blood vessel may produce a massive haemorrhage. Very occasionally, rectal amoebiasis can lead to anorectal abscesses or perianal fistulas. In acute intestinal amoebiasis, there is severe dysentery with numerous small stools containing blood, mucus and necrotic mucosa, accompanied by acute abdominal pain, tenderness and fever. Chronic amoebiasis is characterised by recurrent attacks of dysentery.

The diagnosis of amoebiasis rests upon the identification of the parasite in the faeces or tissues and upon serological studies. On sonography, acute amoebic dysentery is seen as a tender asymmetrically thick-walled caecum. Non-visualisation of a thickened appendix differentiates it from acute appendicitis. Amoebic granuloma (amoeboma) of the caecum or colon is seen as an asymmetrically thick-walled segment of bowel measuring about 8–17 mm in thickness (Hussain and Dinshaw 1990). On transverse scan, there is target, doughnut or pseudo-kidney appearance (Fig. 14.1a,b). This appearance is non-specific. There are no distinctive sonographic features to differentiate amoeboma from Crohn's disease or ulcerative colitis. A concomitant liver abscess strongly suggests an amoebic aetiology. Very occasionally, amoebiasis of the appendix is seen as an enlarged non-tender appendix, either as an isolated finding or along with amoeboma of the caecum (Fig. 14.1c; Oran 2000). Perforation of bowel, essentially the caecum, occurs occasionally in

S. Boopathy Vijayaraghavan, MD, DMRD
SONOSCAN Ultrasonic Scan Centre, 15B Venkatachalam Road, Coimbatore 641 002, Tamil Nadu, India

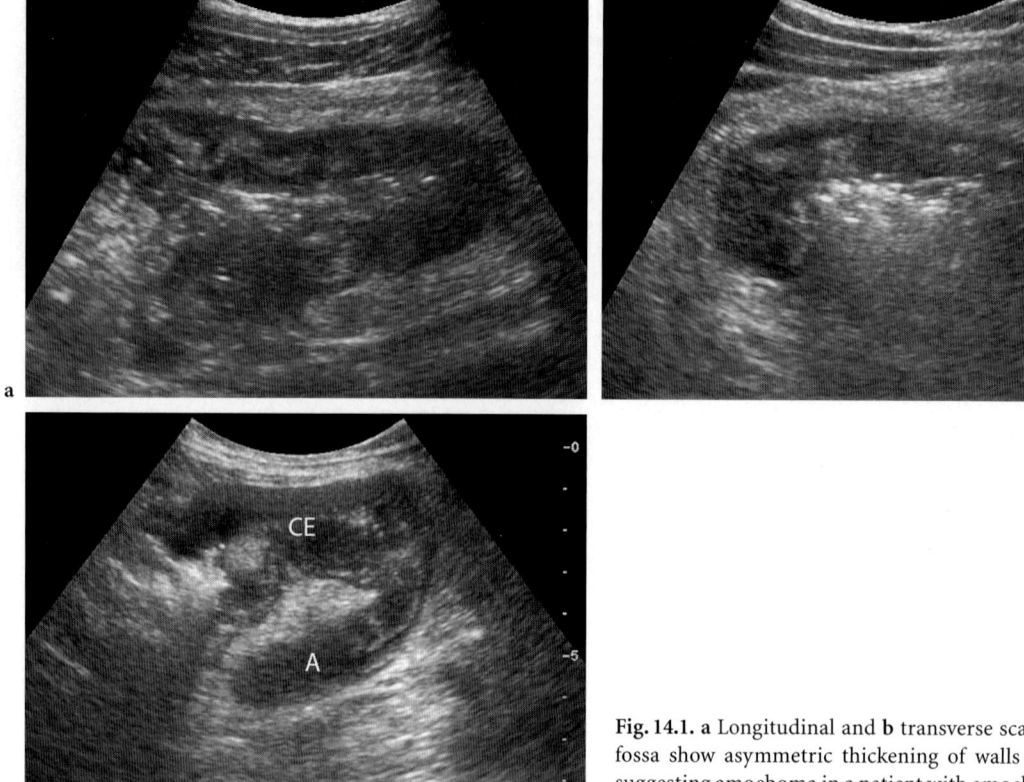

Fig. 14.1. a Longitudinal and b transverse scans of right iliac fossa show asymmetric thickening of walls of the caecum, suggesting amoeboma in a patient with amoebic liver abscess. c Non-tender thickening of appendix (*A*) in amoebiasis. Caecal walls (*CE*) are also slightly thickened

virulent amoebiasis. This results in a retroperitoneal abscess containing air in relation to the caecum and ascending colon that is similar to an appendicular abscess in the same location.

## 14.2
## Ascariasis

Ascariasis is the infestation of humans with the round worm, *Ascaris lumbricoides*. The adult worms normally live in the lumen of the small bowel of an infected individual. The eggs of the worm are passed in the faeces of these individuals and can contaminate water or food. Humans become infected when they ingest contaminated water or food. Gastric juices cause the eggs to hatch in the small bowel. The larvae penetrate the intestinal wall to enter the blood stream and reach the lungs. They migrate, or are carried by the bronchioles to bronchi, ascend the trachea to the glottis and pass down the oesophagus to the small intestine (Neva and Brown 1994). Ascariasis is worldwide in distribution and is more common in tropical countries and is most prevalent where sanitation is poor. It occurs at all ages, but it is most prevalent in children aged 5–9 years. The incidence is approximately the same in both sexes. The usual infection consists of 5–10 worms and often goes unnoticed by the host. The most frequent complaint of patients with ascariasis is vague abdominal pain. When the infestation is heavy, a bolus of worms may cause serious complications such as intestinal obstruction (Malde and Chadha 1993; Wasadikar and Kulkarni 1997; Mahmood et al. 2001), perforation (Hangloo et al. 1990; Chawla et al. 2003), intussusception (Villamizar et al. 1996) or volvulus (Rodriguez et al. 2003). The prognosis of these complications depends on prompt diagnosis and treatment. Delay in diagnosis may give rise to small bowel gangrene. Clinical findings in such cases are those of the complications, which are acute pain in the abdomen, vomiting or signs of peritonitis.

On sonography, the appearance of the round worms varies with the frequency of the transducer

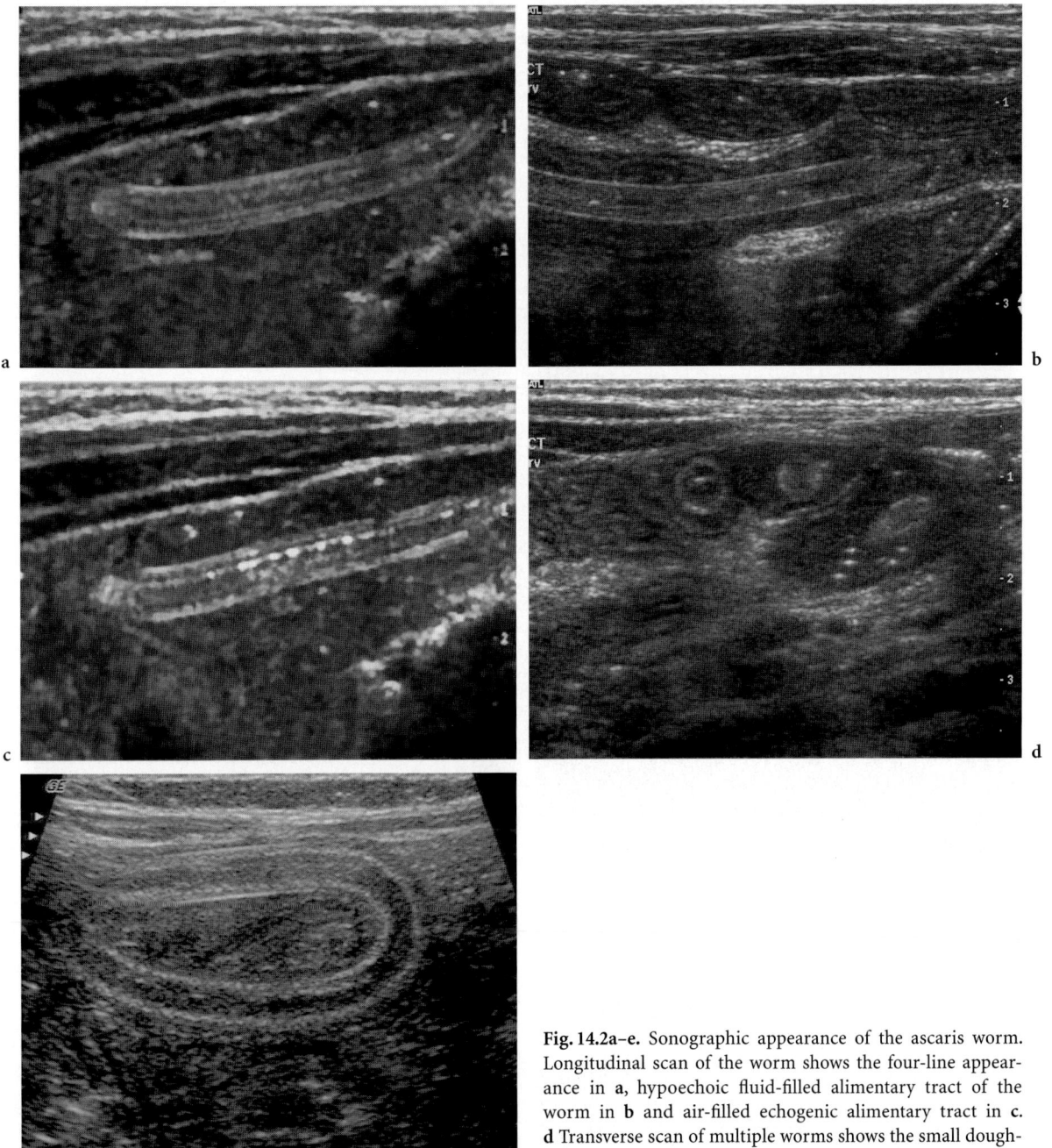

Fig. 14.2a–e. Sonographic appearance of the ascaris worm. Longitudinal scan of the worm shows the four-line appearance in **a**, hypoechoic fluid-filled alimentary tract of the worm in **b** and air-filled echogenic alimentary tract in **c**. **d** Transverse scan of multiple worms shows the small doughnut appearance. **e** On low-frequency scan the worm is seen as two parallel lines

used. When the recent high-resolution probes are used, the ascaris worm is seen as a chord of four echogenic lines in longitudinal scans (Fig, 14.2a,b). These lines represent the reflections from the external walls of the worm and the walls of the alimentary tract of the worm (Mahmood et al. 2001). Sometimes, the alimentary canal appears echogenic when it is filled with air (Fig. 14.2c). On cross section, it appears like a small doughnut (Fig. 14.2d). It is clearly visible if there is fluid around the worm. On low-frequency scans, it is seen as two parallel lines on longitudinal scan (Fig. 14.2e) and a circle on transverse scan. On real-time scan, the worm shows a non-directed curling movement.

In the presence of small bowel obstruction due to a ball of worms, sonography shows signs of small bowel obstruction, namely, dilated small bowel loops with peristalsis. At the site of obstruction, the ball of worms, or helminthoma, appears like spaghetti on longitudinal scan (Fig. 14.3a) and a "shack of cigars" on transverse scan (Fig. 14.3b; MALDE and CHADHA 1993; WASADIKAR and KULKARNI 1997). Sonography is useful in the follow-up of these patients after initiating the treatment. It can reveal resolution of the obstruction or occurrence of other complications such as volvulus or ischaemia of the bowel. In volvulus and ischaemia of the small bowel due to ascariasis, sonography shows multiple loops of unusually dilated, aperistaltic small bowel, containing the ascaris worms with the classical appearance and movement. There is free fluid in the peritoneal cavity. The walls of the bowel are thickened (RODRIGUEZ et al. 2003). Perforation of the bowel due to ascariasis can very occasionally occur because of direct pressure and irritation of the bowel wall by impacted ascaridial masses, leading to ulceration, necrosis and perforation. Lytic secretion from ascarides also probably plays a role (HANGLOO et al. 1990). In perforation, sonography reveals live ascaris worms moving freely within the extraluminal fluid (CHAWLA et al. 2003). Very rarely, the ascariasis worm can enter the appendix and cause appendicitis (MISRA et al. 1999).

## 14.3
## Trichuriasis

Trichuriasis is infestation with the whipworm *Trichuris trichiura*. Man is the principal host. Infection results from ingestion of embryonated eggs via hands, food or drink that have been contaminated by infested soil. When humans ingest the embryonated egg, the activated larva escapes into the upper small bowel. It penetrates a villus and remains there for 3–10 days. Then it passes downward to the caecum, where it usually remains. The worms are also found in the terminal ileum and appendix. Patients with light infection are asymptomatic. Patients with very heavy chronic infection present a characteristic clinical picture consisting of: (a) frequent, small, blood-streaked diarrhoeal stools, (b) abdominal pain, (c) nausea and vomiting, (d) anaemia, and (e) weight loss. *Trichuris* worm may attach itself to the appendiceal mucosa and provide a ground for secondary bacterial infection resulting in acute and sub-acute appendicitis (NEVA and BROWN 1994). On sonography, a thick-walled fluid-distended appendix is seen with the motile worms in the lumen.

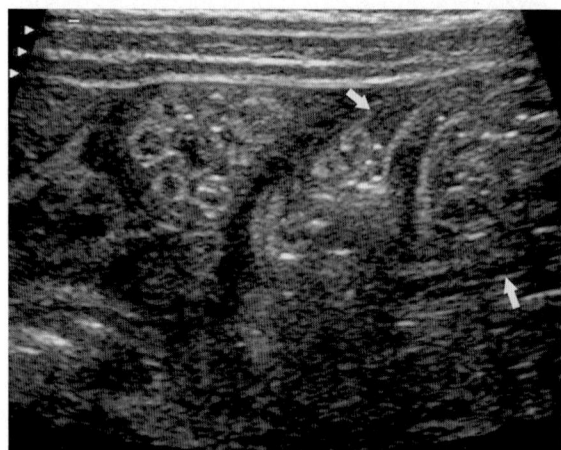

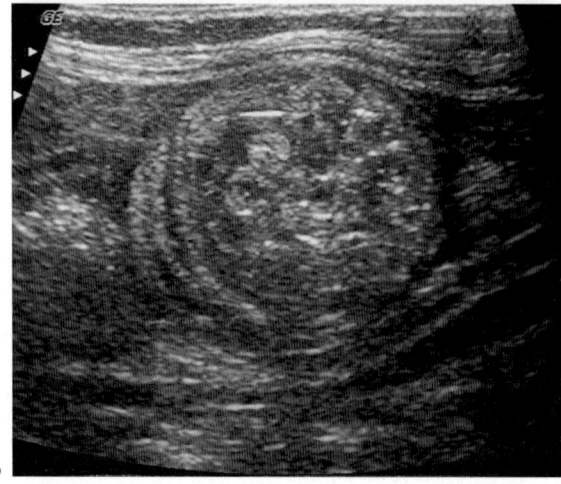

**Fig. 14.3a,b. a** Longitudinal scan of the site of bowel obstruction shows spaghetti appearance (*arrows*) of the curled-up worms. **b** Transverse scan of the same region shows the „shack of cigars" appearance of cross section of multiple worms (Courtesy of R.Subramanian, Sreenivas Ultrasound Scan Centre, Salem,India).

## 14.4
## Oesophagostomiasis

Oesophagostomiasis is infestation with *Oesophagostomum bifurcum*, a human parasitic intestinal helminth. It is endemic in parts of West Africa (POLDERMAN et al. 1991; POLDERMAN et al. 1999). *Oesophagostomum bifurcum* juveniles develop in the colonic wall causing pus-filled granulomas (STOREY et al. 2000). Many people appear to tolerate this histotropic developmental phase of the worm's life cycle; however, there are two distinct clinical presentations of the pathology. Multinodular *Oesophagostomiasis bifurcum* comprises hundreds of pea-sized nodules in the thickened oedematous sub-mucosa and sub-serosa of the colonic wall. These patients present with weight loss, persistent mucosal diarrhoea, diffuse abdominal pain and occasionally rectal bleeding. Urgent surgery may be required for luminal narrowing of the colon or bowel obstructions secondary to inflammatory additions (ANTHONY and MCADAM 1972).

The Dapaong tumour, the uninodular form of the disease, presents as a painful ligneous mass of 30–60 mm in the abdominal wall or within the abdominal cavity (PAGES et al. 1988). It is usually associated with fever. This can lead to cutaneous abscess and fistula, peritonitis due to rupture of nodule, obstruction of bowel due to adhesion and volvulus. Clinical symptoms are often vague and indeterminate. They mimic a lot of other conditions (STOREY et al. 2001).

Sonography shows a long segment of thick-walled right colon displaying target or pseudo-kidney appearance. This is a non-specific appearance seen in most of the colonic pathologies; however, the presence of a distinct nodularity within the thick wall of the colon helps to differentiate it from other conditions in a patient in an endemic area. The Dapaong tumour is seen on sonography as a hypoechoic oval lesion with a well-defined poorly reflective wall in the abdominal wall, or within the abdomen (STOREY et al. 2000).

## References

Anthony PP, McAdam IW (1972) Helminthic pseudotumours of the bowel: thirty-four cases of helminthoma. Gut 13:8–16

Chawla A, Patwardhan V, Maheshwari M, Wasnik A (2003) Primary ascaridial perforation of the small intestine: sonographic diagnosis. J Clin Ultrasound 31:211–213

Hangloo VK, Koul I, Safaya R et al (1990) Primary ascaridial perforations of small intestine and Meckel's diverticulum. Indian J Gastroenterol 9:287–288

Hussain S, Dinshaw H (1990) Ultrasonography in amebic colitis. J Ultrasound Med 9:385–388

Mahmood T, Mansoor N, Quraishy S, Ilyas M, Hussain S (2001) Ultrasonographic appearance of *Ascaris lumbricoides* in the small bowel. J Ultrasound Med 20:269–274

Malde HM, Chadha D (1993) Roundworm obstruction: sonographic diagnosis. Abdom Imaging 18:274–276

Misra SP, Dwivedi M, Misra V, Singh PA, Agarwal VK (1999) Preoperative sonographic diagnosis of acute appendicitis caused by *Ascaris lumbricoides*. J Clin Ultrasound 27:96–97

Neva FA, Brown HW (1994) Basic clinical parasitology, 6th edn. Appleton and Lange, Norwalk, Connecticut

Oran I (2000) Transient appendiceal enlargement in a patient with colonic amebiasis: sonographic detection and follow-up. J Clin Ultrasound 28:368–370

Pages A, Kpodzro K, Boeta S, Akpo-Allavo K (1988) Dapaong "tumor". Helminthiasis caused by oesophagostomum. Ann Pathol 8:332–335

Polderman AM, Krepel HP, Baeta S, Blotkamp J, Gigase P (1991) Oesophagostomiasis, a common infection of man in northern Togo and Ghana. Am J Trop Med Hyg 44:336–344

Polderman AM, Anemana SD, Asigri V (1999) Human oesophagostomiasis: a regional public health problem in Africa. Parasitol Today 15:129–130

Rodriguez EJ, Gama MA, Ornstein SM, Anderson WD (2003) Ascariasis causing small bowel volvulus. Radiographics 23:1291–1293

Storey PA, Anemana S, van Oostayen JA, Polderman AM, Magnussen P (2000) Ultrasound diagnosis of oesophagostomiasis. Br J Radiol 73:328–332

Storey PA, Faile G, Crawley D et al (2001) Ultrasound appearance of preclinical oesophagostomum bifurcum induced colonic pathology. Gut 48:565–566

Villamizar E, Mendez M, Bonilla E, Varon H, de Onatra S (1996) *Ascaris lumbricoides* infestation as a cause of intestinal obstruction in children: experience with 87 cases. J Pediatr Surg 31:201–205

Wasadikar PP, Kulkarni AB (1997) Intestinal obstruction due to ascariasis. Br J Surg 84:410–412

# Neoplasm

# Colorectal Cancer

Jae Hoon Lim

CONTENTS

15.1 Introduction  129
15.2 Pathology  129
15.3 Transabdominal Sonographic Technique  130
15.4 Transabdominal Sonographic Findings of Colon Cancer  130
15.5 Transrectal Sonography  131
References  134

## 15.1 Introduction

Double-contrast barium enema, colonoscopy, and computed tomography (CT) colonography are the procedures of choice for the detection and diagnosis of colorectal cancer; however, abdominal sonography may be the first test that patients with colon cancer undergo because they may present with nonspecific gastrointestinal symptoms and signs (Schwerk et al. 1979). Careful sonographic examination of the colon and rectum may disclose a focal mass or mural thickening, and this may lead a physician to investigate for the diagnosis of colorectal cancer.

Increasing use of sonography in the initial evaluation of patients with abdominal disease may allow detection of unexpected tumors within the abdominal cavity (Schwerk et al. 1979; Price and Metreweli 1988; Rutgeerts et al. 1991). Absence of luminal content in abnormal areas of the colon enabled us to detect a mass or mural thickening by sonographic examination. Sonographic detectability of colorectal cancer, intentionally or unexpectedly, warrants the inclusion of the bowel loops in the abdominal sonographic examination when a patient complains of symptoms suggesting colorectal cancer. In cases with incidentally detected masses or wall thickening of the colon or rectum, an appropriate diagnosis should be made by performing a barium enema, colonoscopy, or CT colonography.

## 15.2 Pathology

Colorectal cancer creates mass or segmental thickening of the wall (Fig. 15.1). Short segmental thickening is much more common than mass formation. Mass

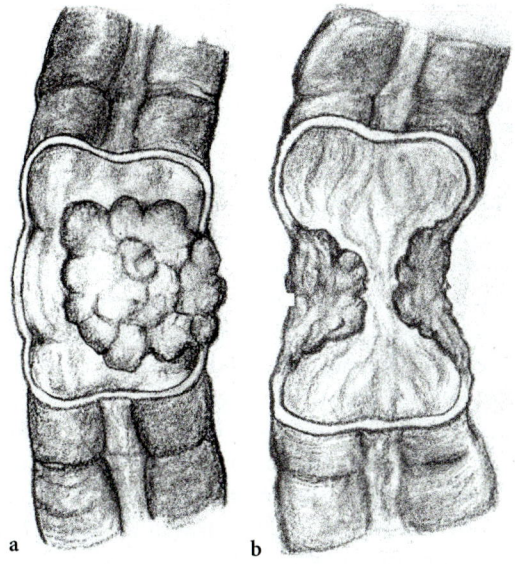

**Fig. 15.1a,b.** Two types of colorectal cancer. **a** Mass-forming colorectal cancer. **b** Short segmental wall thickening

J. H. Lim, MD
Professor of Radiology, Department of Radiology and Center for Imaging Science, Samsung Medical Center, Sungkyunkwan University School of Medicine, 50 Ilwon-dong, Kangnam-ku, Seoul 135-710, Korea

formation is frequent in the right-side colon. Mass may be fungating, intraluminal, or extend outside the colon since it does not cause obstruction. Bowel wall thickening is abrupt and may be symmetrical or asymmetrical, and is usually <5 cm in length. Obstruction and adjacent lymph node involvement are frequent and the liver is the most frequent site of distant metastasis.

## 15.3
### Transabdominal Sonographic Technique

Sonography is performed with 3.5- or 5.0-MHz sector or linear transducers. Sonography of the abdomen and pelvis is performed by moving the transducer slowly over the abdomen with gentle compression to displace adjacent bowel loops. Scanning through the course of the colon proceeds along the length of both flanks of the ascending and descending colon, across the midline of the upper part of the abdomen for the transverse colon, along the left side of the lower part of the abdomen from the descending colon toward the pelvic cavity for the sigmoid colon, and across the midline of the pelvic cavity for the rectum. The colon is differentiated from small bowel loops by the location and course of the bowel loops (Lim et al. 1994a,b).

## 15.4
### Transabdominal Sonographic Findings of Colon Cancer

The normal thickness during the contraction stage is 2–3 mm, and wall thickness >5 mm is considered abnormal. Sonographic appearances of colorectal cancer reflect the pathology, i.e., either a bulky mass or segmental thickening of the colonic wall (Lim 1996). A mass may be small or relatively large, and is usually irregular or lobulated in contour (Fig. 15.2). A large mass can be easily detected using sonography. The cluster of high-amplitude echoes denoting intraluminal gas and fecal content may be visible, centrally or eccentrically located in the mass (Price and Metreweli 1988).

The other common sonographic appearance of colorectal cancer is segmental (Fig. 15.3), eccentric, or circumferential thickening of the colonic wall (Fig. 15.4). The pathological segment usually does not contain feces or gas, making sonographic visualization relatively easy. The mural thickening may be irregular, but not as severe as in a fungating type of carcinoma. The central echo clusters are small (target sign, Figs. 15.3, 15.4), because the pathological lumen is unusually narrow. This type of carcinoma may frequently result in colonic obstruction, and thus the tumor mass can be detected on sonography as a cause of colonic obstruction (Fig. 15.5; Lim et al. 1994a). Adjacent lymph node metastasis can be detected (Fig. 15.4). Sonography of the liver

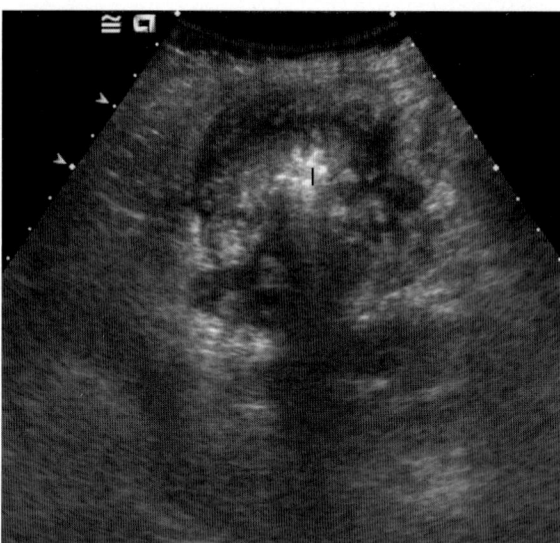

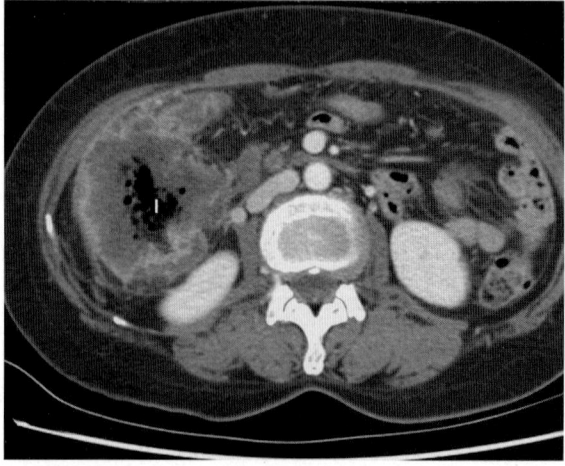

**Fig. 15.2a,b.** Mass-forming colon cancer. **a** Transverse sonogram of the right mid-abdomen shows a well-defined, irregular, large mass, representing adenocarcinoma of the ascending colon. Note high-amplitude echoes denoting gas and fecal content in the lumen (*l*). **b** The CT image shows a large mass with air-containing lumen (*l*)

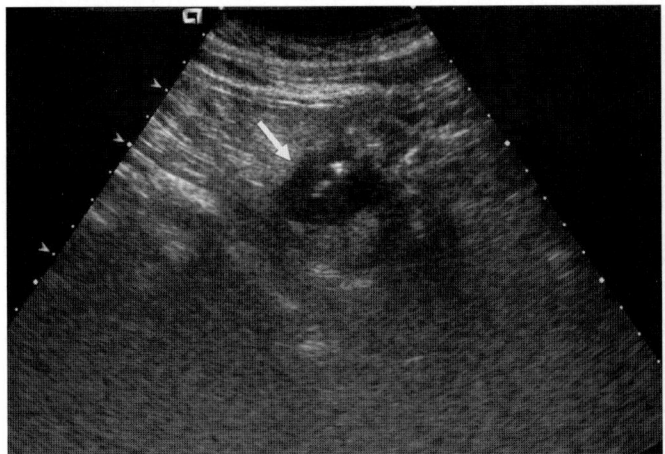
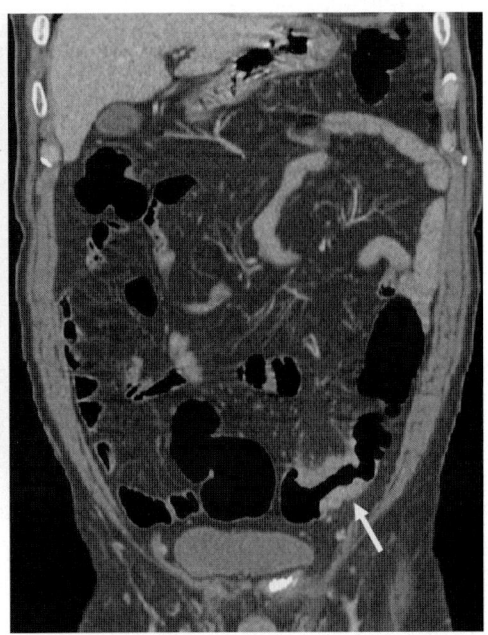

**Fig. 15.3a,b.** Colon cancer with segmental wall thickening. **a** Sonogram of the left lower abdomen shows circumferential thickening of the colon wall, showing target sign (*arrow*). **b** Reformatted CT image of abdomen with a short segmental, symmetrical thickening (*arrow*) of the wall of the sigmoid colon

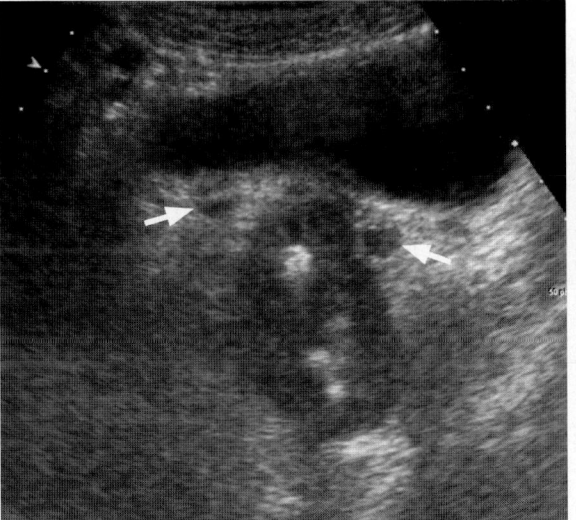
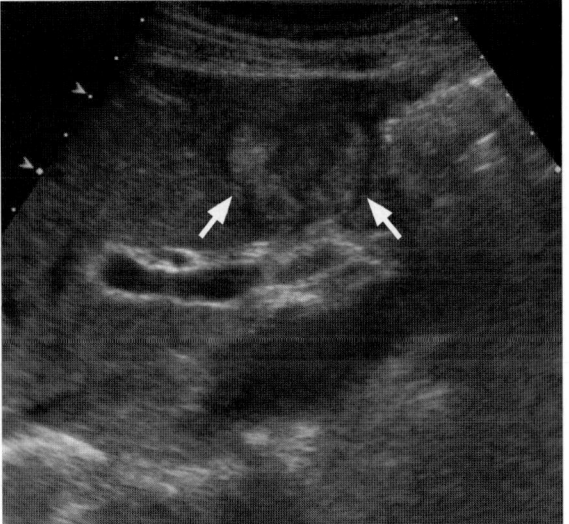

**Fig. 15.4a,b.** Rectal cancer with circumferential thickening of the wall. **a** Transverse sonogram of the pelvis shows circumferential thickening of the rectal wall. Note adjacent small metastatic lymph nodes (*arrows*). **b** Sagittal sonogram of the liver shows a well-defined hepatic mass representing metastasis (*arrow*)

should be performed for the detection of metastasis when a cancer is detected (Fig. 15.4). Inflammatory disease may present with a typical target appearance, but mural thickening in inflammatory disease is usually thinner and more uniform in thickness and involves a longer segment (LIM et al. 1994b). Colon cancer may be detected during the work-up of anemia (Fig. 15.6), nonspecific abdominal symptoms, or in patients with liver metastasis (Fig. 15.4).

## 15.5
## Transrectal Sonography

For treatment of rectal cancer, minimally invasive surgery, such as transanal excision, transanal endoscopic microsurgery, total mesorectal excision, or abdominoperineal resection, are available depending on the location, size, and stage of the tumor (PRICOLO

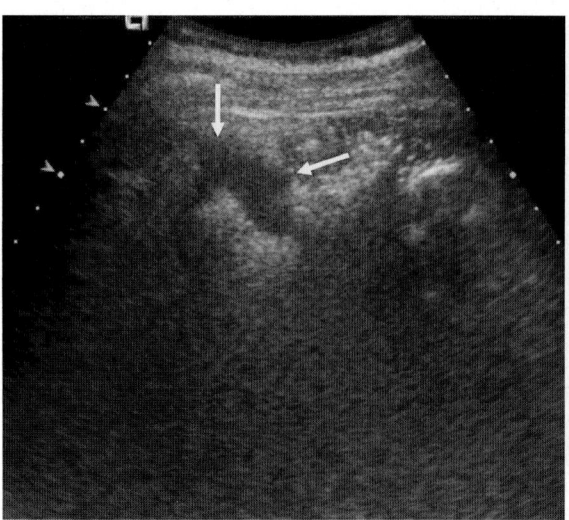 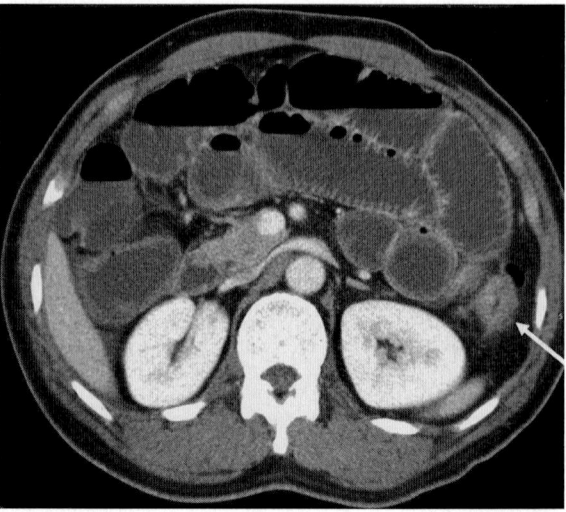

**Fig. 15.5a,b.** Colon cancer with obstruction. **a** Transverse sonogram of the left mid-abdomen shows thickening of the wall of the descending colon (*arrows*) in patient with partial obstruction of the colon. **b** The CT image shows symmetric thickening of the wall of the descending colon (*arrow*) and dilated small bowel loops

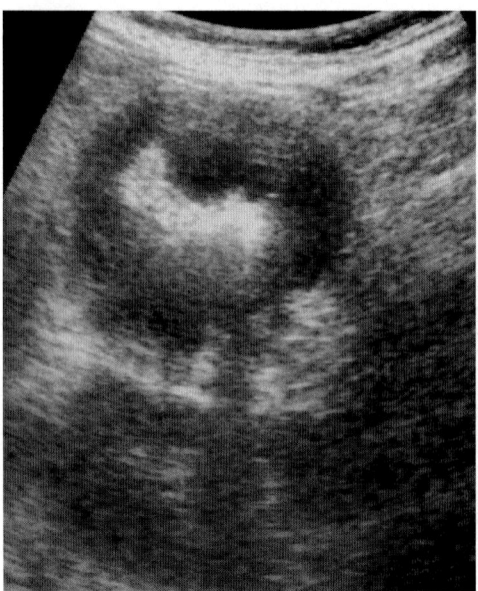

**Fig. 15.6.** Colon cancer detected during the work-up of iron-deficiency anemia. Oblique sagittal sonogram of the right upper abdomen shows a large mass in the hepatic flexure of colon, presenting as a "pseudokidney sign." Note right kidney posterior to the lesion

and POTENTI 2001; ZAGORIA et al. 1997). A sensitive technique for preoperative staging helps in deciding the type of surgery that can be effectively implemented with minimally invasive procedure; therefore, accurate preoperative staging is essential for determining optimal treatment.

Endoscopy and double-contrast enema can demonstrate the intraluminal component of rectal cancer. The extent of the tumor in the bowel layers and the extraluminal component of the tumor can be evaluated with transrectal sonography, CT, and magnetic resonance imaging (MRI). Although CT has been the most widely used method for staging, it has limitations in the evaluation of depth of tumor invasion because of inherent resolution limitation. Transrectal sonography and endorectal coil MRI are known to be superior to CT in assessing tumor depth through the wall, local extension of tumor, and lymph node involvement. The diagnostic accuracy of transrectal sonography was reported to be similar to endorectal coil MRI for determining depth of invasion of rectal carcinoma (ZAGORIA et al. 1997; GUALDI et al. 2000). The major advantages of transrectal sonography, as opposed to MRI, are convenience and shorter examination time.

Transrectal sonographic examination for rectal cancer is performed with a 7- to 10-MHz rigid radial transducer. Patients are asked to perform rectal cleansing 2–3 h prior to the examination with rectal repository pills. Sonographic examination is performed with the patient in the left lateral decubitus position. Before introduction of transducer, 50–150 ml of degassed water is instilled into the rectal lumen by using an enema syringe to improve depiction of the tumor and local staging. As the transducer is slowly pulled back, serial images of the entire length of rectum and anal canal are obtained.

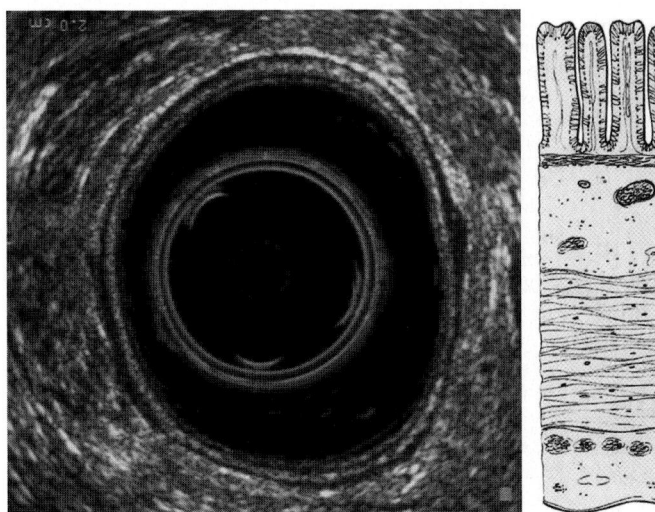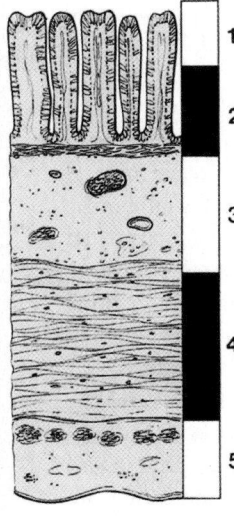

Fig. 15.7. Normal rectal wall. Transrectal sonographic appearances of the normal rectal wall and schematic drawing of histological anatomy and sonographic appearances of the rectal wall. *1* hyperechoic: lumen/mucosal interface and superficial mucosa; *2* hypoechoic: deep mucosa including muscularis mucosa; *3* hyperechoic: submucosa plus submucosa/muscularis propria interface; *4* hypoechoic: muscularis propria minus interface with submucosa; *5* hyperechoic: muscularis propria/perirectal interface and perirectal fat

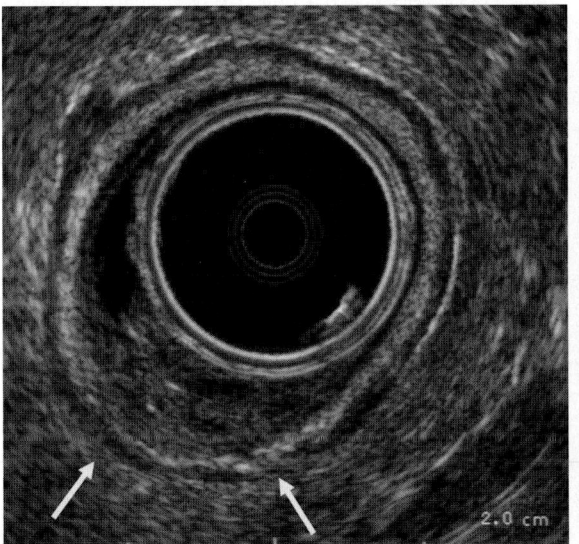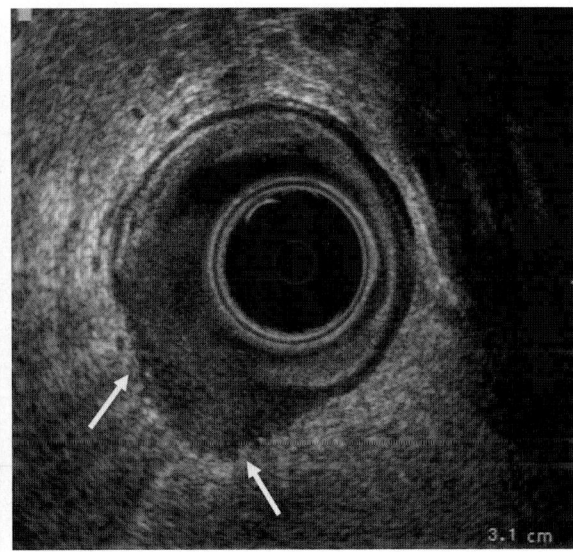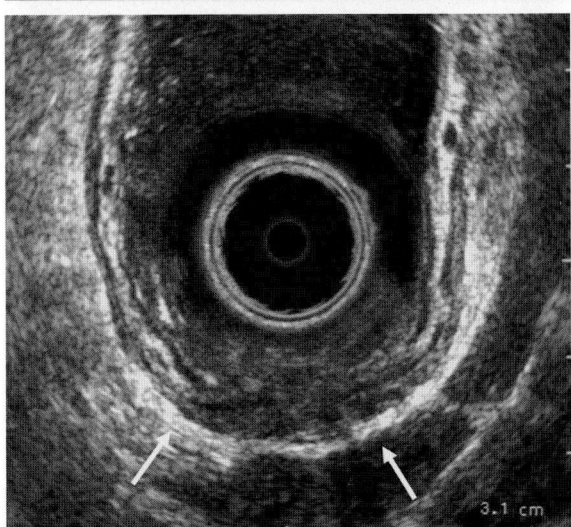

Fig. 15.8. a Rectal cancer confined to the mucosa (T1 cancer). Transrectal sonogram shows a hypoechoic mass (*arrows*) with thinning of the submucosal layer. b Rectal cancer extended to the submucosa (T2 cancer). Transrectal sonogram shows an irregular hypoechoic mass with interruption of the submucosal layer and thickening of the hypoechoic musclolaris propria layer (*arrows*). c Rectal cancer involving the entire wall and perirectal fat (T3 cancer). Transrectal sonogram shows an irregular hypoechoic mass with interruption of the submucosa and muscle layers and serrated hypoechoic lesion in the hyperechoic perirectal fat space (*arrows*)

Transrectal sonography can directly demonstrate whole layers of the rectal wall (Fig. 15.7) and thus make it possible to assess the depth of tumor infiltration. A tumor mass can be imaged clearly by water instillation (Kim et al. 2004). Tumor infiltration onto the muscularis mucosae, submucosa, proper muscle layer, and infiltration onto the perirectal fat can be assessed (Fig. 15.8). The accuracy has been reported as being 81–91% (Kim et al. 2004; Marusch et al. 2002; Bipat et al. 2004). Locoregional lymph node metastasis can be depicted; the accuracy was reported as being 64–88% (Schaffzin and Wong 2004).

Transrectal sonography has limitations in the imaging of tumor located 8–10 cm or above the anal verge when rigid probe is used, in the imaging of stenosing tumor, in depicting lymph nodes that are outside the range of transducer, and the technique is operator dependent.

## References

Bipat S, Glas A, Slors FJM, Zwinderman AH, Bossuyt PMM, Stoker J (2004) Rectal cancer: local staging and assessment of lymph node involvement with endoluminal US, CT, and MR imaging: a meta-analysis. Radiology 232:773–783

Gualdi GF, Casciani E, Guadalaxara A, d'Orta C, Dolettini E, Peppalardo G (2000) Local staging of rectal cancer with transrectal ultrasound and endorectal magnetic resonance imaging. Dis Colon Rectum 43:338–345

Kim SA, Lim HK, Lee SJ et al (2004) Depiction and local staging of rectal tumors: comparison of transrectal US before and after water instillation. Radiology 231:117–122

Lim JH (1996) Colorectal cancer: sonographic findings. Am J Roentgenol 167:45–47

Lim JH, Ko YT, Lee DH et al (1994a) Determining the site and causes of colonic obstruction with sonography. Am J Roentgenol 163:1113–1117

Lim JH, Ko YT, Lee DH et al (1994b) Sonography of inflammatory bowel disease: findings and diagnostic value in differential diagnosis. Am J Roentgenol 163:343–347

Marusch F, Koch A, Schmidt U et al (2002) Routine use of transrectal ultrasound in rectal carcinoma: result of prospective multi-center study. Endoscopy 34:385–390

Price J, Metreweli C (1988) Sonographic diagnosis of clinically non-palpable primary colonic neoplasm. Br J Radiol 61:190–195

Pricolo VE, Potenti FM (2001) Modern management of rectal cancer. Dig Surg 18:1–20

Rutgeerts LJ, Verbanck JJ, Crape AW et al (1991) Detection of colorectal cancer by routine ultrasound. J Belge Radiol 74:11–13

Schaffzin DM, Wong WD (2004) Endorectal ultrasound in the preoperative evaluation of rectal cancer. Clin Colorectal Cancer 4:124–132

Schwerk W, Braun B, Dombrowski H (1979) Real-time ultrasound examination in the diagnosis of gastrointestinal tumors. J Clin Ultrasound 7:425–431

Zagoria RJ, Schlarb CA, Ott DJ et al (1997) Assessment of rectal tumor infiltration utilizing endorectal MR imaging and comparison with endoscopic rectal sonography. J Surg Oncol 64:312–317

# Gastric Cancer

Jiro Hata, Ken Haruma, Noriaki Manabe, Tomoari Kamada,
Hiroaki Kusunoki, Toshiaki Tanaka, and Motonori Sato

CONTENTS

16.1 Introduction 135

16.2 **Sonographic Assessment of the Gastric Wall** 135
16.2.1 Preparation and Equipment 135
16.2.2 Sonographic Image of the Normal Gastric Wall 135

16.3 **Sonographic Features of Gastric Cancer** 136
16.3.1 Early Gastric Cancer 136
16.3.2 Advanced Gastric Cancer 138

16.4 **Staging of Gastric Cancer** 140

16.5 Conclusion 141

References 142

## 16.1
## Introduction

Gastric cancer is still of major importance worldwide despite declining incidence. Endoscopy, radiological examination, and computed tomography are the diagnostic imaging modalities employed for gastric cancer. For early gastric cancers, in particular, endoscopy is the essential diagnostic method of choice; however, with the remarkable improvements in sonographic equipment, transabdominal ultrasonography has recently been reported to be useful in the assessment of gastric cancer. Endoscopic ultrasound is another imaging modality using ultrasound which has not necessarily been as widely used as

---

J. Hata, MD
Department of Clinical Pathology and Laboratory Medicine, Kawasaki Medical School, 577, Matsushima, Kurashiki-city, Okayama, 701-0192, Japan
K. Haruma, MD; N. Manabe, MD; T. Kamada, MD;
H. Kusunoki, MD; T. Tanaka, MD; M. Sato, MD
Division of Gastroenterology, Dept. of Internal Medicine, Kawasaki Medical School, 577, Matsushima, Kurashiki-city, Okayama, 701-0192, Japan

transabdominal ultrasound due to its invasiveness. In this chapter, sonographic imaging of gastric cancer, mainly transabdominal, is described.

## 16.2
## Sonographic Assessment of the Gastric Wall

### 16.2.1
### Preparation and Equipment

For the screening of advanced gastric cancers, special preparations, such as the ingestion of water, and the injection of anticholinergic agents, are not necessary in most cases; however, such preparations are required to visualize smaller lesions. After an overnight fast, the ingestion of approximately 200–400 ml of water makes it easier to detect smaller lesions located in the posterior wall of the gastric circumflex. The injection of spasmolytic agents is seldom necessary.

While a 3–4 MHz curved array scanner is used for routine screening for gastric cancers, detailed examination including the evaluation of wall stratification should be performed with a high-frequency (5–9 MHz) linear probe for its superior spatial resolution. Tissue harmonic imaging is also recommended to reduce noises such as side lobe artifacts (Laing and Kurtz 1982).

### 16.2.2
### Sonographic Image of the Normal Gastric Wall

The abdominal esophagus is visualized between the abdominal aorta and the left lobe of the liver by a left middle subcostal scan. Below the abdominal esophagus lies the gastric fundus. The gastric body is usually located in the left middle upper abdomen. The gastric fold is often observed at the greater curvature of the gastric body (Fig. 16.1). Gastric antrum is located in the right middle upper abdomen. The pylorus is identified as the segmental thickening of the proper muscle (Fig. 16.2). The thickness of the normal gastric wall is usually <5 mm, and wall thickening of >6 mm is considered pathological.

The normal gastric wall is demonstrated as a five-layer structure. The first layer is hyperechoic, and corresponds to the luminal boundary and part of the mucosal layer. The second layer is hypoechoic and includes the remaining part of the mucosa and mucosal muscle layer. The third layer is hyperechoic and corresponds to the submucosal layer. The fourth layer is hypoechoic and corresponds to the proper muscle layer. The fifth layer is hyperechoic and corresponds to the serosa and the extramural boundary.

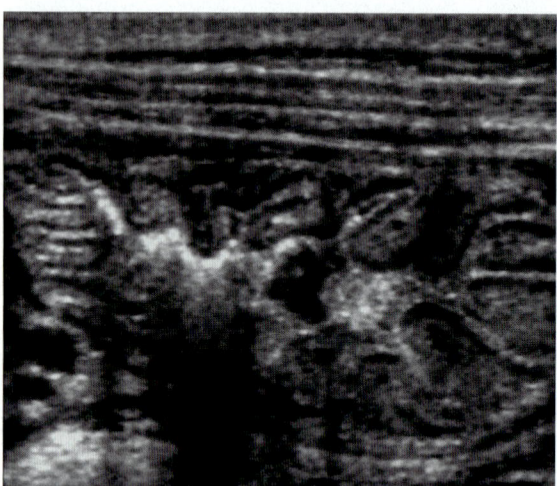

**Fig. 16.1.** Transverse scan of the gastric body. The five-layer structure of the gastric wall and the gastric fold are demonstrated

## 16.3
## Sonographic Features of Gastric Cancer

### 16.3.1
### Early Gastric Cancer

It is not always easy, and often rather difficult, to detect early gastric cancer by means of routine ultrasonographic screening, because both the wall thickening and alteration of wall stratification are too subtle to be detected with transabdominal ultrasound. In this respect, ingestion of water is useful to obtain a clear image of such subtle changes.

Early gastric cancer is usually expressed as focal wall thickening originating in the second layer. No changes of the submucosal layer are shown with intramucosal cancer (Fig. 16.3). When the tumor invades the submucosal layer, the shape and the width of that layer changes (Fig. 16.4) and it finally disappears as the tumor invades the proper muscle; however, the evaluation of cancer invasion becomes difficult when it is complicated by an ulcer, because the fibrosis accompanying ulcer healing is expressed as a hypoechoic area which resembles cancer. The diagnostic accuracy of determination of cancer depth with transabdominal ultrasound is generally thought to be inferior to that with endoscopic ultrasound, which provides a clear image with fewer artifacts and high resolution, although there are several contradictory reports (ISHIGAMI et al. 2004; MEINING et al. 2002). Even with endoscopic ultrasound, however, it is difficult to differentiate fibrotic tissue from cancer.

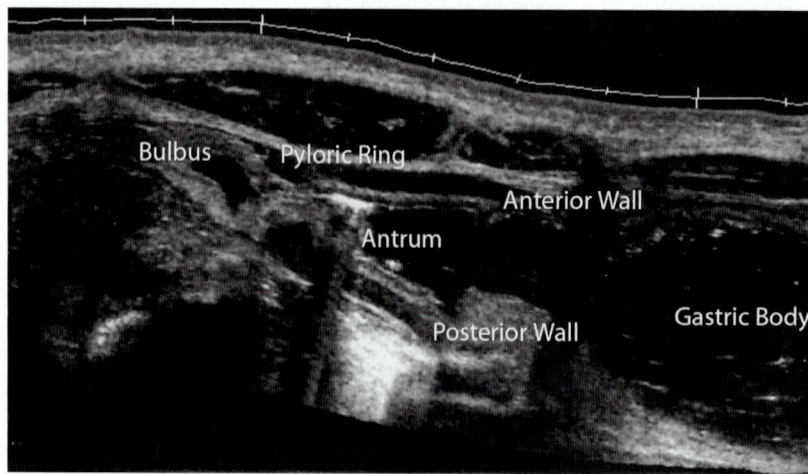

**Fig. 16.2.** Longitudinal scan of the gastric antrum and the duodenal bulb. The gastric lumen is filled with water

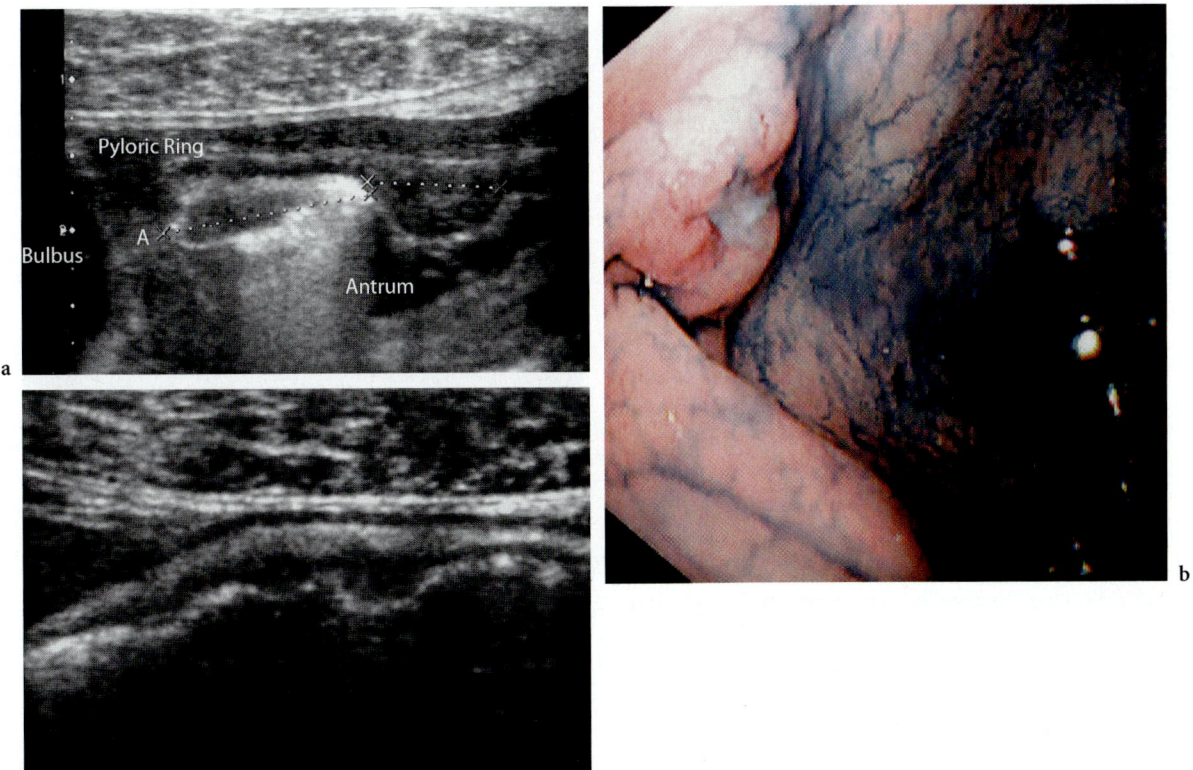

**Fig. 16.3. a** Sonographic image of an early (intramucosal) gastric cancer. Focal wall thickening, which is limited to the mucosal layer, is demonstrated. **b** Endoscopic feature of the same patient as shown in **a**. A focally elevated lesion with an ulcer at the center is visualized. **c** Sonographic image of an early (intramucosal) gastric cancer. Focal wall thickening with an indentation at the center is demonstrated. No narrowing of submucosal layer is observed

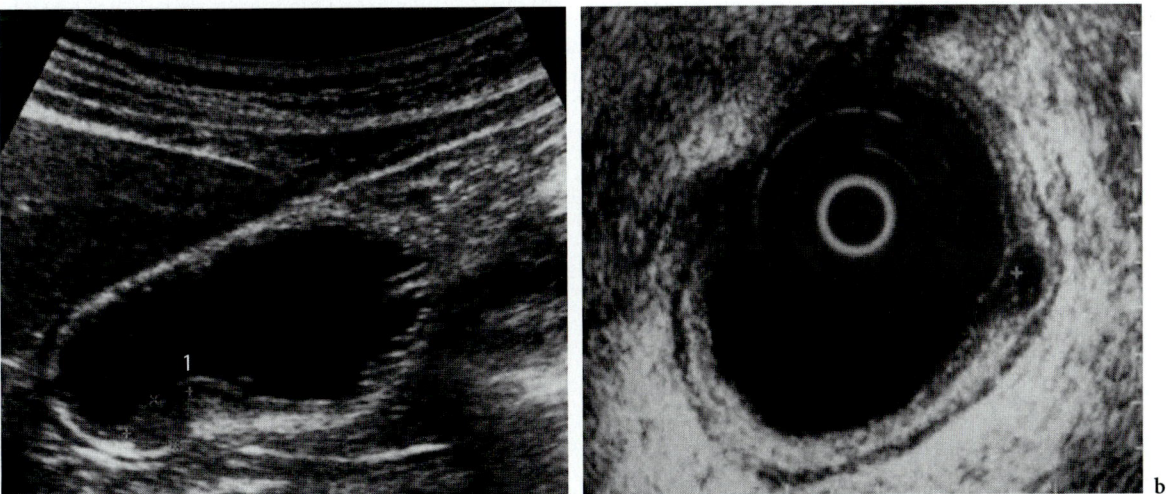

**Fig. 16.4. a** Sonographic image of an early (submucosal invasion) gastric cancer. Narrowing of the submucosal layer is demonstrated. **b** Endoscopic sonography of an early gastric cancer (submucosal invasion). There is narrowing of the submucosal layer beneath the tumor

## 16.3.2
## Advanced Gastric Cancer

Advanced gastric cancer is demonstrated as focal wall thickening without wall stratification (Figs. 16.5, 16.6). The typical sonographic figure is a "pseudokidney sign," i.e., an echogenic area surrounded by a hypoechoic rim that resembles the image of kidney. Exceptionally, in scirrhous cancers, wall stratification is demonstrated, although it is somewhat blurred (Figs. 16.7, 16.8). The lesions of advanced gastric cancer show poor compliance and compressibility, as well as reduced peristalsis or even loss of it. The vascularity on color/power Doppler depends on the nature of cancer and may not necessarily be useful for differentiation between benign and malignant conditions.

Differential diagnoses should be decided among the following: benign gastric ulcer, malignant lymphoma, acute gastric mucosal lesion, and anisakiasis, and ultrasound is useful for this purpose (Okanobu et al. 2003). Benign gastric ulcers show focal wall thickening with a wall defect at the center. Since the wall thickening around the ulcer is due to submucosal edema, wall stratification is basically preserved. Malignant lymphoma also shows focal wall thickening without stratification which resembles advanced gastric cancer, but the thickened wall is characterized by very low echogenicity, often lower than that of gastric carcinoma. Acute gastric mucosal lesions and gastric anisakiasis are characterized by diffuse wall thickening with wall stratification, brought on mainly by submucosal edema, which occasionally resembles scirrhous cancer. In scirrhous cancers, the width of every layer is irregular, and the boundary of each layer is often blurred. Furthermore, the compressibility/compliance is poor and the peristalsis is remarkably reduced.

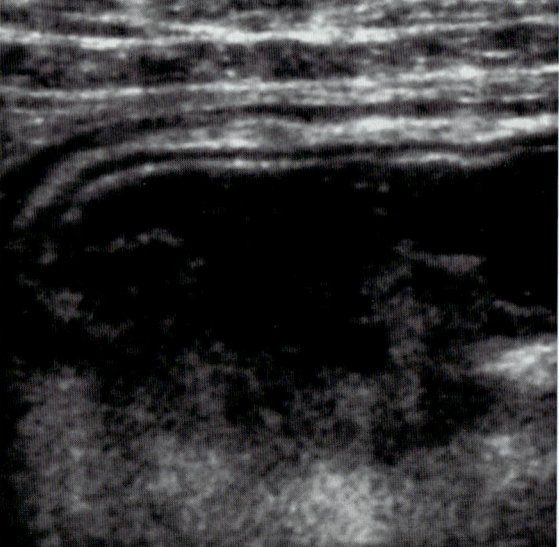
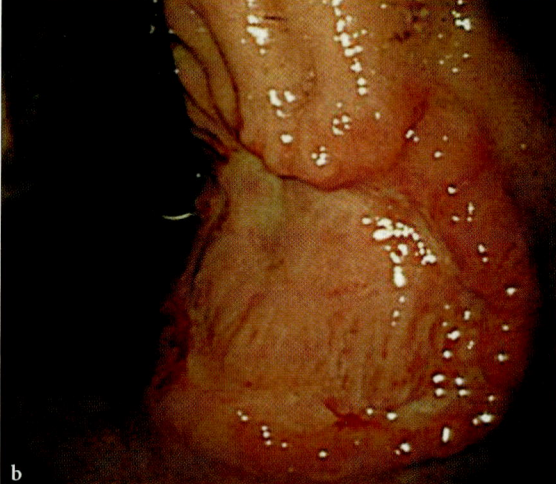
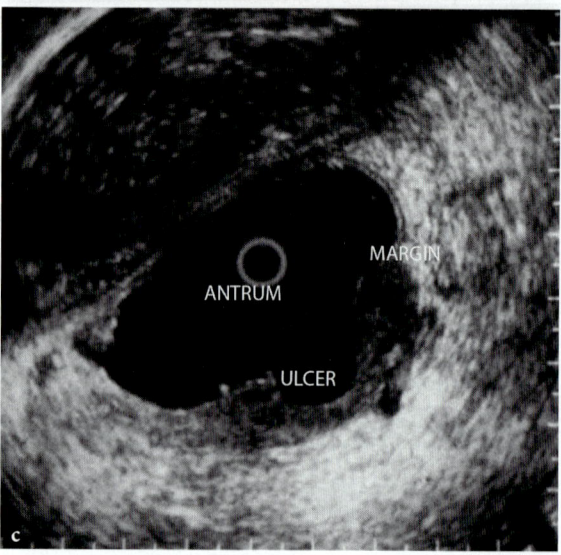

**Fig. 16.5. a** Advanced gastric cancer. Wall stratification has been totally destroyed and the extramural margin is irregular. **b** Endoscopic image of the same case as shown in Fig. 16.5a. **c** Endoscopic ultrasound image of an advanced gastric cancer. Focal wall thickening without wall stratification is observed

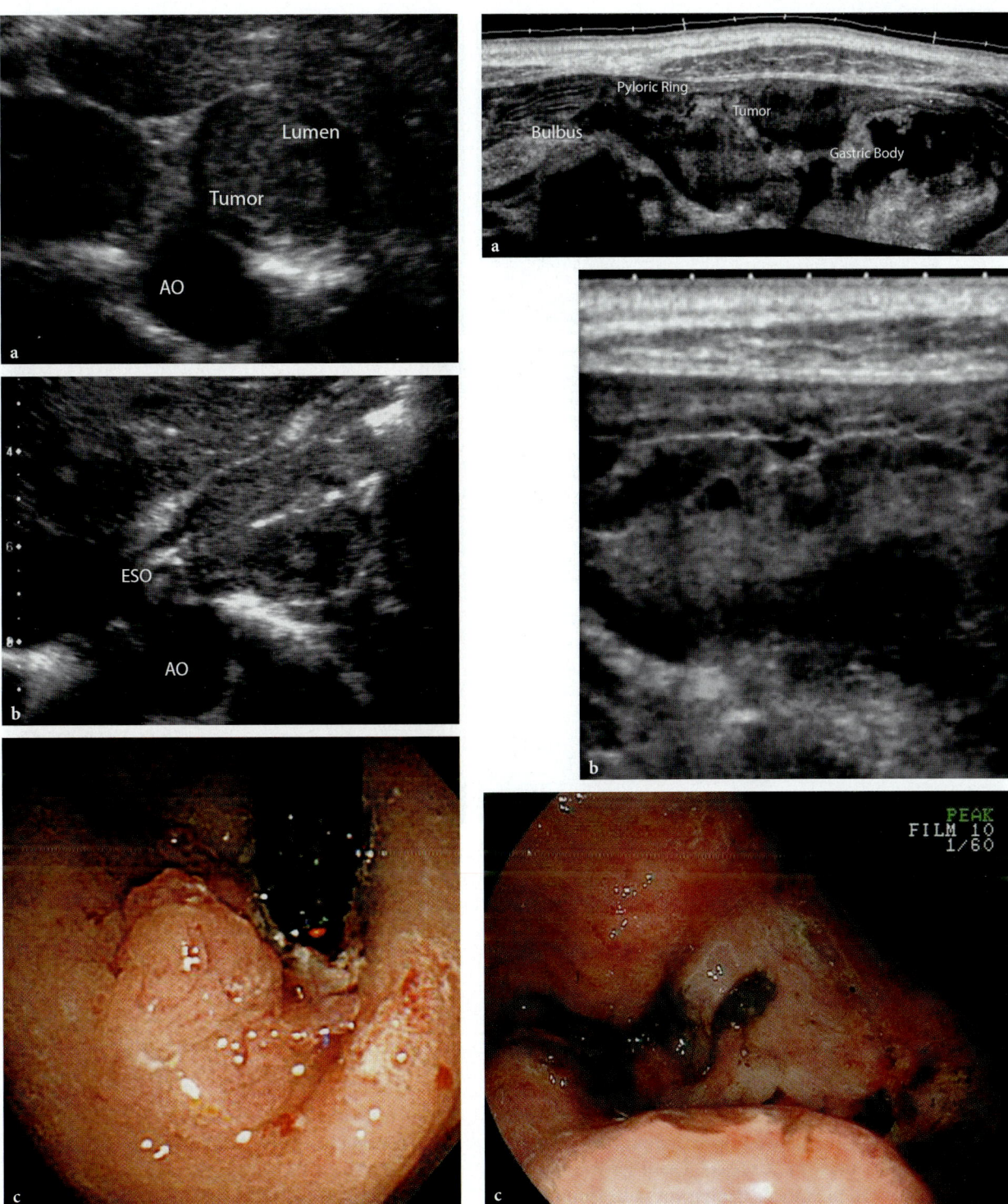

**Fig. 16.6. a** Transverse scan of advanced gastric cancer at the cardia. Wall thickening without stratification is seen in almost all circumferences, accompanied by luminal narrowing. **b** Longitudinal scan of the same lesion as shown in Fig. 16.6a. **c** Endoscopic view of the same case

**Fig. 16.7. a** Longitudinal scan of pyloric stenosis due to an advanced gastric cancer. Diffuse wall thickening of the antrum is demonstrated. **b** Close-up view of the posterior wall of the antrum with a 7-MHz linear probe. Wall stratification has not been completely destroyed. **c** Endoscopy reveals marked luminal narrowing

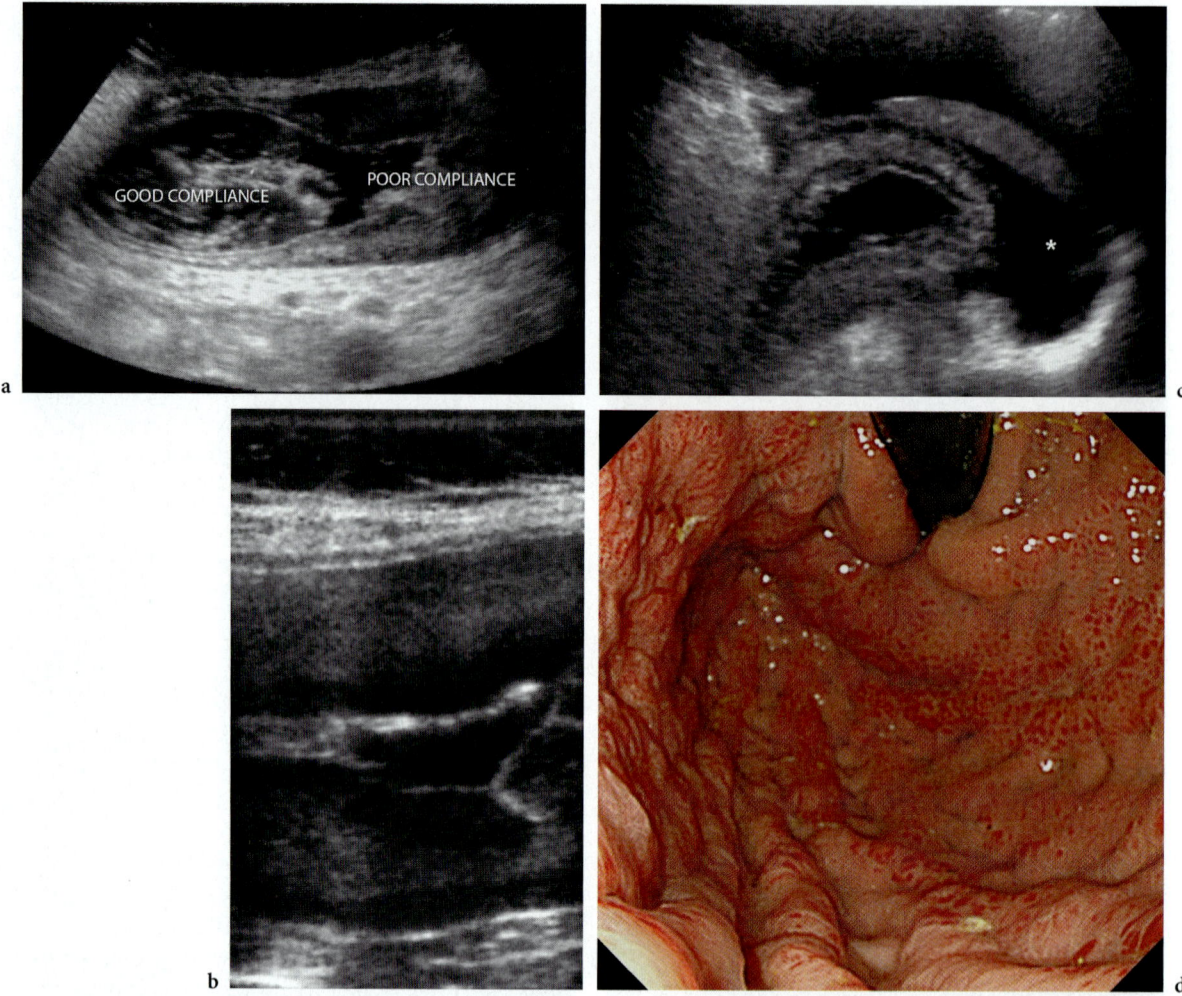

**Fig. 16.8. a** Schirrous-type gastric cancer in the gastric body. Note the difference in gastric compliance at the antrum and the lesion. **b** Close-up view of the lesion with a 7-MHz linear probe. Wall stratification is demonstrated. **c** Schirrous-type gastric cancer at the fornix. Diffuse wall thickening at the fornix and ascites (*asterisk*) are demonstrated. **d** Endoscopic image of giant rugae

## 16.4
## Staging of Gastric Cancer

For the staging of gastric cancer, cancer depth and metastases (to remote organs, lymph nodes, the peritoneum) must be assessed. There have been a few reports on the cancer staging with ultrasound showing high diagnostic ability (Liao et al. 2004; Lim et al. 1994).

The depth of cancer for an early gastric cancer is decided by assessment of alteration of wall stratification. The extension of an advanced gastric cancer is decided by careful evaluation of the tumor margin. When the outer margin of the tumor is smooth and a fat pad or boundary echo is observed between every other contiguous organ and the tumor, the cancer is considered to be within the serosa. Irregularity of the outer margin suggests high risk of the tumor exceeding the serosa. Loss of the boundary echo accompanied by loss of sliding movement between other organs are important findings suspicious of minimal invasion into an adjacent organ. The invasion is obvious when the tumor boundary lies in the contiguous organ and deforms the contour of the organ (Fig. 16.9).

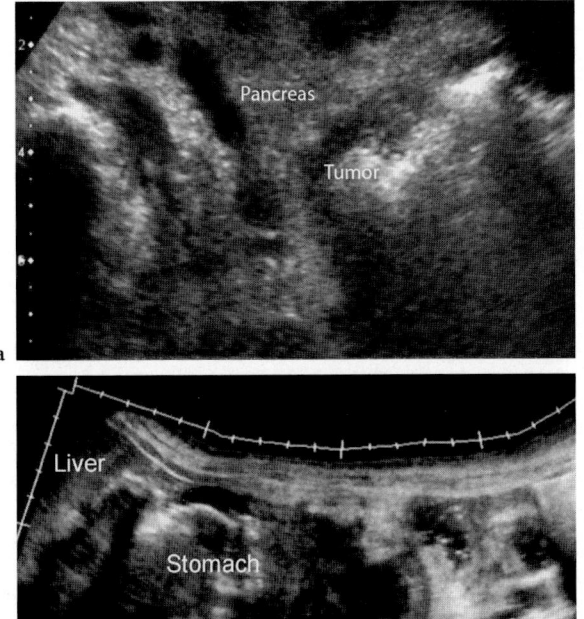

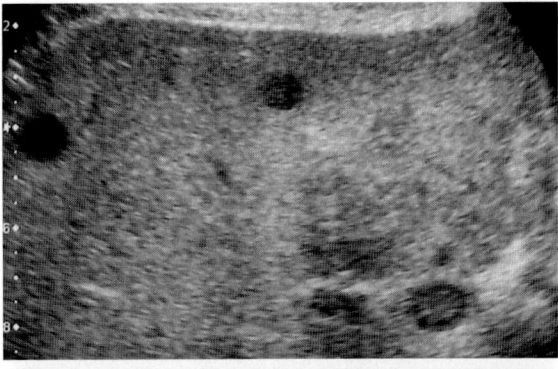

**Fig. 16.9. a** Gastric cancer invasion into the tail of the pancreas is demonstrated. The hypoechoic tumor has altered the contour of the pancreas tail. **b** Gastric cancer invasion into the transverse colon. This hypoechoic tumor is compressing the upper circumference of the transverse colon and the boundary echo between them has disappeared

Typical metastatic liver tumors have a thick hypoechoic rim with a relatively hyperechoic center, known as the "bull's-eye" sign (Fig. 16.10a); however, this finding cannot be applied to all metastatic liver tumors. Penetration of the normal vascular structure through the tumor proven by color/power Doppler, ring-shaped enhancement in the arterial phase, and loss of enhancement in the postvascular phase as determined by contrast ultrasound, are helpful findings for the diagnosis of metastatic liver tumors.

Lymph node metastases are characterized by the round-shaped swelling of lymph nodes (Fig. 16.10b). One must be careful in the differentiation from inflammatory swelling of lymph nodes caused by a benign gastric ulcer, which is more elliptical in shape than that of metastatic lymph nodes.

Tumor seeding is demonstrated as a hypoechoic nodule on the visceral or parietal peritoneum (Fig. 16.10c). Often ascites with floating echogenic particles accompanies tumor seedings, indicating peritonitis carcinomatosa.

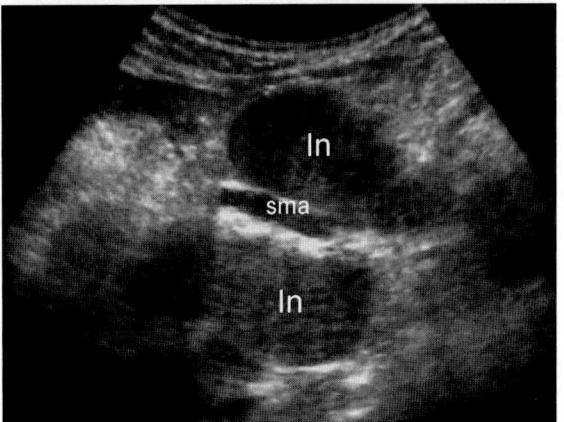

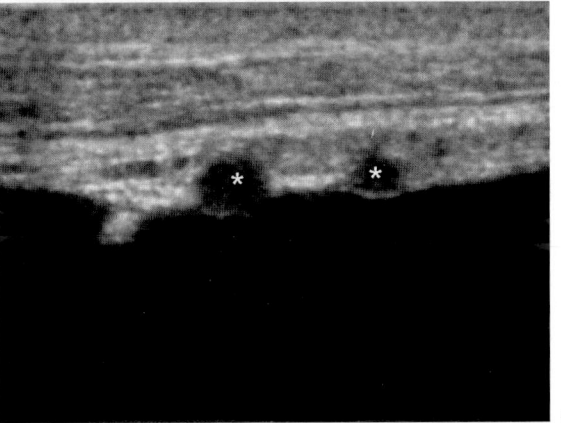

**Fig. 16.10. a** Metastatic liver tumors are demonstrated. **b** Metastatic lymph nodes (*ln*) around the superior mesenteric artery (*sma*) are demonstrated. **c** A seeding nodule (*asterisks*) seen in a patient with advanced gastric cancer

## 16.5
## Conclusion

Although influenced by the patients' constitution and the skill of the operator, transabdominal ultrasound can be a useful diagnostic tool for the evaluation of gastric cancer.

## References

Ishigami S, Yoshinaka H, Sakamoto F et al (2004) Preoperative assessment of the depth of early gastric cancer invasion by transabdominal ultrasound sonography (TUS): a comparison with endoscopic ultrasound sonography (EUS). Hepatogastroenterology 51:1202–1205

Laing FC, Kurtz AB (1982) The importance of ultrasonic sidelobe artifacts. Radiology; 145:763–8

Liao SR, Dai Y, Huo L et al (2004) Transabdominal ultrasonography in preoperative staging of gastric cancer. World J Gastroenterol 23:3399–3404

Lim JH, Ko YT, Lee DH (1994) Transabdominal US staging of gastric cancer. Abdom Imaging 19:527–531

Meining A, Dittler HJ, Wolf A et al (2002) You get what you expect? A critical appraisal of imaging methodology in endosonographic cancer staging. Gut 50:599–603

Okanobu H, Hata J, Haruma K et al (2003) Giant gastric folds: differential diagnosis at US. Radiology 228:986–990

# Gastrointestinal Lymphoma

Severin Daum, Jörg C. Hoffmann, and Martin Zeitz

CONTENTS

17.1 Introduction 143
17.2 **Endoscopic Ultrasound** 143
17.2.1 Gastric Non-Hodgkin Lymphoma 143
17.2.2 Differentiation from Gastric Cancer 144
17.2.3 Primary Staging 144
17.2.4 Follow-Up 147
17.2.5 Other Locations of Gastrointestinal Non-Hodgkin Lymphoma 147
17.2.6 Ultrasonic Miniprobes and New Generation Radial Ultrasound Probes 148

17.3 **Transabdominal Ultrasound** 148

References 149

## 17.1 Introduction

The incidence of gastrointestinal non-Hodgkin lymphoma (NHL) is about 1.1/100,000, which is low in comparison to other gastrointestinal malignancies, such as colorectal carcinoma with about 14–17/100,000 (D'Amore et al. 1994; Scheiden et al. 2005). Because of this low incidence and the fact that small intestinal NHL often presents as an emergency, there are no prospective studies dealing with primary diagnosis by transabdominal ultrasound. Transabdominal ultrasound was considered less sensitive than computed tomography for the diagnosis of abdominal malignancies in the 1970s. However ultrasound techniques are now essential for the accurate diagnosis and follow-up of mainly gastric malignancies following the introduction of endoscopic ultrasound (EUS) in 1976 (Lutz and Rosch 1976). Today, EUS forms the main diagnostic tool in early cancer of the upper gastrointestinal tract, as well as in early stages of mucosa-associated lymphoid tissue (MALT)-NHL of the stomach. Based on the diagnostic accuracy of EUS, the concepts of endoscopic treatment in early malignancies have been delineated. Data on transabdominal ultrasound in gastrointestinal NHL are still based on case reports. Differentiation of underlying diseases is not possible without histology (Table 17.1).

Table 17.1. Differential diagnosis to intestinal NHL

| |
|---|
| Crohn's disease |
| (Ulcerative) colitis |
| Intestinal ischaemia |
| Intestinal tuberculosis |
| Intestinal invagination |
| Diverticulitis |
| Post-radiation enteritis |
| Adenocarcinoma |
| Gastrointestinal stromal tumour |
| Intestinal metastases |
| Appendicitis |
| Intramural haematoma |

## 17.2 Endoscopic Ultrasound

### 17.2.1 Gastric Non-Hodgkin Lymphoma

The stomach is the most common site of gastrointestinal NHL and is seen in 70–80% of patients (Domizio et al. 1993; D'Amore et al. 1994; Radaszkiewicz

S. Daum, MD
J. C. Hoffmann, MD
M. Zeitz, MD
Medizinische Klinik und Poliklinik I, Gastroenterologie, Infektiologie und Rheumatologie, Charité – Universitätsmedizin Berlin, Campus Benjamin Franklin, Hindenburgdamm 30, 12200 Berlin, Germany

et al. 1992). MALT-NHL without aggressive histology comprises about 40–50% of gastric NHL, while aggressive subtypes are found in about 50–60%, but show low-grade components simultaneously in about 30% (KOCH et al. 2001). Stage is the most important prognostic factor in both low- and high-grade NHL (RADASZKIEWICZ et al. 1992; D'AMORE et al. 1994; RUSKONE-FOURMESTRAUX et al. 2001). In the case of *Helicobacter pylori*-associated gastric MALT-NHL, distinction between stage $I_{1/2}$ and $II_1$ is of utmost importance, as stage predicts response to antibiotic treatment (RUSKONE-FOURMESTRAUX et al. 2001; CHEN et al. 2001; SACKMANN et al. 1997; NAKAMURA et al. 2001; CALETTI et al. 2002). For this purpose, EUS has proven to be a simple and highly valuable investigation.

### 17.2.2
### Differentiation from Gastric Cancer

Involvement of the gastric wall in lymphomatous disease is similar to gastric cancer: disruption of the normal layer pattern by diffuse thickening of the layers or a change in echogenicity of the layers indicate infiltration (KIMMEY et al. 1989); echo-poor lesions being most commonly described (PÜSPÖK et al. 2002), but also echo-intense lesions may be seen (Fig. 17.1). In contrast to gastric cancer, lymphomatous involvement is preceded mainly by longitudinal infiltration within the wall instead of vertical growth (BOLONDI et al. 1987; CALETTI and BARBARA 1993). Also, wall infiltration may be seen far distal to endoscopic alterations like ulcerations (BOLONDI et al. 1987). BOLONDI et al. (1987) also reported that gastric cancer appears more echogenic, infiltration of the gastric wall is more often transmural and involvement of extramural structures and perigastric lymph nodes are more frequent than in gastric lymphoma. However, the diagnosis of an infiltrative lesion may not be based on EUS alone and is often inconclusive.

### 17.2.3
### Primary Staging

Most studies have used the Ann Arbor classification modified by Musshoff and Radaszkiewicz, which summarizes infiltration of mucosa and submucosa into I1 and further involvement into stage I2 (Table 17.2, Fig. 17.2) (MUSSHOFF and SCHMIDT-VOLLMER 1975; RADASZKIEWICZ et al. 1992; SACKMANN et al. 1997; KOCH et al. 2001). Lymph node involvement has been further subdivided into regional (II1) and non-regional (II2) infiltration (Fig. 17.3) (RADASZKIEWICZ et al. 1992).

The modified Ann Arbor classification has proved to be relevant for prognosis and feasible. In the Lugano classification stage I is not divided into stages I1 and I2 and stage III has been omitted and included in stage IV (Table 17.3). The Lugano classification may bring sufficient information, but, in most studies, the modified Ann Arbor classification has been used

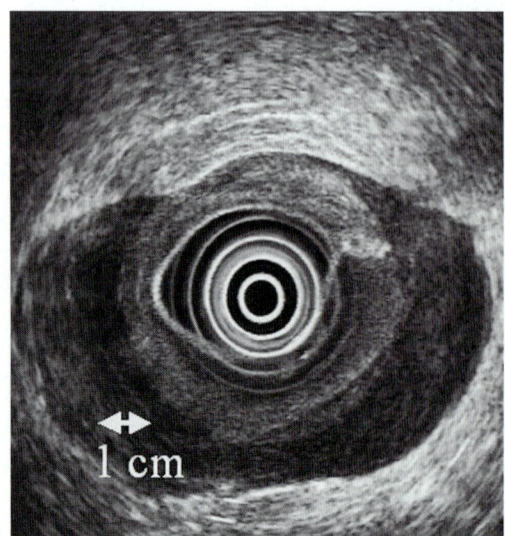
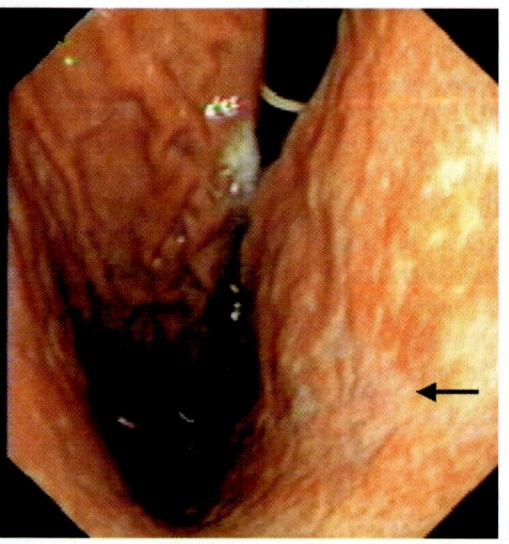

**Fig. 17.1. a** Disruption of the normal layer pattern by diffuse thickening of the layers (*arrow*) and an increased echogenicity in a patient with low grade gastric MALT-NHL stage I2. **b** Endoscopic loss of gastric folds and an ulceration was detected (*arrow*), harbouring the NHL

Table 17.2. Staging of primary gastrointestinal lymphoma. [According to the staging system of Ann Arbor (1971) modified by Musshoff and Schmidt-Vollmer (1975) and Radaszkiewicz et al. (1992)]

| Stage | |
|---|---|
| I | Localized or non-localized involvement of the GI-tract without involvement of lymph nodes and without infiltration of other organs |
| I1 | Involvement of mucosa and submucosa |
| I2 | Infiltration beyond submucosa |
| II | Localized or non-localized involvement of the GI-tract of every depth and involvement of infradiaphragmal lymph nodes |
| II1 | Regional infradiaphragmal lymph nodes |
| II2 | Non-regional infradiaphragmal lymph nodes |
| III | Localized or non-localized involvement of the GI-tract of every depth. Additional involvement of infra- und supradiaphragmal lymph nodes including further localized GI organ involvement, spleen (IIIS) or both |
| IV | Disseminated involvement of extra GI organs with or without lymph node involvement |

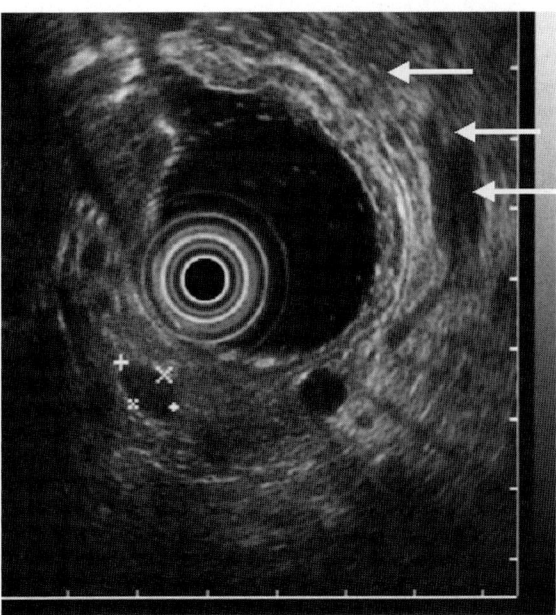

Fig. 17.3. Thickening of the gastric layers up to 7 mm without disruption of the layers (*arrows*) and paragastric lymph node with a diameter of 9 mm with normal echogenic pattern (*crosses*) seen in a patient with low-grade gastric MALT-NHL

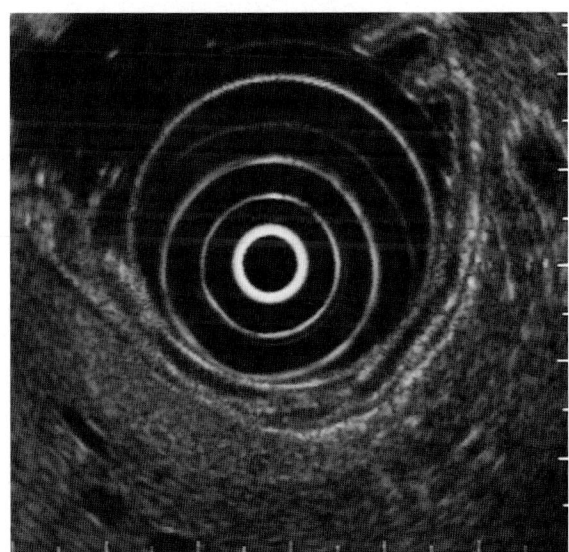

Fig. 17.2. Thickening of the submucosa with preserved layers of the gastric wall in a patient with MALT-NHL stage I1

(Sackmann et al. 1997; Radaszkiewicz et al. 1992; Koch et al. 2001). Unresolved problems are that a disseminated and incurable infiltration of the gastrointestinal tract can be staged as stage I or II according to the modified Ann Arbor staging (Table 17.2).

To address these problems, several different recommendations for the staging system have been made. The Paris staging system published in 2003, presented by several European specialists, introduced a differentiation of distant lymphoma manifestations depending on the involved organ, as well as a further subdivision of lymph node involvement (Table 17.4) (Ruskone-Fourmestraux et al. 2003). In this classification further non-continuous gastrointestinal tract involvement is stated separately. It also made further distinction of early stages of gastric NHL into T1m and T1sm similar to gastric cancer which had been proposed by Caletti et al. (1996) (Ruskone-Fourmestraux et al. 2003).

In spite of new and more differentiated staging systems, questions in clinical daily work are in most cases sufficiently answered by the Ann Arbor staging system modified by Musshoff and Radaszkiewicz (Musshoff and Schmidt-Vollmer 1975; Radaszkiewicz et al. 1992). The Paris staging system may be used in forthcoming studies to permit accurate staging and comparison of patient cohorts (Ruskone-Fourmestraux et al. 2003).

In clinical gastrointestinal practice, relevant questions to be answered in primary staging include depth of wall infiltration and involvement of the paragastric lymph nodes (Radaszkiewicz et al.

Table 17.3. Staging of primary gastrointestinal lymphoma according to the Lugano conference (ROHATINER et al. 1994)

| Stage | |
|---|---|
| I | Tumor confined to GI tract |
| II | Tumor extending into abdomen from primary GI site |
| | Nodal involvement |
| II1 | Local (paragastric in cases of gastric lymphoma and para-intestinal for intestinal lymphoma) |
| II2 | Distant (mesenteric in the case of an intestinal primary, otherwise: para-aortic, paracaval, pelvic, inguinal) |
| IIE | Penetration of serosa to involve adjacent organs or tissues (enumerate actual site of involvement, e.g. IIE (pancreas), IIE (large intestine) or IIE (post-abdominal wall) |
| IV | Disseminated extranodal involvement, or a GI tract lesion with supra-diaphragmatic nodal involvement |

E, infiltrative (per continuitatem) growth into neighboring structures

Table 17.4. Paris staging system for primary gastrointestinal lymphomas. [See also RUSKONÉ-FOURMESTRAUX et al. (2003)]

| Stage | |
|---|---|
| TX | Lymphoma extent not specified |
| T0 | No evidence of lymphoma |
| T1 | Lymphoma confined to the mucosa/submucosa |
| T1m | Lymphoma confined to mucosa |
| T1sm | Lymphoma confined to submucosa |
| T2 | Lymphoma infiltrates muscularis propria or subserosa |
| T3 | Lymphoma penetrates serosa (visceral peritoneum) without invasion of adjacent structures |
| T4 | Lymphoma invades adjacent structures or organs |
| NX | Involvement of lymph nodes not assessed |
| N0 | No evidence of lymph node involvement |
| N1 | Involvement of regional lymph nodes |
| N2 | Involvement of intra-abdominal lymph nodes beyond the regional area |
| N3 | Spread to extra-abdominal lymph nodes |
| MX | Dissemination of lymphoma not assessed |
| M0 | No evidence of extranodal dissemination |
| M1 | Non-continuous involvement of separate site in gastrointestinal tract (e.g. stomach and rectum) |
| M2 | Non-continuous involvement of other tissues (e.g. peritoneum, pleura) or organs (e.g. tonsils, parotid gland, ocular, adnexa, lung, liver, spleen, kidney, breast, etc.) |
| BX | Involvement of bone marrow not assessed |
| B0 | No evidence of bone marrow involvement |
| B1 | Lymphomatous infiltration of bone marrow |
| TNM | Clinical staging: status of tumour, node, metastasis, bone marrow |
| pTNMB | Histopathological staging: status of tumour, node metastasis, bone marrow |
| pN | The histological examination will ordinarily include six or more lymph nodes |

1992; D'AMORE et al. 1994). Only two studies comparing computed tomography with EUS in primary local staging have been conducted. TIO et al. (1986) tested EUS versus non-helical computed tomography, whereas VORBECK et al. (2002) applied an up-to-date computed tomography technique. VORBECK et al. (2002) demonstrated superiority in the detection rate of mucosal wall thickening for EUS compared to hydro-spiral computed tomography; the detection of enlarged lymph nodes was comparable for both techniques (TIO et al. 1986; VORBECK et al. 2002). Thus, the only indication for computed tomography in gastric NHL is assessment of the more distant lymph node status. However, a report in 1999 revealed that EUS was applied in only about 50% of centres treating gastric-NHL and results seemed strongly dependent on the investigator's experience (DE JONG et al. 1999).

Accurate estimation of staging depends on consecutive operation as the "gold standard" for staging and has been conducted in only a limited number of studies. In the prospective multicenter study with the largest patient numbers, preoperative EUS staging showed only a 67% sensitivity in stage I1, 83% in stage I2 and 71% in stage II1 (FISCHBACH et al. 2002). This study mirrors the reality in clinical practice as 34 centres took part with differing experience in EUS. Standardized regimens for staging are missing as demonstrated by a high interobserver disagreement for early lesions (T1 submucosa) and T2 lesions, but good results in staging of local lymph nodes before *Helicobacter pylori* eradication (FUSAROLI et al. 2002).

As *Helicobacter pylori* eradication is the treatment of choice in early stages I1 and I2 and even under regular control in stage II1, sensitivity of EUS seems to be sufficient. Local response controls in short term intervals are mandatory and 3-month intervals are recommended initially (FISCHBACH et al. 2004).

In single cases, EUS-guided needle aspiration for differentiation of lymph node involvement, for example of coeliac lymph nodes, may be necessary. In these cases, a linear scanner is used (ELOUBEIDI et al. 2004).

## 17.2.4
## Follow-Up

In spite of its high accuracy in primary staging of gastric MALT-NHL, EUS has limitations with regard to predicting treatment response during follow-up. In comparison to histological response, changes seen by EUS occur later than histological changes: in a study by PÜSPÖK et al. (2002), endosonographic remission was reached after 41.7 weeks in comparison to 29.1 weeks using histological criteria (PÜSPÖK et al. 2002). Endosonographic remission was defined as restoration of a five-layer structure of the gastric wall, measuring ≤ 4 mm in thickness without enlarged lymph nodes. This prolonged response to treatment can be understood in view of the corresponding histology: here gastric layers often remain thickened with increased fibrous tissue after eradication of lymphoma (Fig. 17.4). PÜSPÖK et al. (2002) also tested prediction of histological remission by endosonographic criteria: neither decrease in gastric wall thickness nor increase in echogenicity correlated with complete histological remission (PÜSPÖK et al. 2002).

In several studies, hypoechoic wall changes have been attributed to preceding radiotherapy and might correspond to inflammatory changes (NATTERMANN et al. 1993; TOYODA et al. 2001a). These changes were mainly found in the third wall layer, but may also occur in other regions.

In case of histological relapse, EUS often does not demonstrate the recurrence of lymphoma: in a case report by NOBRE-LEITAO et al. (1998) and in the study by PÜSPÖK et al. (2002) only one out of five patients with histological relapse also had EUS changes indicative of recurrent lymphoma. Occasionally, however, EUS changes can, indeed, precede histological features: HOEPFFNER et al. (2003) detected two patients presenting with an endosonographically demonstrable relapse before histological detection.

EUS may be useful in detecting lymphoma tissue in deeper layers of the gastric wall not responding to treatment; however, EUS is quite inaccurate in demonstrating early response or detecting minimal residual disease (PÜSPÖK et al. 2002; BAYERDÖRFFER et al. 1995). EUS, nevertheless, should remain part of the follow-up investigation for gastric MALT-NHL patients, as it may detect relapse earlier than histology in certain patients.

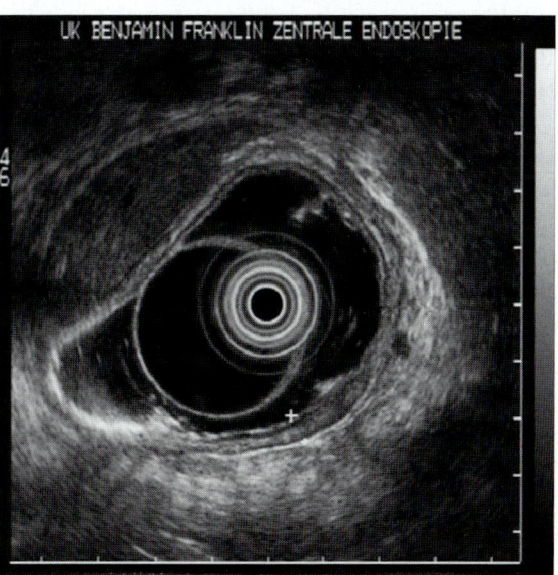

Fig. 17.4. Preserved gastric wall layers with an echo-intense thickening of the submucosal layer measuring 5.2 mm (*crosses*) after antibiotic treatment for *Helicobacter pylori* in a patient with low-grade gastric MALT-NHL

## 17.2.5
## Other Locations of Gastrointestinal Non-Hodgkin Lymphoma

EUS has been applied in patients with NHL of the duodenum, the ampulla of Vater and rectum (HORI et al. 2002; TOYODA et al. 2001b). One case report describes primary diagnosis and follow-up staging of a NHL of the ampulla of Vater with endoscopic ultrasound (TOYODA et al. 2001b). In this patient, computed tomography was unable to detect the lymphoma. In rectal disease, endoscopic ultrasound may be employed just as in gastric disease. Incidence data on rectal lymphoma are limited: in a letter, GAVIOLI et al. (2000) describe a 45-year-old patient with rectal low-grade NHL, in whom local staging was well established by endoscopic ultrasound. Due to the limited number of rectal lymphoma cases, there are no prospective studies on comparison of EUS versus computed tomography or magnetic resonance imaging. However, local wall involvement may be assessed more precisely with EUS and may be easily followed up.

## 17.2.6
### Ultrasonic Miniprobes and New Generation Radial Ultrasound Probes

In some cases of small malignant lesions which may not be found by conventional endoscopic ultrasound, ultrasonic miniprobes have been developed (RÖSCH and CLASSEN 1990). The ultrasonic miniprobe technique enables scanning under parallel endoscopic visualisation. These radial scanners have a diameter of 2.5 mm and rotating transducers of 12 MHz or 20 MHz and can be introduced through the instrument channel of a standard endoscope (MENZEL et al. 1996). In gastric NHL LÜGERING et al. (2001) compared endosonography with miniprobes to standard techniques. They showed that endosonography with miniprobes is feasible and results are comparable to those of standard EUS. However, miniprobes have limitations with regard to markedly thickened gastric walls due to insufficient depth visualisation in comparison to standard EUS. Therefore, lymph node involvement cannot be described with sufficient accuracy. Due to the higher costs and longer working time, this method is indicated for the investigation of lymphoma only in special situations, like gastrointestinal stenoses, which cannot be passed by conventional endoscopes or localized lymphoma (Fig. 17.5). To overcome the limited depth of visualisation, new generation mechanical radial probes and, in particular, electronic radial ultrasound endoscopes have been developed, which provide high resolution of the gastrointestinal wall, as well as excellent visualisation of more distant structures (YASUDA et al. 2004). One major advantage of electronic radial ultrasound endoscopes is that colour Doppler is also available, helping to distinguish lymph nodes from blood vessels.

## 17.3
## Transabdominal Ultrasound

Transabdominal ultrasound has its limitations due to the inter-observer variability and patient characteristics, e.g. severe obesity. However, abdominal ultrasound constitutes the first and most easily available method for abdominal abnormalities including investigation of mesenteric lymph nodes and liver abnormalities. Only retrospective studies and case reports exist with regard to the detection of gastrointestinal lymphoma by ultrasound (GOERG et al. 1990, 1992; STUCKMANN and ZOLLIKOFER 1996). In gastric NHL, optimal conditions require water-filling of the stomach (WORLICEK 1986). Thickness of the gastric wall should not exceed 5 mm in the corpus and proximal antrum, while the wall may reach 8 mm in thickness in the distal antrum and pylorus. Intestinal wall thickness above 3 mm is suspect for inflammatory or malignant involvement. In gastrointestinal lymphoma, lesions are echo poor, infiltrating the gastrointestinal wall with dissolution of the characteristic layers (GOERG et al. 1990; GOERG et al. 1992) (Fig. 17.6). The lumen may be narrowed and the wall asymmetrically infiltrated. Stenosis and hypervascularisation may be detected.

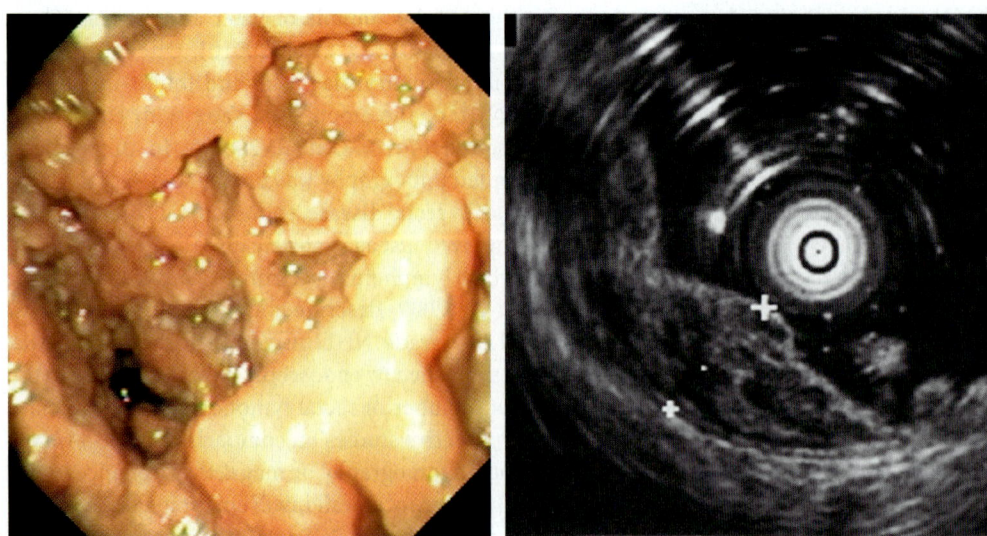

Fig. 17.5a,b. Duodenal NHL showing multiple nodules in the descending duodenum (a) and a thickened mucosa (b)

Loss of peristalsis is a late sign of lymphoma (GOERG et al. 1990). In high-grade lymphoma, ultrasound most often showed large-nodular lesions (Fig. 17.7), whereas low-grade lymphomas showed a tendency towards small-nodular or diffuse lesions (see Ch. 2) (GORG et al. 1996). In intestinal NHL the occurrence of pathological circumferential wall thickening is a classic sign: it is defined by a hypoechogenic circular structure with a central hyperechogenic structure. However, discrimination between inflamed bowel or infiltrative disease is not easy with ultrasound and computed tomography has definite advantages in that the technique is less user dependent, documentation of the primary lesion is well standardized and the technique is more sensitive for the detection of distant lymph nodes. Another alteration seen on ultrasound in intestinal NHL has been described as "white bowel" (HOLLERWEGER and DIETRICH 2005). This syndrome describes a hyperechogenic small bowel wall in patients with several different underlying diseases like Whipple's disease, HIV-associated Mycobacterium avium-intracellulare enteropathy and also coeliac disease and complicating intestinal T-NHL. Lymph oedema of the bowel wall caused by enlarged mesenteric lymph nodes or mesenteric vein thrombosis may be the underlying mechanism (HOLLERWEGER and DIETRICH 2005). Future studies need to demonstrate the role of oral contrast media like polyethylene glycol for transabdominal bowel ultrasound (PARENTE et al. 2004).

### Acknowledgements

Authors thank Dr. S. Faiss for providing a number of the figures.

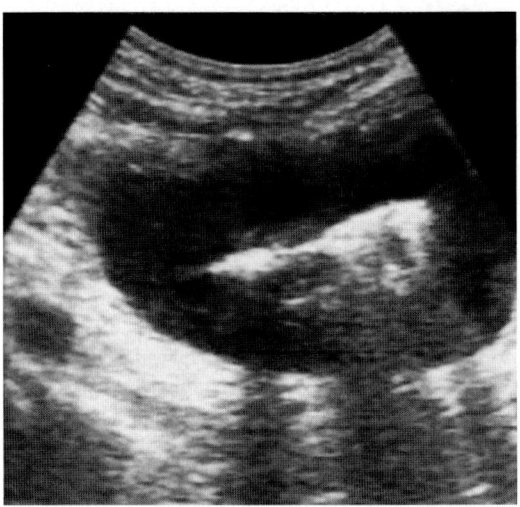

**Fig. 17.6.** Transverse sonogram shows marked hypoechoic thickening of bowel wall and loss of normal stratification. (Courtesy of I. De Sio, University of Naples, Italy)

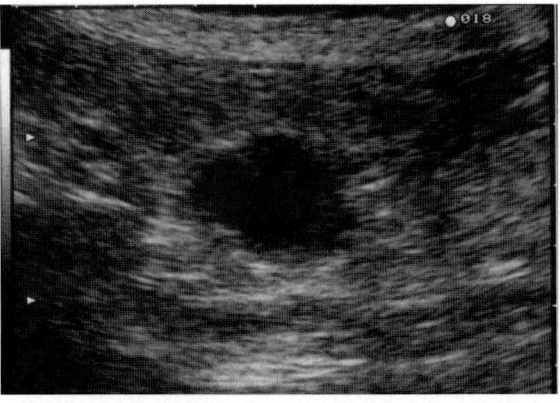

**Fig. 17.7.** Large, round and hypoechoic mesenteric lymph node, with smooth margins, in patient with non-Hodgkin lymphoma

### References

Bayerdörffer E, Neubauer A, Rudolph B et al (1995) Regression of primary gastric lymphoma of mucosa-associated lymphoid tissue type after cure of Helicobacter pylori infection. MALT Lymphoma Study Group. Lancet 345:1591–1594

Bolondi L, Casanova P, Caletti GC, Grigioni W, Zani L, Barbara L (1987) Primary gastric lymphoma versus gastric carcinoma: endoscopic US evaluation. Radiology 165:821–826

Caletti G, Barbara L (1993) Gastric lymphoma: difficult to diagnose, difficult to stage? Endoscopy 25:528–530

Caletti GC, Ferrari A, Bocus P, Togliani T, Scalorbi C, Barbara L (1996) Endoscopic ultrasonography in gastric lymphoma. Schweiz Med Wochenschr 126:819–825

Caletti G, Zinzani PL, Fusaroli P et al (2002) The importance of endoscopic ultrasonography in the management of low-grade gastric mucosa-associated lymphoid tissue lymphoma. Aliment Pharmacol Ther 16:1715–1722

Chen LT, Lin JT, Shyu RY et al (2001) Prospective study of Helicobacter pylori eradication therapy in stage IE high-grade mucosa-associated lymphoid tissue lymphoma of the stomach. J Clin Oncol 19:4245–4251

d'Amore F, Brincker H, Gronbaek K et al (1994) Non-Hodgkin's lymphoma of the gastrointestinal tract: a population-based analysis of incidence, geographic distribution, clinicopathologic presentation features, and prognosis. J Clin Oncol 12:1673–1684

de Jong D, Aleman BM, Taal BG, Boot H (1999) Controversies and consensus in the diagnosis, work-up and treatment of gastric lymphoma: an international survey. Ann Oncol 10:275–280

Domizio P, Owen RA, Shepherd NA, Talbot IC, Norton AJ (1993) Primary lymphoma of the small intestine – a clinicopathological study of 119 cases. Am Surg Pathol 17:429–442

Eloubeidi MA, Vilmann P, Wiersema MJ (2004) Endoscopic ultrasound-guided fine-needle aspiration of celiac lymph nodes. Endoscopy 36:901–908

Fischbach W, Goebeler-Kolve ME, Greiner A (2002) Diagnostic accuracy of EUS in the local staging of primary gastric lymphoma: results of a prospective, multicenter study comparing EUS with histopathologic stage. Gastrointest Endosc 56:696–700

Fischbach W, Goebeler-Kolve ME, Dragosics B, Greiner A, Stolte M (2004) Long term outcome of patients with gastric marginal zone B cell lymphoma of mucosa associated lymphoid tissue (MALT) following exclusive Helicobacter pylori eradication therapy: experience from a large prospective series. Gut 53:34–37

Fusaroli P, Buscarini E, Peyre S et al (2002) Interobserver agreement in staging gastric malt lymphoma by EUS. Gastrointest Endosc 55:662–668

Gavioli M, Bagni A, Garoia C, Piccagli I, Biscardi A, Natalini G (2000) Role of endosonography in rectal lymphoma. Haematologica 85:882–883

Goerg C, Schwerk WB, Goerg K (1990) Gastrointestinal lymphoma: sonographic findings in 54 patients. AJR Am J Roentgenol 155:795–798

Goerg C, Schwerk WB, Neumann K (1992) Gastric lymphoma: ultrasound appearance due to isolated mucosal infiltration. J Clin Ultrasound 20:59–61

Gorg C, Weide R, Schwerk WB (1996) Sonographic patterns in extranodal abdominal lymphomas. Eur Radiol 6:855–864

Hoepffner N, Lahme T, Gilly J, Koch P, Foerster EC, Menzel J (2003) Endoscopic ultrasound in the long-term follow-up of primary lymphomas of the stomach under conservative therapy. Z Gastroenterol 41:1151–1156

Hollerweger A, Dietrich CF (2005) "White bowel". A sonographic sign of intestinal lymph edema? Ultraschall Med 26:127–133

Hori K, Nishigami T, Chiba T, Matsushima Y, Kojima T (2002) Regression of MALT lymphomas coexisting in the duodenal bulb and the stomach by eradication of Helicobacter pylori. J Gastroenterol 37:288–292

Kimmey MB, Martin RW, Haggitt RC, Wang KY, Franklin DW, Silverstein FE (1989) Histologic correlates of gastrointestinal ultrasound images. Gastroenterology 96:433–441

Koch P, del Valle F, Berdel WE et al (2001) Primary gastrointestinal non-Hodgkin`s lymphoma: II. Combined surgical and conservative or conservative management only in localized gastric lymphoma – results of the prospective German Multicenter study GIT NHL 01/92. J Clin Oncol 19:3874–3883

Lügering N, Menzel J, Kucharzik T et al (2001) Impact of miniprobes compared to conventional endosonography in the staging of low-grade gastric malt lymphoma. Endoscopy 33:832–837

Lutz H, Rosch W (1976) Transgastroscopic ultrasonography. Endoscopy 8:203–205

Menzel J, Domschke W, Brambs HJ et al (1996) Miniprobe ultrasonography in the upper gastrointestinal tract: state of the art 1995, and prospects. Endoscopy 28:508–513

Musshoff K, Schmidt-Vollmer H (1975) Prognosis of non-Hodgkin´s lymphomas with special emphasis on the staging classification. Z Krebsforsch 83:323–341

Nakamura S, Matsumoto T, Suekane H et al (2001) Predictive value of endoscopic ultrasonography for regression of gastric low grade and high grade MALT lymphomas after eradication of Helicobacter pylori. Gut 48:454–460

Nattermann C, Katz L, Dancygier H (1993) Endoscopic ultrasound in the demonstration and staging of non-Hodgkin's lymphomas of the stomach. Dtsch Med Wochenschr 118:567–573

Nobre-Leitao C, Lage P, Cravo M et al (1998) Treatment of gastric MALT lymphoma by Helicobacter pylori eradication: a study controlled by endoscopic ultrasonography. Am J Gastroenterol 93:732–736

Parente F, Greco S, Molteni M et al (2004) Oral contrast enhanced bowel ultrasonography in the assessment of small intestine Crohn's disease. A prospective comparison with conventional ultrasound, X-ray studies, and ileocolonoscopy. Gut 53:1652–1657

Püspök A, Raderer M, Chott A, Dragosics B, Gangl A, Schofl R (2002) Endoscopic ultrasound in the follow up and response assessment of patients with primary gastric lymphoma. Gut 51:691–964

Radaszkiewicz T, Dragosics B, Bauer P (1992) Gastrointestinal malignant lymphomas of the mucosa-associated lymphoid tissue: factors relevant to prognosis. Gastroenterology 102:1628–1638

Rohatiner A, d'Amore F, Coiffier B et al (1994) Report on a workshop convened to discuss the pathological and staging classifications of gastrointestinal tract lymphoma. Ann Oncol 5:397–400

Rosch T, Classen M (1990) A new ultrasonic probe for endosonographic imaging of the upper GI-tract. Preliminary observations. Endoscopy 22:41–46

Ruskone-Fourmestraux A, Lavergne A, Aegerter PH et al (2001) Predictive factors for regression of gastric MALT lymphoma after anti-Helicobacter pylori treatment. Gut 48:297–303

Ruskone-Fourmestraux A, Dragosics B, Morgner A, Wotherspoon A, Dd Jong D (2003) Paris staging system for primary gastrointestinal lymphomas. Gut 52:912–913

Sackmann M, Morgner A, Rudolph B et al (1997) Regression of gastric MALT lymphoma after eradication of Helicobacter pylori is predicted by endosonographic staging. MALT Lymphoma Study Group. Gastroenterology 113:1087–1090

Scheiden R, Pescatore P, Wagener Y, Kieffer N, Capesius C (2005) Colon cancer in Luxembourg: a national population-based data report, 1988–1998. BMC Cancer 5:52

Stuckmann G, Zollikofer C (1996) Gastrointestinal lymphomas: ultrasonic aspects. Schweiz Med Wochenschr 126:813–818

Tio TL, den Hartog Jager FC, Tytgat GN (1986) Endoscopic ultrasonography in detection and staging of gastric non-Hodgkin lymphoma. Comparison with gastroscopy, barium meal, and computerized tomography scan. Scand J Gastroenterol Suppl 123:52–58

Toyoda H, Nomoto Y, Ii N et al (2001a) Endosonographic images of low-grade lymphoma of mucosa-associated lymphoid tissue after radiotherapy. J Clin Gastroenterol 33:237–240

Toyoda H, Yamaguchi M, Nakamura S et al (2001b) Regression of primary lymphoma of the ampulla of Vater after eradication of Helicobacter pylori. Gastrointest Endosc 54:92–96

Vorbeck F, Osterreicher C, Puspok A et al (2002) Comparison of spiral-computed tomography with water-filling of the stomach and endosonography for gastric lymphoma of mucosa-associated lymphoid tissue-type. Digestion 65:196–199

Worlicek H (1986) Sonographic diagnosis of the fluid-filled stomach. Ultraschall Med 7:259–263

Yasuda K, Ogawa M, Sato A et al (2004) Newly developed ultrasound endoscope with an electronic radial array transducer. Dig Endo 16 [Suppl]:219–222

# Peritoneal Metastasis

Ilario de Sio, Loredana Tibullo, and Camillo Del Vecchio-Blanco

CONTENTS

18.1 Introduction  151
18.2 **Ultrasonographic Findings**  151
18.2.1 Ascites  152
18.2.2 Omental Involvement  153
18.2.3 Peritoneal Parietal and Serosal Implants  154
18.2.4 Accessory Findings  154
18.3 **Differential Diagnosis and Role of Ultrasound-Guided Biopsy of Peritoneal Masses**  156
References  157

## 18.1 Introduction

Metastatic involvement of peritoneum (peritoneal carcinomatosis) is by far the most common peritoneal tumor (Walsh and Williams 1971; Bell and Scully 1990). Tumors that preferentially metastasize to the peritoneum include the following adenocarcinomas: stomach; intestine (colon–rectum); gallbladder or biliary tree; pancreas; breast; lung; ovary; and uterus (Runyon et al. 1988); as well as lymphoma and other tumors, such as the sarcomas (Runyon and Hoefs 1986). About two-thirds of women with ovarian cancer present abdominal dissemination of the disease (Johnson 1993; Longatto Filho et al. 1997), whereas sarcomas account for only 3% of metastatic peritoneal malignant tumors (Walsh and Williams 1971). Neoplastic diffusion of cancer to peritoneum occurs both due to contiguity and lymphatic or hematic spreading. Pseudomyxoma peritonei is a special case in metastatic peritoneal tumors: it derives from the rupture of an ovary or appendix tumor with accumulation of mucin in the peritoneal cavity (Mann et al 1990). Its malignancy is variable and diagnosis is usually made when jelly-like material is observed during surgery, at laparoscopy, or is aspired by interventional procedure such as guided ultrasound (US) and/or computed tomography (CT; Novell and Lewis 1990). Clinical presentation of peritoneal carcinomatosis includes abdominal pain and distension, early satiety, important ascites (usually bloody), abdominal masses which determine bowel obstruction, and weight loss. Prognosis is generally poor (Yamada et al. 1983). Ultrasonography is the first choice procedure in evaluation of patients with abdominal pain, distension, and palpable masses. It is used as a guide for cyto-histological evaluation of ascites and abdominal masses, thus avoiding either laparoscopy or laparotomy for diagnosis.

I. de Sio, MD
Gastroenterology Unit, Ultrasonography Section, II University of Naples, Via S. Pansini 5, 80131 Naples, Italy
L. Tibullo, MD, PhD
Department of Internal Medicine and Gastroenterology Ultrasonography Section, II University of Naples, Via S. Pansini 5, 80131 Naples, Italy
C. Del Vecchio-Blanco, MD
Department of Internal Medicine and Gastroenterology, II University of Naples, Via S. Pansini 5, 80131 Naples, Italy

## 18.2 Ultrasonographic Findings

Presence of ascites, omental involvement, serosal implants, mesenteric involvement, peritoneal implants, and interruption of the anterior peritoneal line are the most frequently described ultrasonographic findings in patients with peritoneal metastasis. Accessory findings are represented by liver metastasis, lymphadenopathies, and gallbladder wall thickening (RIOUX and MICHAUD 1995). Ultrasonography is also useful in detecting primary cancer in patients without known malignancy: in fact, in a consecutive series on 37 patients, ultrasonography revealed a primary tumor in 16 (57%) out of 28 patients with no clinical or imaging signs of primary cancer (RIOUX and MICHAUD 1995).

Table 18.1 summarizes the prevalence of ultrasonographic signs in peritoneal carcinomatosis.

Table 18.1. Prevalence of ultrasonographic findings in peritoneal carcinomatosis. (From RIOUX and MICHAUD 1995)

| Ultrasonographic finding | Prevalence (%) |
| --- | --- |
| Omental involvement | 97 |
| Ascites | 49 |
| Serosal implants | 19 |
| Mesenteric involvements | 16 |
| Peritoneal implants | 54 |
| Interruption of the anterior peritoneal line | 16 |
| Liver metastasis | 38 |
| Lymphadenopathies | 24 |
| Gallbladder wall thickening | 32 |

## 18.2.1
## Ascites

Ultrasonography is a highly sensitive test in detecting ascites of small volume (BRANNEY and WOLFE 1995), e.g., 5–10 ml ascites are clearly detectable; however, ascites is common in many benign conditions such as liver cirrhosis, portal hypertension, nephrotic syndrome, cardiac insufficiency, etc. (RUNYON et al. 1988). Even if ultrasonography is often unable to distinguish between benign and malignant ascites, its presence in patients with known neoplasia is highly indicative of neoplastic involvement of the peritoneum, and its presence in the lesser omentum (in absence of pancreatitis) is also highly indicative of malignancy (DODDS et al. 1985). Some ultrasonographic characteristics may be helpful in differentiating benign from malignant ascites.

Frequently, in malignant ascites, the fluid is echogenic (due to the presence of blood and/or neoplastic cells; Fig. 18.1), septa are often present (Fig. 18.2), bowel loops are fixed and smashed for mesenteric involvement (Fig. 18.3), and serosal and parietal peritoneal implants are often visible. Indeed, abun-

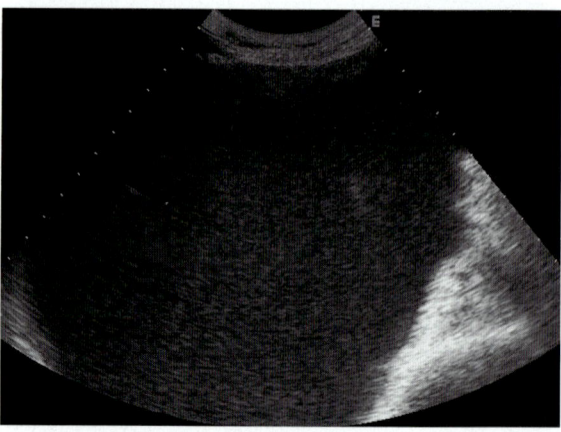

Fig. 18.1. Echogenic malignant ascites in a case of ovarian cancer. The fluid is echogenic with fine corpusculated echoes and declivous sediment

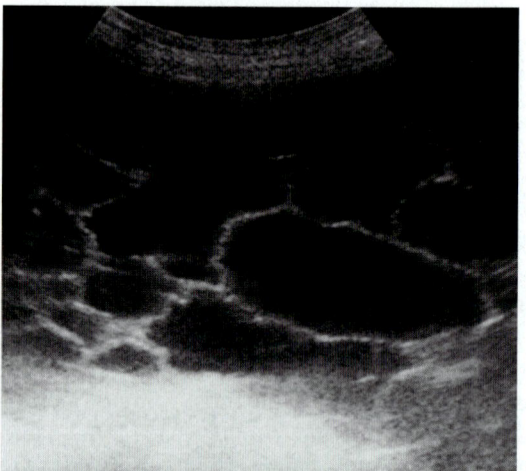

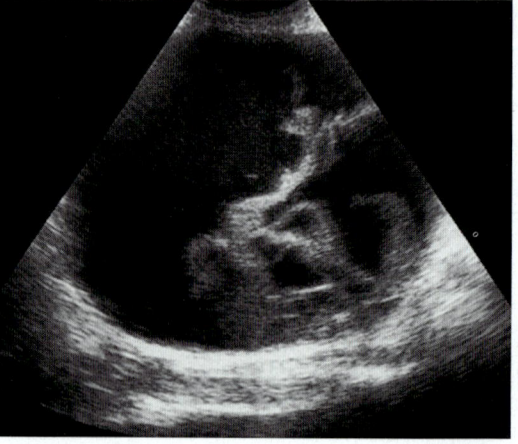

Fig. 18.2. a Ascites with fine hyperechogenic septa are clearly visible in malignant ascites due to pancreatic cancer. b More evident thickened hyperechogenic septa in malignant ascites due to gastric cancer

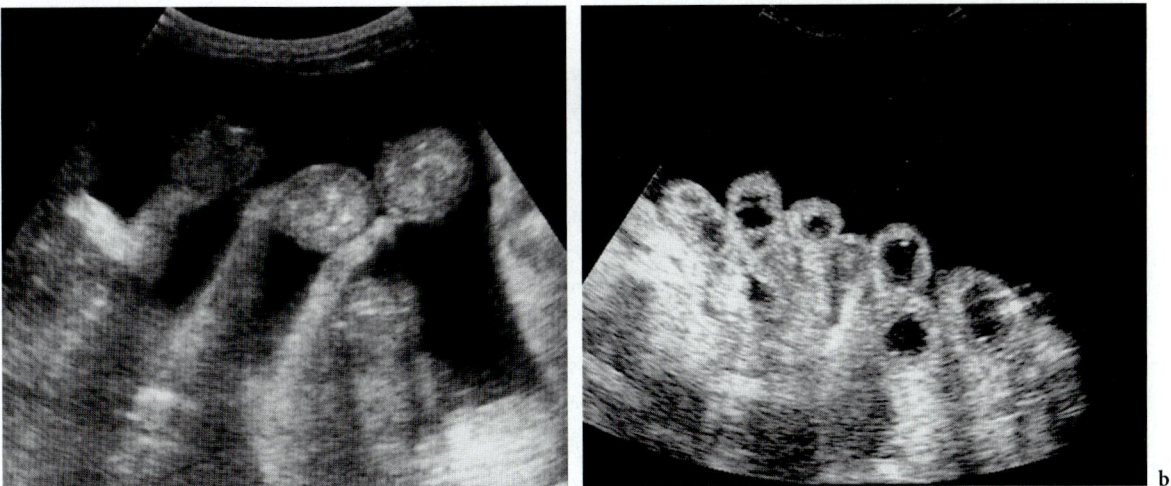

**Fig. 18.3. a** A case of benign ascites. Note the bowel loops free in the anechoic fluid. **b** Contrary to what is seen in **a**, the intestinal loops are fixed and smashed in malignant ascites

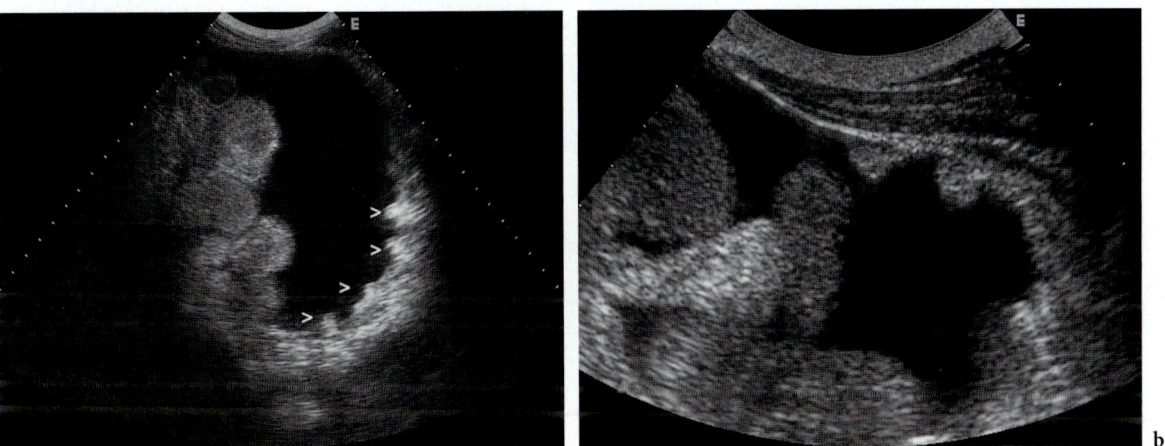

**Fig. 18.4. a** Very small nodules (>) are clearly visible on the posterior abdominal wall in a case of peritoneal involvement (colon cancer). **b** Small solid nodules adhering to the anterior abdominal wall in a patient with ovarian cancer

dant ascites facilitates visualization of small nodules infiltrating the parietal peritoneum, since it acts as a means of contrast (Fig. 18.4; GOERG and SCHWERK 1991).

Table 18.2 summarizes differential ultrasonographic characteristics between benign and malignant ascites; however, significant ascites is present in about 50% of patients with peritoneal metastasis (RIOUX and MICHAUD 1995).

Diagnosis of peritoneal metastatic involvement is often based on fluid analysis and ultrasound-guided aspiration of ascites is frequently used in patients with small amounts of liquid (Fig. 18.5).

Combined with repeated cytological examination of fluid, ultrasound offers 92% sensitivity in the diagnosis of peritoneal carcinomatosis, thus avoiding laparotomy or laparoscopy (GERBES 1991; RUNYON et al. 1988).

## 18.2.2
## Omental Involvement

STEIN (1977) clearly described the omental band as a new sign of peritoneal metastasis. Neoplastic infiltration of the great omentum is visualized by

Table 18.2. Ultrasonographic differential diagnosis between benign and malignant ascites

| Ultrasonographic finding | Benign ascites | Malignant ascites |
|---|---|---|
| Echogenic ascites | ± | +++ |
| Septa | Absent | Present |
| Peritoneal line | Regular | Irregular; interruption; evidence of nodules |
| Omentum | Thin | "Omental cake" |
| Mesentery | Free | Fixed |
| Intestinal loops | Free | Fixed/smashed |
| Liver metastasis | Absent | Present |
| Lymphadenopathies | Absent | Present |
| Other US signs | Liver cirrhosis Pancreatitis Cardiac failure | Absent |

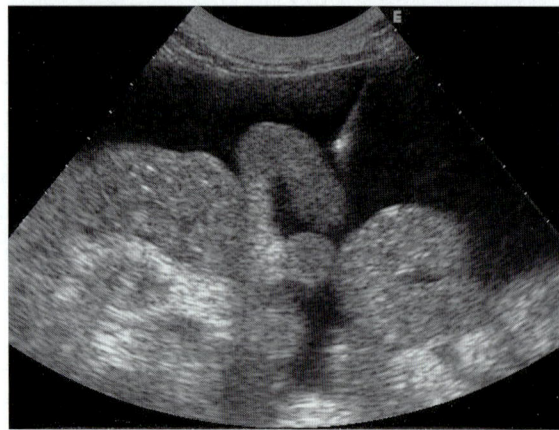

Fig. 18.5. Ultrasound-guided percutaneous fine-needle aspiration of ascitic fluid. Note the tip of the needle clearly visible in the fluid

ultrasound as a uniformly thick, hyposonic band-shaped structure adjacent to the anterior and lateral walls of the abdomen, following the contour of the abdominal convexity and containing low-level non-structural internal echoes (omental cake) (Fig. 18.6). From this finding, a diffuse metastatic involvement of the omentum can probably be inferred with a high degree of reliability.

Omental involvement is present in about 97% of patients with peritoneal metastasis (RIOUX and MICHAUD 1995).

## 18.2.3
## Peritoneal Parietal and Serosal Implants

Peritoneal parietal and serosal implants are visible on ultrasound as soft tissue masses or nodules adhering to the peritoneum, as irregularity or interruption of the anterior hyperechoic peritoneal line (Fig. 18.7). Visualisation is facilitated by the presence of ascites. The ultrasonographic study of the peritoneal line is facilitated by the use of high frequency ultrasound probes, which allow also visualization of very small peritoneal implants (Fig. 18.8; LORENZ et al. 1990). Peritoneal implants, serosal implants, and interruption of the anterior hyperechoic peritoneal line are present at the rates of about 54, 19, and 16%, respectively in patients with peritoneal carcinomatosis (RIOUX and MICHAUD 1995).

## 18.2.4
## Accessory Findings

Liver metastases are found in about 38% of patients with peritoneal carcinomatosis, but represent a non-specific finding. In fact, liver metastases are frequently found even in the absence of peritoneal involvement. Lymphadenopathies are present in about 24% of cases, but like liver metastases, they do not represent a specific sign of peritoneal carcinomatosis (RIOUX and MICHAUD 1995).

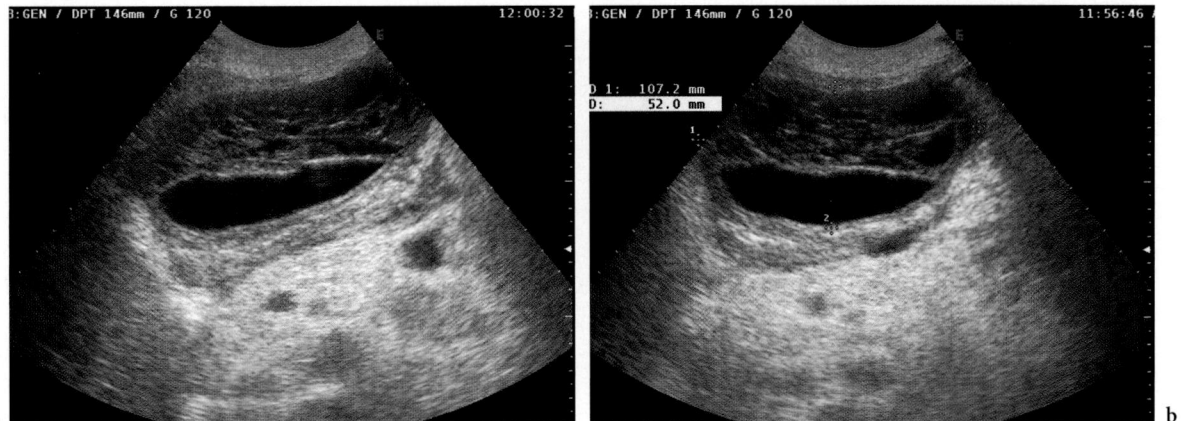

**Fig. 18.6a,b.** The "omental cake sign": neoplastic infiltration of the great omentum is visualized by ultrasound as uniformly thick, hyposonic band-shaped structure adjacent to the anterior and lateral walls of the abdomen, following the contour of the abdominal convexity and containing low-level non-structural internal echoes

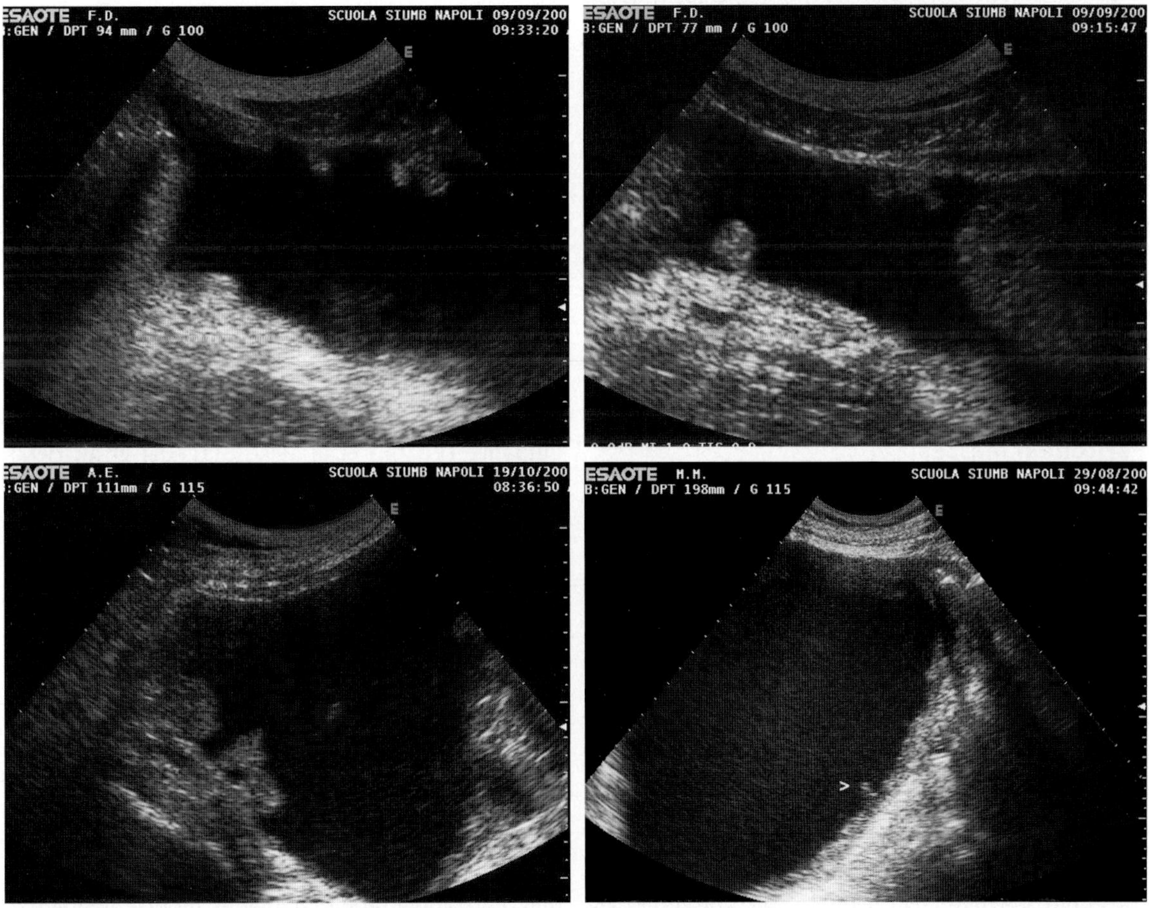

**Fig. 18.7.** Small peritoneal implants are clearly visible as hypoechoic nodules on the peritoneal line (**a–c**) or as irregularity (>) of the peritoneal line (**d**). **d** Echogenic ascites is also clearly visible

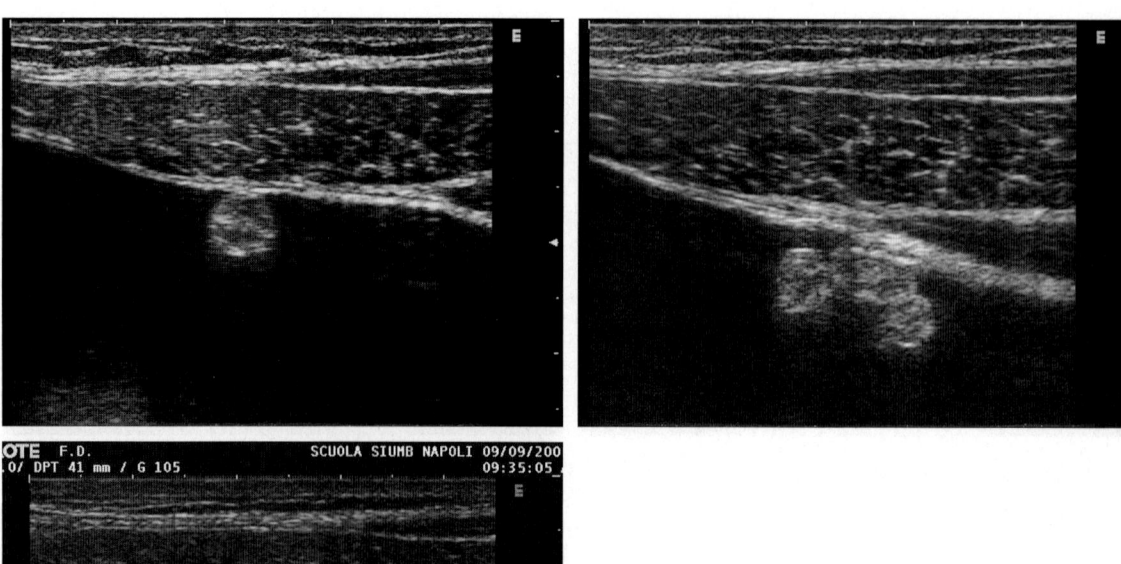

**Fig. 18.8a–c.** The ultrasonography study with high-frequency probes (cases shown in Fig.18.7a–c) clearly documented the peritoneal metastatic implants

## 18.3
## Differential Diagnosis and Role of Ultrasound-Guided Biopsy of Peritoneal Masses

The definitive diagnosis of metastatic peritoneal carcinomatosis and its differentiation from peritoneal mesothelioma may be difficult on account of the clinical, macroscopic, and microscopic variability of the latter. Conventionally, these criteria may be established only after surgical exploration and extensive sampling. Recent imaging literature shows excellent correlation between CT or ultrasound, and operative or autopsy findings. These imaging modalities have shown soft tissue masses or nodules, thickened omentum (omental cake), peritoneum, mesentery, bowel wall thickening, pleural plaques, and usually disproportionately small, if any, ascites. The latter two observations may be useful in differentiating macroscopically mesothelioma from peritoneal carcinomatosis (RAPTOPOULOS 1985). Furthermore, fine-needle aspiration biopsy, after performing wide sampling of the tumors in different locations under US or CT guidance (POMBO et al 1997; SISTROM et al. 1992), produced diagnostic cytological specimens; thus, the need for exploratory surgery may be reduced, and the differential diagnosis between peritoneal metastasis and peritoneal mesothelioma may be made prospectively and relatively non-invasively at the same time using computed tomography or ultrasound and fine-needle aspiration biopsy.

Ultrasound-guided needle biopsy in peritoneal masses has been mostly performed using a fine needle (i.e., needle with an outer diameter <1 mm to 20 G), but very little experience exists regarding the use of a large needle with core biopsy. In the experience of RIOUX and MICHAUD (1995), sonographic findings, confirmed by percutaneous biopsy, avoided 24 unnecessary exploratory laparotomies. SPENCER et al. (2001) performed image-guided peritoneal biopsy in

35 women using an 18-G core biopsy in omental cake (25 cases), peritoneal (7 cases), and adnexal (3 cases) sites. A correct diagnosis was obtained in 77% of cases with no false positives and only one false-negative result without significant complications, leading the authors to conclude that image-guided peritoneal biopsy is a simple, safe, and accurate technique for providing site-specific diagnosis in women with undiagnosed peritoneal carcinomatosis.

GOTTLIEB et al (1998) determined the effectiveness of sonographically guided biopsies, of extra-visceral masses, in the peritoneal cavity (outside solid organs). They retrospectively reviewed the results of sonographically guided biopsies of extra-visceral masses found in the peritoneal cavity of 52 patients, 51 of whom underwent biopsy through the abdominal wall. Placement of the biopsy needle within the lesion was successful in all patients. Biopsy results were true positive for malignancy in 37 patients (no false positives), true negative for benign masses in 10 patients, and false negative for malignancy in 3 patients (sensitivity 93%, specificity 100%, accuracy 94%). Non-diagnostic samples were obtained only in 2 patients (4%). Treatment was based on diagnostic biopsy results in 43 patients (86%). The authors concluded that sonography is an effective alternative to CT in guiding the biopsy of extra-visceral masses in the peritoneal cavity.

## References

Bell DA, Scully RE (1990) Serous borderline tumors of peritoneum. Am J Surg Pathol 14:230–234
Branney SW, Wolfe RE (1995) Quantitative sensitivity of ultrasound in detecting free intraperitoneal fluid. J Trauma 39:375–380
Dodds WJ, Foley WD, Lawson TL et al. (1985) Anatomy and imaging of the lesser peritoneal sac. Am J Roentgenol 144:567–575
Gerbes A (1991) Ascitic fluid analysis for the differentiation of malignancy-related and non-malignant ascites. Cancer 68:1808–1812
Goerg C, Schwerk WB (1991) Malignant ascites: sonographic signs of peritoneal carcinomatosis. Eur J Cancer 27:720–723
Gottlieb RH, Tan R, Widjaja J et al (1998) Extravisceral masses in the peritoneal cavity: sonographically guided biopsies in 52 patients. Am J Roentgenol 171:697–701
Johnson RJ (1993) Radiology in the management of ovarian cancer. Clin Radiol 48:75–82
Longatto Filho A, Bisi H, Alves VA et al (1997) Adenocarcinoma in females detected in serous effusions. Cytomorphologic aspects and immunocytochemical reactivity to cytokeratins 7 and 20. Acta Cytol 41:961–971
Lorenz R, Krestin GP, Neufang KF (1990) Diagnosis and differential diagnosis of a peritoneal carcinosis. Conventional techniques, sonography, computed tomography, magnetic resonance tomography. Radiologe 30:477–480
Mann WJ, Wagner J, Chumas J et al (1990) The management of pseudomyxoma peritonei. Cancer 66:1636–1640
Novell R, Lewis A (1990) Role of surgery in the treatment of pseudomyxoma peritonei. J R Coll Surg Edinb 35:21–26
Pombo F, Rodriguez E, Martin R et al (1997) CT guided core needle biopsy in omental pathology. Acta Radiol 38:978–981
Raptopoulos V (1985) Peritoneal mesothelioma. Crit Rev Diagn Imaging 24:293–328
Rioux M, Michaud C (1995) Sonography detection of peritoneal carcinomatosis: a prospective study of 37 cases. Abdom Imaging 20:47–51
Runyon B, Hoefs JC (1986) Peritoneal lymphomatosis with ascites: a characterization. Arch Intern Med 146:887–889
Runyon B, Hoefs JC, Morgan TR (1988) Ascitic fluid analysis in malignancy related ascites. Hepatology 8:1104–1109
Sistrom CL, Abbitt PL, Feldman PS (1992) Ultrasound guidance for biopsy of omental abnormalities. J Clin Ultrasound 20:27–31
Spencer JA, Swift SE, Wilkinson R et al (2001) Peritoneal carcinomatosis: image-guided peritoneal core biopsy for tumor type and patient care. Radiology 221:173–177
Stein MA (1977) Omental band: new sign of metastasis. J Clin Ultrasound 5:410–412
Walsh D, Williams G (1971) Surgical biopsy studies of omental and peritoneal nodules. Br J Surg 58:428–431
Yamada S, Takeda T, Matsumoto K (1983) Prognostic analysis of malignant pleural and peritoneal effusions. Cancer 51:136–139

# Carcinoid and Submucosal Tumors

Jiro Hata, Ken Haruma, Noriaki Manabe, Tomoari Kamada,
Hiroaki Kusunoki, Toshiaki Tanaka, and Motonori Sato

CONTENTS

19.1 Introduction  159

19.2 Preparations for Sonographic Assessment of Submucosal Tumors  159

19.3 Carcinoid Tumor  159

19.4 Submucosal Tumor  161
19.4.1 Cyst and Lymphangioma  161
19.4.2 Lipoma  161
19.4.3 Ectopic Pancreas  161
19.4.4 Hemangioma  161
19.4.5 Gastrointestinal Stromal Tumor  161
19.4.6 Schwannoma  161
19.4.7 Extramural Compression  161
19.4.8 Pneumatosis Cystoides Intestinalis  161

19.5 Conclusion  165

References  165

## 19.1 Introduction

The diagnosis of carcinoid and submucosal tumors by endoscopy or barium contrast studies is not easy since these tumors are usually covered with a normal mucosal layer. To determine the main portion of the wall stratification in the gastrointestinal wall in which the tumors lie is the most important part of diagnostic imaging of submucosal tumors. For this purpose, endoscopic ultrasound (EUS), including the use of an EUS-guided fine-needle aspiration biopsy (FNA), is the best choice (Arantes et al. 2004; Vandernoot et

J. Hata, MD
Department of Clinical Pathology and Laboratory Medicine, Kawasaki Medical School, 577, Matsushima, Kurashiki-city, Okayama, 701-0192, Japan
K. Haruma, MD; N. Manabe, MD; T. Kamada, MD;
H. Kusunoki, MD; T. Tanaka, MD; M. Sato, MD
Division of Gastroenterology, Dept. of Internal Medicine, Kawasaki Medical School, 577, Matsushima, Kurashiki-city, Okayama, 701-0192, Japan

al. 2004); however, not all institutions have the equipment or experienced staff to easily perform EUS in all cases with submucosal tumors. Transabdominal ultrasound, with the remarkable improvement of equipment, can be used as an alternative method (Polkowski et al. 2002; Futagami et al. 2001; Tsai et al. 2000). There have been several reports on transabdominal ultrasound as an acceptable alternative for the diagnosis of submucosal tumors. In this chapter, the sonographic images of carcinoid and submucosal tumors are discussed.

## 19.2 Preparations for Sonographic Assessment of Submucosal Tumors

For the evaluation of gastroduodenal lesions, an overnight fast and the ingestion of water (200–400 ml) are useful. However, for the small bowel lesions, such preparations are not so advantageous for better visualization; therefore, intestinal lesions, especially when they are small in size, are not easy to detect with transabdominal ultrasound. The retrograde water filling method is effective for the assessment of colonic lesions, but it requires total clearance of colonic contents before the examination, which makes its routine use difficult.

## 19.3 Carcinoid Tumor

Since carcinoid tumors usually originate in the deep mucosa, they appear as a focal mass with a clear margin and smooth contour located in the second layer (Figs. 19.1, 19.2). The echogenicity of the tumor is homogenous and relatively low compared with that

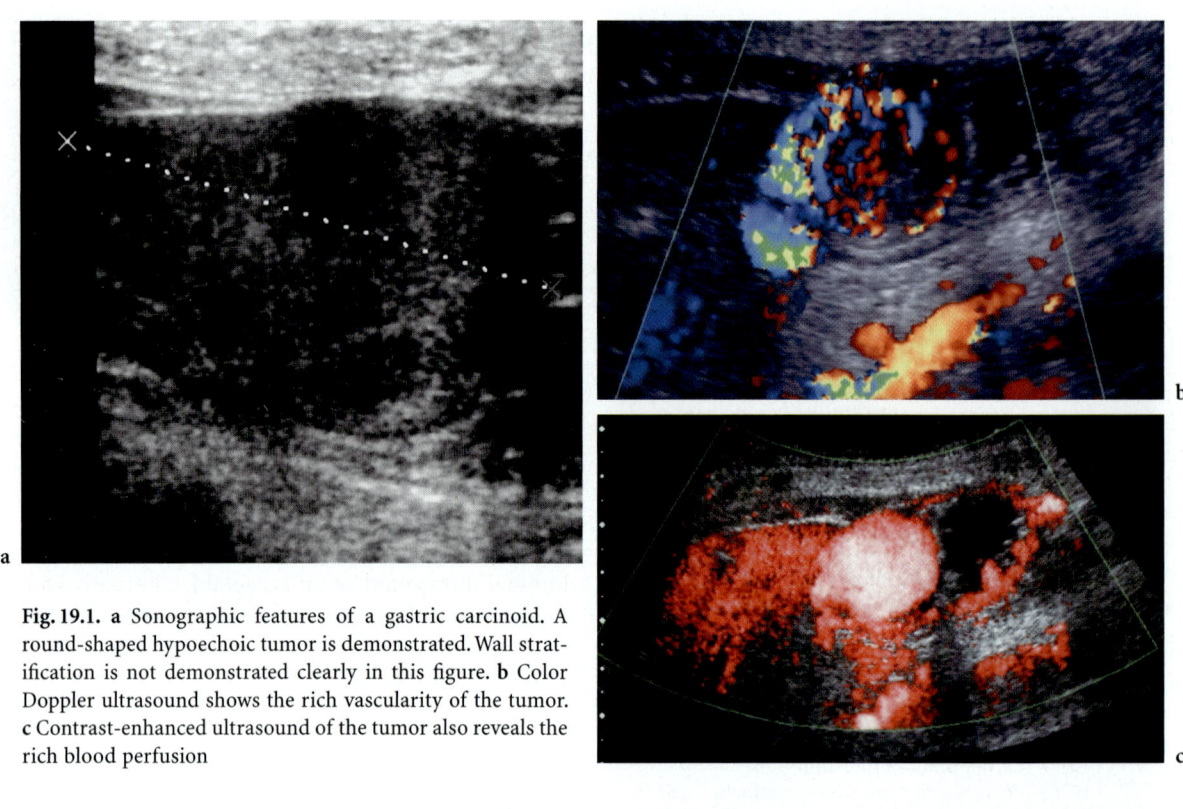

**Fig. 19.1. a** Sonographic features of a gastric carcinoid. A round-shaped hypoechoic tumor is demonstrated. Wall stratification is not demonstrated clearly in this figure. **b** Color Doppler ultrasound shows the rich vascularity of the tumor. **c** Contrast-enhanced ultrasound of the tumor also reveals the rich blood perfusion

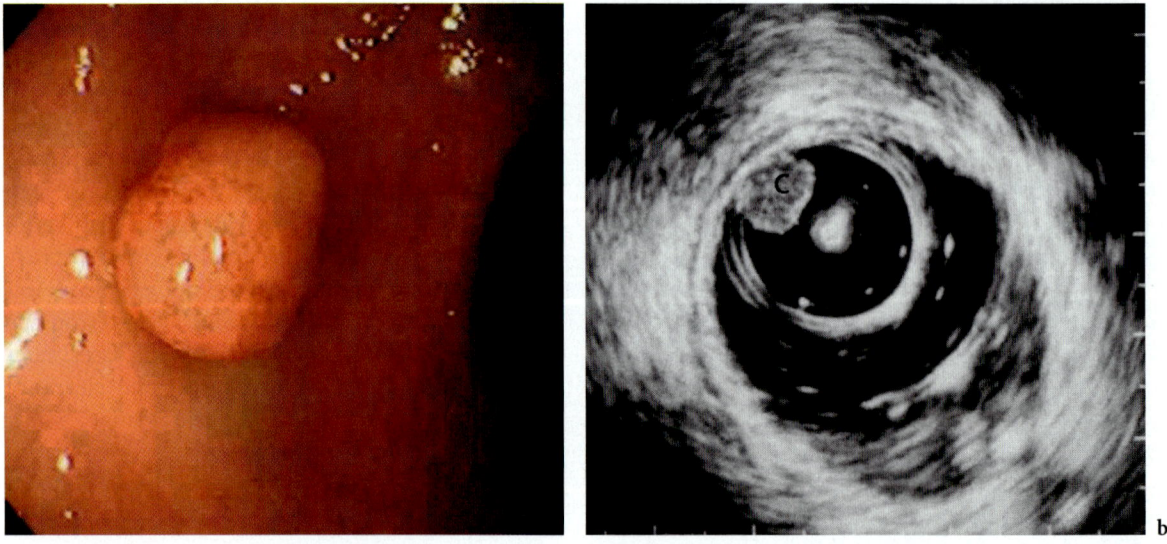

**Fig. 19.2. a** Endoscopic feature of rectal carcinoid. A small (5 mm in diameter) submucosal tumor is demonstrated. **b** Endosonography with a miniature ultrasound probe (12 MHz). A small round-shaped tumor (*C*) is demonstrated beneath the first layer and no changes in submucosal layer are seen

of the surrounding mucosal layer. As the gastrointestinal wall is invaded more deeply by the tumor, the stratification of the wall is deformed, and it is finally destroyed when the tumor grows transmurally. Even with endoscopic ultrasound, the differentiation of a carcinoid tumor from a myogenic tumor arising from the muscularis mucosae or a granular cell tumor is often difficult.

## 19.4
## Submucosal Tumor

### 19.4.1
### Cyst and Lymphangioma

Cysts and lymphangiomas are located in the submucosal layer (Figs. 19.3, 19.4). They are well demarcated by a thin wall and are anechoic. Posterior echo enhancement as an artifact is a characteristic figure. They show good compressibility and change their shapes with external compression. Color Doppler does not reveal any vascular structure inside. Often septal structures are seen inside the tumor.

### 19.4.2
### Lipoma

Lipomas also lie in the submucosal layer (Fig. 19.5). They are very soft, and their shape can be changed easily by external compression or peristalsis. Their internal echoes are generally equivalent or slightly lower than those of the adjacent submucosal layer. Vascular signals are seldom detected with color Doppler. Usually no changes are seen in the mucosal and proper muscle layers.

### 19.4.3
### Ectopic Pancreas

An ectopic pancreas is characterized as a hypoechoic tumor located mainly in the submucosal layer with thickening of the adjacent proper muscle layer (Fig. 19.6). A tiny cystic area representing the ductal structure may be demonstrated.

### 19.4.4
### Hemangioma

A hemangioma is demonstrated as a hyperechoic tumor in the submucosal layer. Calcification is occasionally seen inside the tumor (Fig. 19.7). Since the blood flow of the capillaries making up the tumor is extremely slow, it is difficult to detect blood flow signals using the conventional color Doppler method.

### 19.4.5
### Gastrointestinal Stromal Tumor

Gastrointestinal stromal tumors (GISTs) are demonstrated as focal hypoechoic nodules originating in the proper muscle layer (Figs. 19.8, 19.9). They are usually well demarcated and round shaped. In accordance with the tumor growth, the internal echo tends to be more heterogenic with hyper/hypoechoic nodules inside representing the focal degeneration of the tumor. With color Doppler, rich vascular structures running toward the center of the tumor (centripetal) are visualized. Although there is a study showing that heterogenous echotexture, size >3 cm, and irregular margins are the risks for presence of malignancy (BRAND et al. 2002), it is not easy to decide the malignant potential of each GIST with ultrasound preoperatively (ROSCH et al. 2002). GISTs exceeding 5 cm in diameter generally require surgical resection following FNA.

### 19.4.6
### Schwannoma

A schwannoma usually lies in the proper muscle layer and is demonstrated as a well-demarcated round tumor with a smooth contour (Fig. 19.10). It is difficult to differentiate this tumor from GIST, since the main layer in which the tumor lies and the shape and echogenicity of both tumors are very similar.

### 19.4.7
### Extramural Compression

The most frequently encountered condition mimicking submucosal tumors is extramural compression. Diagnosis is achieved by demonstrating the normal five-layer structure in the elevated portion and the cause of compression, such as the adjacent spleen (Fig. 19.11).

### 19.4.8
### Pneumatosis Cystoides Intestinalis

Pneumatosis cystoides intestinalis is not actually a submucosal tumor, but the endoscopic features resemble those of a submucosal tumor. Endoscopic ultrasound shows an echogenic spot with a comet-tail artifact in the submucosal layer, which represents the air bubble (Fig. 19.12).

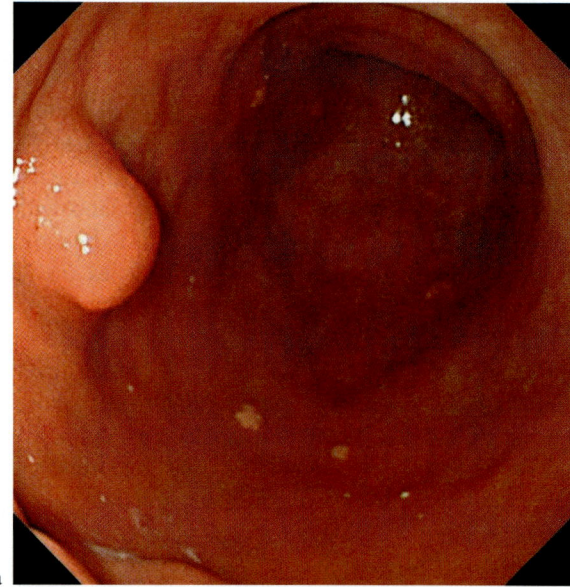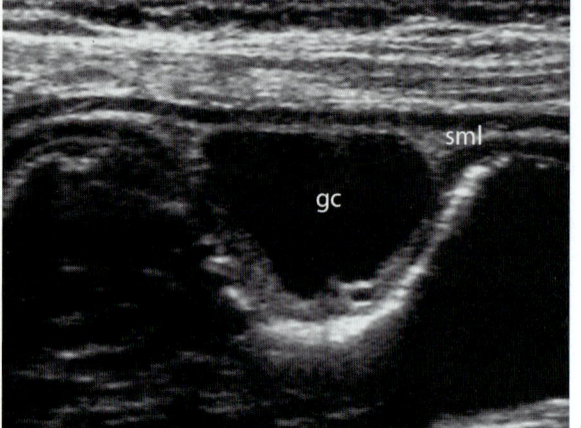

Fig. 19.3. a Endoscopy of a gastric cyst. The lesion is located in the anterior wall of the antrum and is covered with normal mucosa without indentation or erosion. b Sonography with a convex probe (3 MHz) of the gastric cyst (*gc*). A small anechoic lesion is demonstrated, although the main layer where it lies is not clear. c Scanning with a high-frequency linear probe (7 MHz) revealed that the lesion (*gc*) lies in the submucosal layer (*sml*). *S* stomach

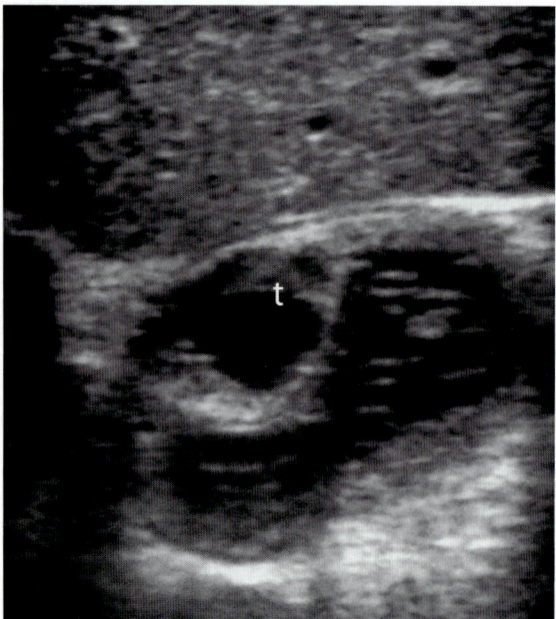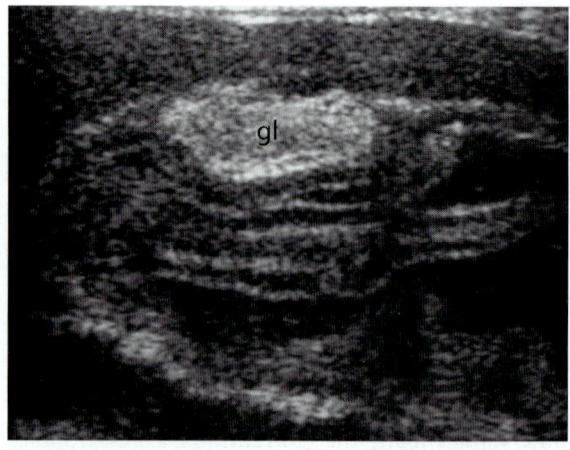

Fig. 19.4. Lymphangioma at the duodenal bulb. A cystic tumor (*t*) with septa is seen in the submucosal layer

Fig. 19.5. Sonographic feature of a gastric lipoma (*gl*). A hyperechoic tumor located in the submucosal layer is demonstrated

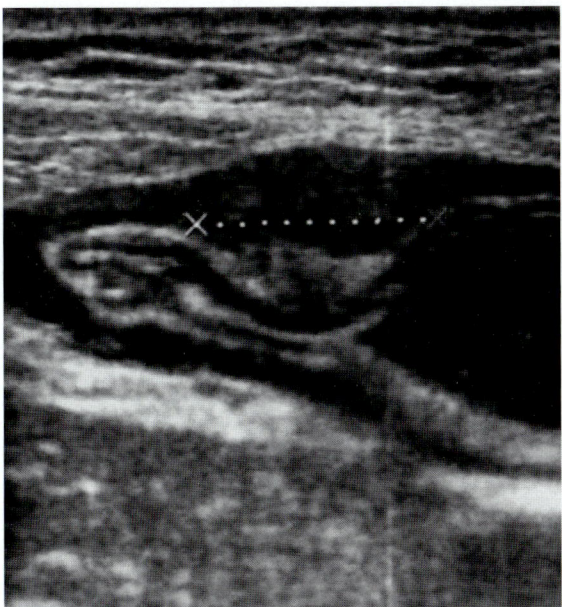

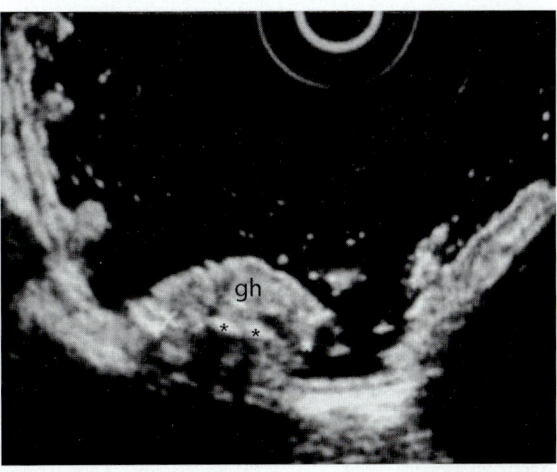

**Fig. 19.6.** Aberant pancreas. A hypoechoic tumor located mainly in the submucosal layer accompanied by focal thickening of the proper muscle layer is observed

**Fig. 19.7.** Endosopic ultrasound of a gastric hemangioma (*gh*). The tumor lies in the submucosal layer and calcifications inside the tumor are seen (*asterisks*)

**Fig. 19.8. a** Sonography of a gastrointestinal stromal tumor (GIST; *st*). A well-demarcated hypoechoic tumor is demonstrated. The tumor is strongly connected to the proper muscle layer (*ml*). **b** Color Doppler ultrasound shows the rich vascularity of the tumor (*st*)

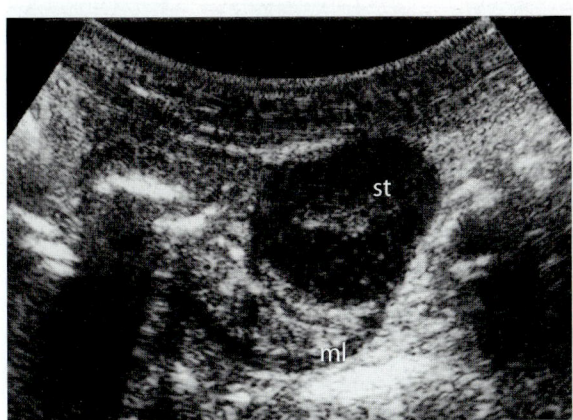

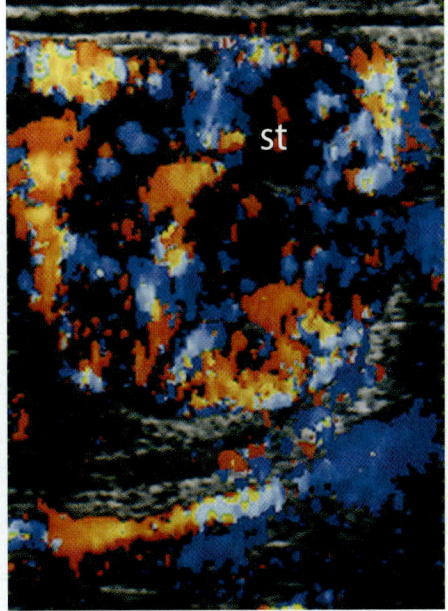

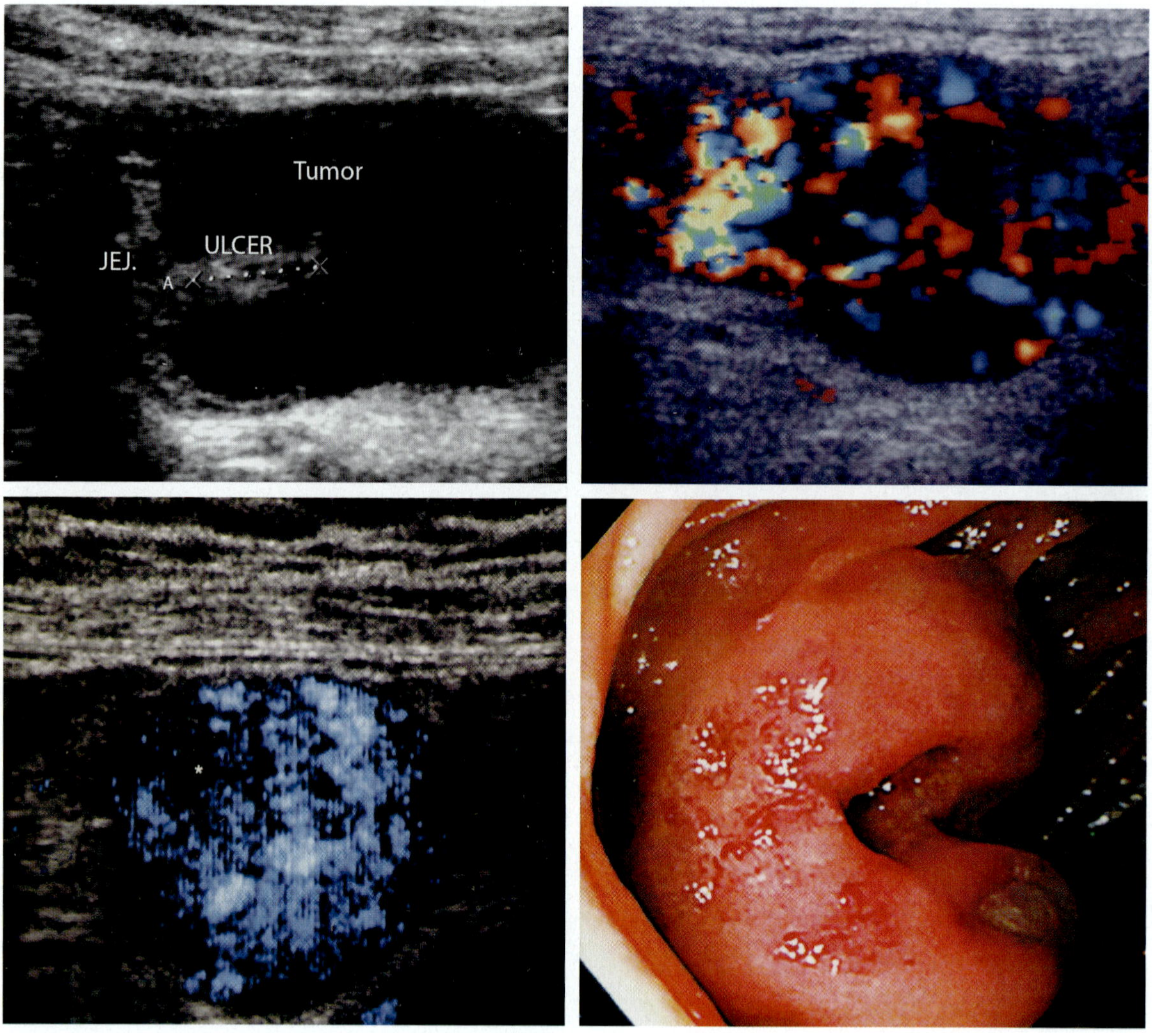

**Fig. 19.9. a** Sonography of the jejunal GIST. An oval-shaped tumor with a deep ulcer is demonstrated. The tumor is well demarcated and the contour of the tumor is smooth. **b** Color Doppler ultrasound of the tumor shows the rich vascularity. **c** Contrast-enhanced ultrasound reveals the rich perfusion with a focal perfusion defect inside the tumor (*asterisk*). **d** Endoscopic feature of the tumor. A submucosal tumor with a deep ulcer at the center is demonstrated

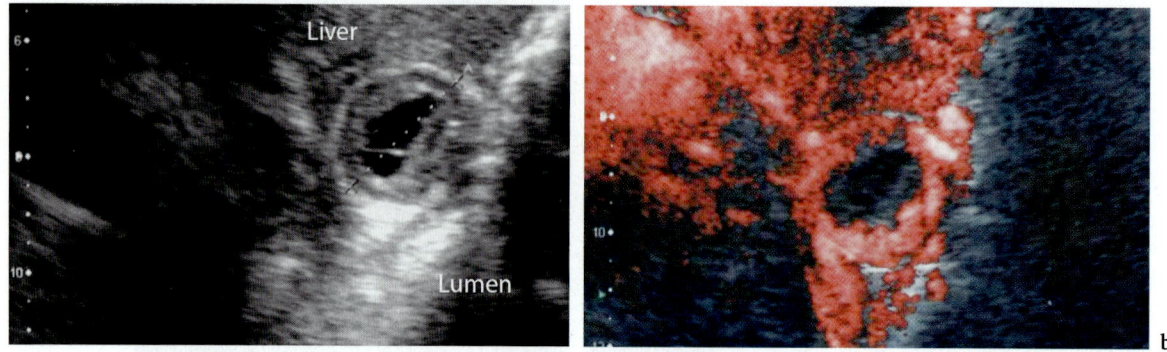

**Fig. 19.10. a** Sonography of a gastric schwannoma with massive central necrosis. A hypoechoic tumor with a cystic area inside is demonstrated at the anterior wall of the gastric body. **b** Contrast ultrasound reveals loss of perfusion in the cystic area

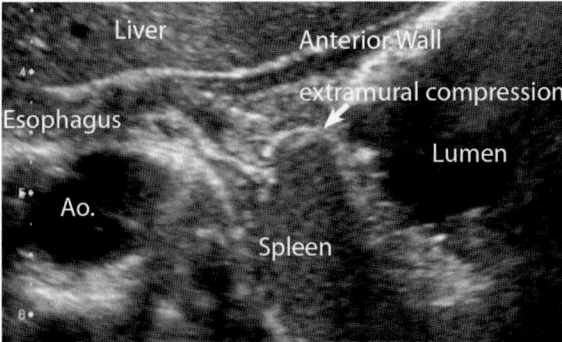
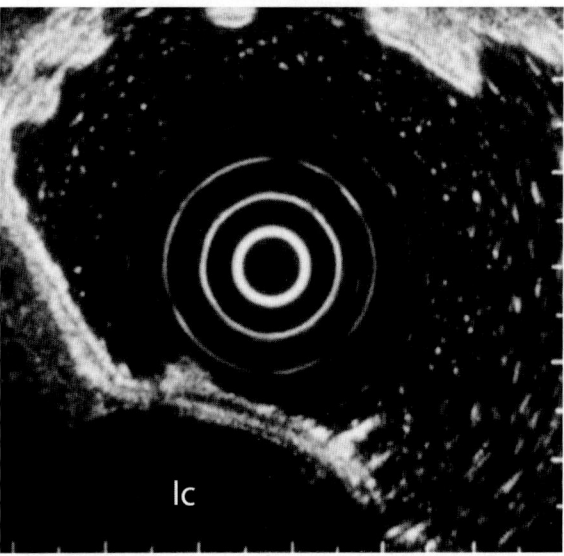

Fig. 19.11. a Extramural compression of the gastric wall by the spleen. An elevated area due to compression of spleen is shown. b Endosonographic feature of the extramural compression by a liver cyst (*lc*). The normal five-layer structure is observed at the elevated area. *Ao* aorta

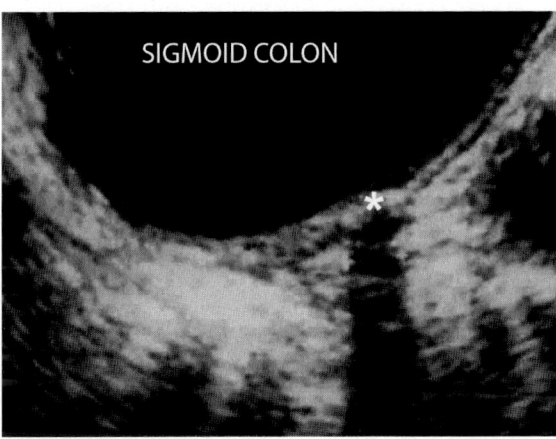

Fig. 19.12. Endosonographic feature of pneumatosis cystoides intestinalis. A strong echo (*asterisk*) with a comet-tail echo is demonstrated in the submucosal layer of the colon wall

## 19.5 Conclusion

Transabdominal ultrasonography can be a useful alternative modality to EUS in the assessment of carcinoid or submucosal tumors.

## References

Arantes V, Logrono R, Faruqi S et al (2004) Endoscopic sonographically guided fine-needle aspiration yield in submucosal tumors of the gastrointestinal tract. J Ultrasound Med 23:1141–1150

Brand B, Oesterhelweg L, Binmoeller KF et al (2002) Impact of endoscopic ultrasound for evaluation of submucosal lesions in gastrointestinal tract. Digest Liver Dis 34:290–297

Futagami K, Hata J, Haruma K et al (2001) Extracorporeal ultrasound is an effective diagnostic alternative to endoscopic ultrasound for gastric submucosal tumours. Scand J Gastroenterol 36:1222–1226

Polkowski M, Palucki J, Butruk E (2002) Transabdominal ultrasound for visualizing gastric submucosal tumors diagnosed by endosonography: Can surveillance be simplified? Endoscopy 34:979–983

Rosch T, Kapfer B, Will U et al (2002) Accuracy of endoscopic ultrasonography in upper gastrointestinal submucosal lesions: a prospective multicenter study. Scand J Gastroenterol 37:856–862

Tsai TL, Changchien CS, Hu TH et al (2000) Demonstration of gastric submucosal lesions by high-resolution transabdominal sonography. J Clin Ultrasound 28:125–132

Vander Noot MR III, Eloubeidi MA, Chen VK et al (2004) Diagnosis of gastrointestinal tract lesions by endoscopic ultrasound-guided fine-needle aspiration biopsy. Cancer 102:157–163

# Procedures
# and Technical Developments

# Intravenous Contrast-Enhanced Bowel Ultrasound

Doris Schacherer and Jürgen Schölmerich

CONTENTS

20.1 Introduction  169
20.2 Bowel Sonography (B-Mode, Doppler and Power Doppler Sonography)  169
20.2.1 Limitations of Colour and Power Doppler Sonography  170

20.3 Intravenous Contrast Agents  170
20.3.1 History  170
20.3.2 Types  171
20.3.2.1 SHU-563-A  172
20.3.3 Indications/Applications  172
20.3.4 Safety  173

20.4 Contrast Harmonic Imaging  173

20.5 Instrumentation Technology  174

20.6 Intravenous Contrast-Enhanced Bowel Sonography  174
20.6.1 General  174
20.6.2 Inflammatory Bowel Diseases  174
20.6.3 Bowel Ischaemia  176
20.6.4 Appendicitis  176
20.6.5 Other Indications  177

20.7 Future Prospects  178
References  178

## 20.1 Introduction

Several imaging methods are available to evaluate gastrointestinal tract disorders. With respect to sonography, important progress in equipment technology has improved its diagnostic capabilities in the last few years. Compared with other imaging modalities, ultrasound has multiple advantages; these include real-time imaging, relatively low costs, portability, wide availability, non-invasiveness and lack of ionizing radia-

tion. For these reasons, many patients with abdominal symptoms are referred for an ultrasound study as their initial diagnostic evaluation; however, optimal imaging by sonography is often limited by artefacts arising from gas in the stomach and the adjacent bowel. The sound beam is almost totally reflected at soft tissue–gas interfaces due to the marked differences in acoustic impedance and the high compressibility and low density of gas. As a consequence, the results of this examination are often inconclusive, leading to supplementary imaging by means of more expensive imaging modalities, such as computed tomography (CT) or magnetic resonance imaging (MRI).

In this chapter, we first describe the role of ultrasound in the case of gastrointestinal disorders. We then illustrate the historical development and different types of contrast agents and their advantages, limitations and applications with respect to bowel diseases.

## 20.2 Bowel Sonography (B-Mode, Doppler and Power Doppler Sonography)

Already in the 1970s, the grey-scale ultrasound examination was performed in patients with Crohn's disease (CD; Holt and Samuel 1979). At present, the principal tools for the diagnosis of inflammatory bowel disease are colonoscopy with multiple biopsies and radiological examinations; however, colonoscopy, barium enema and enteroclysis cannot assess the transmural extent of the inflammation or extraintestinal involvement of the disease, and CT is associated with a certain radiation dose. Consequently, a non-invasive test which avoids radiation, such as ultrasound, would be preferable. Brightness mode (B-mode) represents an early diagnostic tool for almost all entities of intestinal disease and is able to investigate the localization of intestinal disease, length of the intestinal segments involved, loss of

D. Schacherer, MD; J. Schölmerich, MD
Department of Internal Medicine I, University of Regensburg, Franz-Josef-Strauss-Allee 11, 93042 Regensburg, Germany

stratification, intestinal obstruction or stenoses and mesenterial changes, as well as associated complications such as abscesses, fistulas, perforation, ascites and stenoses. B-mode imaging is always a prerequisite for the useful application of Doppler and ultrasound contrast imaging techniques (SCHLOTTMANN et al. 2005b). In B-mode sonography, five layers of the normal bowel wall can be visualised by high-resolution sonography: superficial mucosa; deep mucosa; submucosa; muscularis propria; and serosa with serosal fat. If any pathology of the bowel is suspected, special attention should be paid to the distal ileum in the right iliac fossa and all areas of tenderness or localised pain. In experienced hands, B-mode sonography helps to assess wall thickening, free intraperitoneal fluid and mesenteric masses (phlegmon, abscess, lymph nodes).

According to data in literature, transabdominal ultrasonography has a high sensitivity (up to 85%) and specificity (95%) in the initial assessment of inflammatory bowel disorders, and has diagnostic values similar to those of CT (PARENTE et al. 2003; TARJAN et al. 2000). B-mode together with Doppler sonography can visualize transmural bowel inflammation in Crohn's disease, discriminate Crohn's disease from ulcerative colitis, determine the extent and anatomical location of lesions and detect complications such as strictures/stenoses, fistulas and absesses (TARJAN et al. 2000). Of stenoses, 90% documented by small bowel enema and subsequently confirmed at surgery are correctly diagnosed by the use of high-resolution ultrasound (PARENTE et al. 2002). In addition, the use of Doppler sonography has been shown to be able to discriminate between active and inactive disease by measuring the superior mesenteric artery blood flow (LUDWIG et al. 1999).

In general, the greatest advantages of combining power Doppler imaging and ultrasound contrast agents are the ability to better visualise smaller vessels, and vessel continuity (i.e., length; Table 20.1). The possibility to improve the visualisation of complex neovascularity is of particular importance in tumour diagnosis. Comparing colour Doppler imaging and power Doppler imaging in combination with ultrasound contrast agents, the latter improved visualisation both of normal and abnormal blood flow in 70% of all cases (GOLDBERG et al. 1996). Due to the fact that this mode is more susceptible to colour artefacts, it is not suitable for the evaluation of flow in structures with significant motion. Motion artefacts caused by peristalsis or heartbeat often disturb the measurement of Doppler signals, but such artefacts do not impair contrast-enhanced sonography at low mechanical index (MI).

### 20.2.1
### Limitations of Colour and Power Doppler Sonography

No objective parameters exist permitting definition of the type of echo structure or flow patterns (such as the Hounsfield scale in CT). The vascular flow signal is often too weak because of beam attenuation or signal absorption or distortion and power Doppler sonography fails to assess blood flow direction (Table 20.2).

Table 20.2. Characteristics of power Doppler sonography. (From FORSBERG and GOLDBERG 1997)

| Advantages | Disadvantages |
| --- | --- |
| Increases display dynamic range (increased sensitivity) | Susceptible to tissue motion artefacts |
| No multiple-angle artefact | No direction information |
| No aliasing | No velocity information |
| Limited angle dependence | Limited temporal resolution |
| Better functional lumen/vessel wall definition | |

## 20.3
## Intravenous Contrast Agents

### 20.3.1
### History

Echocardiographers recognized by chance in the 1960s that the tiny air bubbles incidentally introduced into the circulation after intravenous injections produce transient echo enhancement in the right side of the heart. Such bubbles do not pass through the normal pulmonary circulation, but systemic enhancement

Table 20.1. Advantages of contrast-enhanced power Doppler ultrasound. (From SALLOMI 2003)

| |
| --- |
| High sensitivity and specificity in the detection and evaluation of inflammatory abdominal masses |
| Detection of small inflammatory abdominal masses of 1 cm and above is possible |
| Absence of radiation; repeated examinations are possible |

effects can be used to test for a right-to-left shunt (BLOMLEY and COSGROVE 1997).

The first microbubble agents were described by GRAMIAK and SHAH in 1968. They were discovered during the injection of indocyanine green as M-mode echocardiography was being developed. More precisely, their first encounter with the contrast phenomenon came in late April 1967 in the cardiac catheterization laboratory during study of a patient with aortic regurgitation. Contrast injections were decisive in identifying the walls of the aortic root, distinguishing it from the left ventricular outflow tract and detailing normal cusp motion. The resulting publication was the first report of the use of ultrasonic contrast agents (GRAMIAK and SHAH 1968). Serious attempts to develop intravenous contrast agents for ultrasound began in the late 1970s and early 1980s. It was subsequently surmised that bubbles were responsible for the contrast effect.

In the early 1980s, clinical echocardiography was performed with a sector scanner, a stand-alone Doppler unit capable of a pulsed and continuous-wave mode operation, a spectral analyser with high temporal resolution and an in-house "black box" which allowed EKG display along with the spectra (GRAMIAK and HOLEN 1984). Due to the fact that small gas bubbles dissolve rapidly in blood, the next aim was the production of agents small enough to traverse the pulmonary capillary bed.

SMITH et al. (1984) used a galactose-based contrast agent called SHU-454 (Echovist, Schering, Berlin, Germany), whereas successful transpulmonary delivery of microbubbles was achieved by using an agent similar to SHU-454 with the addition of palmitic acid surfactant called SHU-508A (Levovist, Schering, Berlin, Germany; SMITH et al. 1989).

In the late 1980s, the systematic development of contrast media started. Nearly all of them consisted of gas bubbles, since gas has, for physical reasons, the optimum pre-requisites for an ultrasound contrast agent. Due to the high efficacy and low specific density of gas, only small amounts of a foreign substance have to be administered (OPHIR and PARKER 1989). To make the contrast-giving gas bubbles suitable for transpulmonary passage after intravenous injection, the bubbles were surrounded with a thin film to prevent dissolution of the bubbles in the blood stream. The material of the protective layer around the microbubble is, in most cases, a highly flexible structure which does not reduce the acoustic response by limiting the oscillation of the bubble. Transpulmonary passage was now possible and, therefore, the arterial part of the vascular system could be assessed. For imaging of different organs, contrast agents which are concentrated in organs were necessary; therefore, there was a need for agents which can survive cellular uptake without losing their acoustic properties.

Although backscatter is highly dependent on bubble size, microbubbles must have a limited size range. If the bubble is too small, it will be short-lived (i.e., it will collapse under cardiac and systemic pressures). If the bubble is too large (>10 μm), the pulmonary capillaries will trap it or the bubbles may transiently obstruct the capillaries and act as gas emboli; therefore, microbubble size is limited from 1 to 5 μm in diameter. At present, all microbubble contrast agents which have been developed for ultrasound are small, gas-filled microbubbles, about 3 μm in size, and all commercial ultrasound contrast media for human applications are encapsulated microbubbles. So, microbubbles are too large to escape the capillaries and, contrary to most X-ray and MRI contrast media, which are rapidly distributed to the extravascular, extracellular space, most microbubbles are confined to the vascular bed. The increase in Doppler signal intensity they produce is linearly proportional to relative microbubble concentration.

## 20.3.2
## Types

Levovist (Schering, Berlin, Germany) is an agent like those described above, made of galactose microparticles and palmitic acid. The microparticles adsorb the gas dissolved in the water, forming micrometre-sized air bubbles that remain stable for several minutes, thanks to the palmitic acid additive. After transit through the pulmonary circulation, the bubbles reach the systemic circulation where they enhance the backscattering of signals from blood vessels (BOUAKAZ et al. 1998).

The main mechanisms for signal enhancement are backscattering, bubble resonance and bubble rupture. These mechanisms are highly dependent on the acoustic power of the transmitted ultrasound, which is reflected by the MI. Backscattering means that ultrasound is reflected whenever there is a change in acoustic impedance. The larger the change, the more ultrasound is reflected. Bubble resonance means that at intermediate acoustic power (MI between 0.1 and 0.5) gas microbubbles may show strong oscillatory motion, provided the frequency of the ultrasound beam is close to the resonant frequency of the microbubbles. Small bubbles (<5 μm) will have resonance frequencies in the frequency range used in medical ultrasound imaging. The bubbles are more easily expanded than compressed, and this non-linear behaviour creates harmonics, which are exploited in non-linear imaging. At a mechanical index >0.5, the microbubble resonance frequency will cause the bubbles to rupture.

In summary, microbubbles work by resonating in an ultrasound beam, rapidly contracting and expanding in response to the pressure changes of the sound wave. By coincidence, they vibrate particularly strongly at the high frequencies used for diagnostic ultrasound imaging. This makes them several thousand times more reflective than normal body tissues. In this way, they enhance both grey-scale images and Doppler signals (by raising the intensity of weak signals to a detectable level; BLOMLEY et al. 2001).

### 20.3.2.1
### SHU-563-A

With SHU-563-A microbubbles are protected by a biodegradable polymeric shell. Polybutyl-2-cyanoacrylate was the material to build up the shell of the microparticles. Although the polymer membrane has only a thickness of approximately 100 ηm, it is stable enough to protect the enclosed gas bubble from dissolution in the blood stream, and also allows the particle to be phagocytosed; however, the shell is thin and elastic enough to oscillate in the ultrasound field. The vascular phase can be used for imaging of venous and arterial vascular systems as well as tumour vascularization and organ perfusion. This can be done using conventional B-mode or Doppler techniques.

SonoVue (Bracco, Milan, Italy) is a second-generation ultrasound contrast agent. It contains sulphur hexafluoride (SF6), a gas with low solubility in blood for the gaseous phase of the microbubbles, and of a phospholipidic monolayer for the shell. Due to the high flexibility of the shell, the microbubbles are strongly echogenic in a wide range of frequencies and acoustic pressure. The mean microbubble diameter is 2.5 μm. The concentration of the microbubbles is between 100 and 500 million per millilitre. Contrast agents of the second generation, e.g. SonoVue, are of diagnostic value even at very low transmission power (MI<0.3) because of their physical behaviour during insonation. The high molecular weight gas with low solubility in water was selected since laboratory tests showed that it confers to the bubbles a good resistance to pressure changes such as those that occur in the left ventricle, in the pulmonary capillaries, or in the coronary circulation (SCHNEIDER 1999); therefore, continuous real-time sonography can be performed without destruction of the microbubbles, which is a benefit for the dynamic analysis of contrast-enhancement in the early phase. The microbubbles circulate in vessels, crossing the pulmonary and systemic capillary circulation. During low-MI imaging, the SonoVue microbubbles have a much higher non-linear behaviour than native tissue, resulting in detectable echoes. Due to the long persistence of the microbubbles, SonoVue is also potentially useful in the assessment of myocardial perfusion, as well as microcirculatory disorders. Real-time observation of microbubbles allows the detection of all parts of the vascular system. Even single microbubbles slowly traversing tissue, which is indicative of the presence of capillaries, can be shown. In comparison with Levovist, SonoVue has the advantage that its microbubbles are stable against the ultrasound beam, which allows continuous real-time observation of microbubble signals (VON HERBAY et al. 2004). In contrast, analysis of Levovist enhancement has to be performed with the interval delay technique because the rupture of Levovist microbubbles does not allow real-time scanning.

### 20.3.3
### Indications/Applications

Levovist as an intravenous microbubble contrast agent is particularly useful in the detection of small vessel flow, especially in those areas in which Doppler sensitivity limits performance, including Doppler examinations, in which the signal-to-noise ratio determines detectability. Intravenous administration of Levovist is an effective method of markedly enhancing cardiac, femoral arterial and transcranial Doppler signal intensity (CAMPANI et al. 1998; MEAIRS et al. 2000), in the evaluation of breast tumours (DUDA et al. 1993), and in the detection of liver metastases (BLOMLEY et al. 1999). Concerning the role of microbubble contrast agents in cardiology, they help in assessing the left ventricular function, and they can estimate the ejection fraction, assess the wall motion and detect left ventricular thrombus. Emerging roles of microbubbles in cardiology include assessing myocardial perfusion (MULVAGH et al. 2000). Contrast agents represent a useful and safe method in the case of an insufficient native signal in transcranial Doppler investigation, where the skull greatly attenuates the ultrasound signal (RIES et al. 1993). Microbubbles can also be administered into body cavities, allowing simple functional tests to be performed. For example, vesicoureteric reflux in children can be revealed by injecting them into the bladder cavity and scanning the kidneys and ureters (DARGE et al. 1999). Colour-mode sonography can show the angioarchitecture of superficial lymph nodes to detect vessel abnormalities, a possible feature of malignancy. Although more intranodal flow patterns can be detected in such lymph nodes with contrast-enhanced sonography, the use of these agents does not improve the diagnostic accuracy in identifying malignant lymph nodes (SCHULTE-ALTEDORNEBURG et al. 2003). Contrast-enhanced sonography is used in several other clinical settings, to the point of assessing ophthalmic tumour perfusion (SCHLOTTMANN et al. 2005a).

Perhaps the most promising clinical application of contrast-enhanced sonography is the imaging of the liver. The main practical importance is that many focal liver lesions, particularly metastases and hepatocellular carcinoma, appear as defects. Scanning in pulse-inversion mode after Levovist improves the detection of liver metastases and reveals more lesions of smaller size than conventional ultrasonography and computed tomography (HARVEY et al. 2000). The method seems particularly useful in detecting small lesions (<1 cm diameter), for which all imaging methods lack sensitivity. Contrast agents may also increase specificity in liver imaging since some lesions can be characterized by their enhancement patterns. Because the bubbles are destroyed by ultrasound, e.g. liver enhancement lasts for one or two frames as the transducer is swept across the bubble-filled liver. Because space-occupying lesions lack sinusoids and reticulo-endothelial cells, they appear hypoechoic relative to the enhanced background of the liver. Even biopsies of liver lesions under real-time continuous contrast harmonic imaging at low MI are feasible (SCHLOTTMANN et al. 2004); however, one limitation of this imaging modality is the difficulty in accessing the whole liver.

Concerning the bowel wall, contrast enhancement of defined layers of the wall can be shown even though B-mode visualization of small vessels in the bowel wall is impossible. The more or less homogenous enhancement of particular layers will increase with the level of hyperperfusion of the intestinal wall (SCHLOTTMANN et al. 2005b).

In general, the non-linear harmonic echoes generated by the SHU-508 bubbles are visualised at high transmit power. This high-MI technique is used more widely to analyse tissue perfusion and hepatic metastases rather than perfusion of visceral vessels (SCHLOTTMANN et al. 2005b).

Using the contrast agent SonoVue, the microbubbles act as reflectors for the ultrasound beam enhancing backscatter beam. The agents remain in the circulation and, according to the perfusion phase (arterial, capillary, portal venous), lead to enhancement of different structures. This imaging modality allows an analysis of tumour perfusion under real-time conditions.

### 20.3.4
### Safety

Injecting a gas into the circulation may seem potentially hazardous, but extensive clinical experience has shown that the tiny volume of the air or gas given (<200 µl) is not dangerous, and the safety of microbubbles compares well with that of conventional agents in radiography and MRI (NANDA and CARSTENSEN 1997). At the moment, the use of SonoVue is not permitted in mechanically ventilated intensive care unit patients and in patients with heart failure, right-to-left shunts of the heart, uncontrolled hypertension and adult respiratory distress syndrome.

## 20.4
## Contrast Harmonic Imaging

The observation that insonation of microbubbles induces non-linear harmonic echoes caused by the oscillation or disruption of the microbubbles was followed by the development of imaging techniques which visualised the non-linear harmonic signals of bubble oscillation and disruption (contrast harmonic imaging). Contrast harmonic imaging utilizes the non-linear properties of contrast agents by transmitting at the fundamental frequency but receiving at the second harmonic. The advantage of this processing scheme lies in the difference in backscattering for tissue and contrast agent at two frequencies. The extent of the backscattered contrast-enhanced signal at the harmonic frequency is much greater than that of the tissue. This technology works in grey-scale imaging as well as in Doppler sonography. The harmonic response of the agent is strong and, in combination with the high stability of the microparticles, blood flow in small vessels can be directly visualised. This method is not influenced by attenuation.

## 20.5
## Instrumentation Technology

The other area of significant expansion in this field was brought by the instrumentation technology, where specific pulsing and post-processing techniques have been developed to take advantage of the presence of microbubbles in the circulation.

Pulse inversion sonography (also called second harmonic) is a technique that works by sending two separate pulses, 180° out of phase, and summing the reflected echoes to form the final sonographic signal.

Increasingly sophisticated, broadband or multiple focusing transducers also play an important role. Contrast-enhanced sonography can be performed not only with 3.5-MHz transducers usually used in abdominal ultrasound, but also with 5- to 12-MHz transducers which offer a higher spatial resolution.

## 20.6
## Intravenous Contrast-Enhanced Bowel Sonography

### 20.6.1
### General

In general, the major indication for organ imaging with contrast agents is the enhancement of perfused tissues, which allows the detection of perfusion defects or alterations in perfusion.

### 20.6.2
### Inflammatory Bowel Diseases

Crohn's disease (CD) manifests with highly variable signs and symptoms, and the assessment of the status of the disease, in the single patient, can be difficult. Being a chronic inflammatory bowel disease, it is characterized by an inflammatory process that involves the full thickness of the bowel wall, including the mesentery and the lymph nodes. Many clinical and laboratory parameters have been proposed to indicate disease activity; however, none of these indices can provide a fully reliable assessment of disease status. As mentioned above, in recent years, transabdominal bowel sonography has become increasingly important as a reliable and non-invasive tool in the diagnosis and follow-up of patients with CD. Ultrasonography is able to diagnose and locate transmural bowel inflammation in CD, discriminate it from ulcerative colitis (UC) and detect complications such as fistulas, strictures and abscesses; however, small intraperitoneal abscesses may remain unidentified (KOLKMAN et al. 1996). Nevertheless, the early detection of intestinal complications in CD is probably one of the most important aspects of the management of these patients. The detection of such complications in the initial stages of disease allows effective medical therapy to control their progression, thus avoiding surgical treatment in some cases.

Intestinal hyperaemia is a sign of active disease in the inflamed intestine, which can be detected by Doppler sonography. Tissue motion artefacts (peristalsis) sometimes make the assessment difficult, but visualisation of vessels by using contrast harmonic imaging at a low MI is not restricted by peristalsis (Fig. 20.1).

Few studies have been performed to detect bowel wall hyperaemia in inflammatory bowel disease. Contrast harmonic imaging at a low MI is technically feasible for the demonstration of increased intestinal perfusion in inflammatory bowel disease by using high-frequency ultrasound transducers (PLIKAT et al. 2004). One of the conclusions of a study by RAPACCINI et al. (2004) was that intestinal loops with thickened walls should be subjected to colour power Doppler sonography, and if intramural flow signals are absent, the examination should be repeated with echo enhancement since the presence of colour flow signals shows good agreement with clinical and laboratory indices of active disease. In patients with active disease, power Doppler signals emerged in the intestinal wall. In other words, the utilization of echo-enhancer media improves the diagnostic sensitivity of intestinal wall power Doppler scan (Table 20.3).

ROBOTTI et al. (2004) evaluated intestinal wall vascularisation in 52 patients with CD after intravenous injection of SonoVue and compared their results with those from clinical and laboratory tests and follow-up. They demonstrated that the US examination was most useful in the follow-up of the affected patients. The results of DI SABATINO et al. (2002) demonstrate that the use of a bubble-disrupting mode in the diagnosis of CD can increase the sonographic sensitivity from 70.9 to 96.7% (Table 20.4). Moreover, Doppler signal enhancement after Levovist injection seems to be indicative of subclinical ongoing disease activity

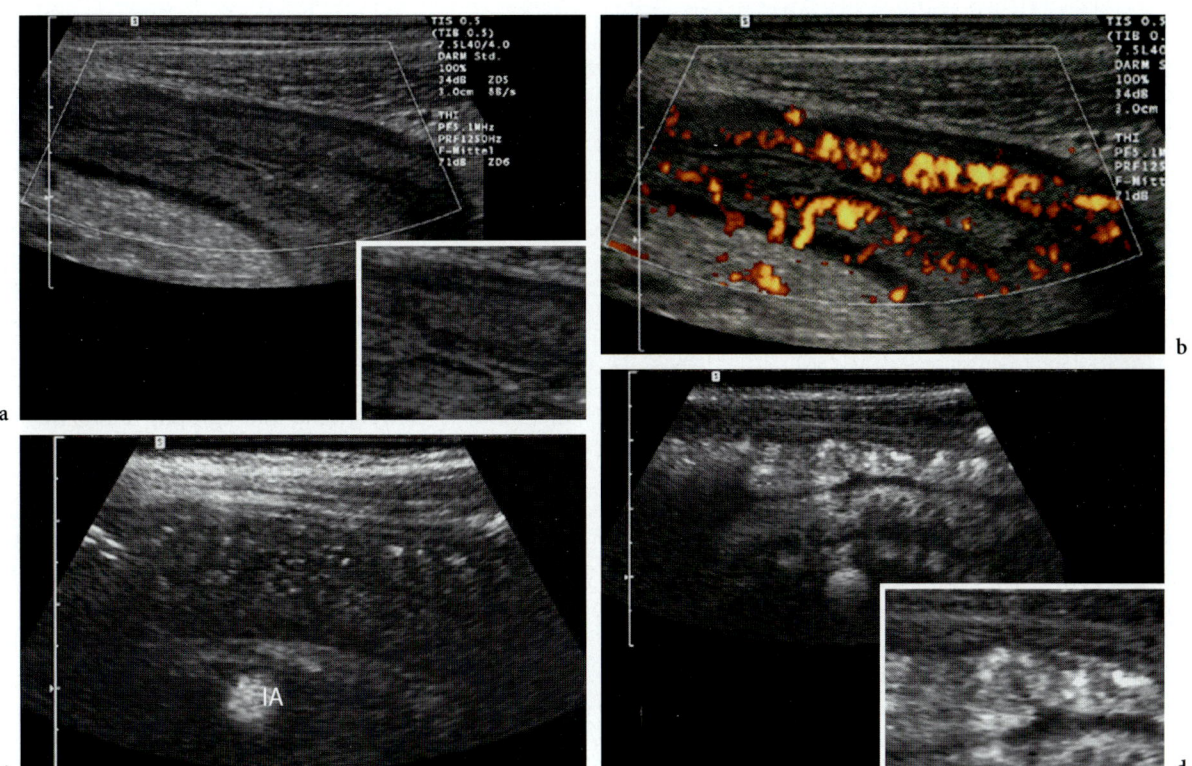

Fig. 20.1a–d. Sigmoid colon of a patient with ulcerative colitis. In B-mode sonography, three different layers of the muscularis propria, including the outer and inner muscle layer, as well as a separating layer, are discernible. a The adjacent prominent submucosal layer is thickened. b Power Doppler sonography shows a massive hyperaemia of the colon wall, with a maximum within the submucosal layer. c Fifteen seconds after injection of SonoVue: contrast enhancement with microbubbles visible mainly in the iliac artery (*IA*) as well as in the bowel wall. The different bowel layers cannot be demarcated at a mechanical index of 0.1. d Sixty seconds after injection of SonoVue: maximum of contrast enhancement in the submucosal layer (view magnification) and only faint perfusion of the muscularis propria (From SCHACHERER and SCHLOTTMANN 2005)

Table 20.3. Characteristics of patient subgroups with active and quiescent Crohn's disease. (From RAPACCINI et al. 2004)

|  | Quiescent disease | Active disease | Significance (p) |
|---|---|---|---|
| No. of patients | 26 | 22 | – |
| Intestinal wall thickness[a] | 6.8±1.3 mm | 7.5±1.3 mm | 0.11 |
| SMA RI[b] | 0.83±0.02 | 0.81±0.01 | 0.001 |
| Intramural flow signals in affected intestinal loops (power Doppler sonography) | 5 of 26 (20%) | 11 of 22 (50%) | 0.052 |
| Intramural flow signals in affected intestinal loops (contrast-enhanced power Doppler sonography) | 8 of 26 (31%) | 22 of 22 (100%) | <0.001 |

[a] Maximal thickness measured in affected loops on B-mode sonography
[b] Resistance index of the superior mesenteric artery

with early relapse in patients with quiescent CD (DI SABATINO et al. 2002).

ESTEBAN et al. (2003) have demonstrated for the first time the usefulness of contrast agents in the detection and follow-up of inflammatory abdominal masses associated with CD. The use of power Doppler was combined with the intravenous administration of Levovist. The premise of this study was that the earlier abdominal masses are detected in CD patients, the greater is the chance of the patient

Table 20.4. Sensitivity and specificity of transabdominal bowel sonography (*TABS*), colour Doppler, and contrast-enhanced colour Doppler sonography (From DI SABATINO et al. 2002)

|  | Sensitivity (%) | Specificity (%) |
| --- | --- | --- |
| TABS | 70.9 | 95.0 |
| Colour Doppler | 45.1 | 100 |
| Contrast-enhanced colour Doppler | 74.1 | 100 |
| TABS + colour Doppler | 77.4 | 100 |
| TABS + contrast-enhanced colour Doppler | 96.7 | 100 |

responding to conservative treatment. Grey-scale, Doppler and pulse-wave ultrasound were undertaken with additional contrast-enhanced power Doppler examination. These findings were correlated with each other and with contrast-enhanced CT as the gold standard. After Levovist injection, all the lesions showed intense vascularization in the interior and/or the peripheral soft tissue. The use of a contrast-enhancing agent increased the number and intensity of the colour signals in those lesions with previously detected vascularity. It also produced colour signals in some lesions that had shown no detectable vascularity in the baseline examination, thus allowing the diagnosis of inflammatory masses in doubtful cases. The authors could show that contrast-enhanced power sonography more abdominal masses than CT (ESTEBAN et al. 2003).

KRATZER et al. (2002) investigated 11 patients with confirmed CD and sonographically visualized stenoses of small bowel. Contrast-enhanced power Doppler sonography was repeated after application of SHU-508 (Levovist). Semi-quantitative evaluation based on sonography indicated that the degree of vascularisation led to the presumptive diagnosis of either inflammatory or cicatricial intestinal obstruction. Sonographic diagnoses were compared with the findings of surgery and subsequent histological examination or with patients' response to conservative therapy. The authors concluded that contrast-enhanced power Doppler sonography appears to be effective in the recognition of predominantly cicatricial stenoses in patients with CD (KRATZER et al. 2002).

On the one hand, the accurate and early detection of intestinal complications is a major issue in the management of patients with CD. On the other hand, contrast-enhanced sonography in this context can be repeated at regular intervals, which allows the early detection of complications and the monitoring of patients' response to treatment.

## 20.6.3
### Bowel Ischaemia

To our knowledge, only one study has been performed that deals with contrast agents in patients with bowel ischaemia. In this study, by HATA et al. (2005), 51 patients with evidence of small bowel dilatation at conventional radiography underwent contrast-enhanced ultrasound with SHU-508. The authors demonstrated that this method is able to depict microperfusion of the gastrointestinal wall as a strong signal produced by the destruction of microbubbles. By pooling diminished and absent colour signals together as a diagnostic indicator of bowel ischaemia against normal colour signals, the sensitivity was 85% and the specificity was 100%. Although some limitations of this study exist (subjective assessment of colour signals without evaluation of interobserver agreement, small number of patients), this method constitutes a promising tool for the assessment of bowel ischaemia (HATA et al. 2005).

## 20.6.4
### Appendicitis

In grey-scale ultrasound, the normal appendix can be visualized as a blind-ending, tubular, compressible intestinal loop, continuous with the caecum with a diameter <6 mm. The normal appendix seldom shows Doppler signals, because normal appendiceal vessels are small and the blood flow in the vessels is slow. In acute appendicitis, the feeding vessels and the vessels in the periappendicular soft tissues enlarge due to inflammation, and the blood flow as well as appendix diameter increases. High-resolution real-time sonography with graded compression has shown a sensitivity up to of 89% and a specificity up to 95% in the diagnosis of acute appendicitis (JEFFREY et al. 1987; KEYZER et al. 2005).

INCESU et al. (2004) demonstrated that power Doppler sonography has a sensitivity of 74% and contrast-enhanced power Doppler US a sensitivity of 100%, respectively, in the diagnosis of acute appendicitis (Table 20.5). In their study, feeding vessels of all inflamed appendices were visible. They concluded that contrast-enhanced power Doppler sonography is a promising method in the diagnosis of acute appendicitis and determination of inflammation stage (INCESU et al. 2004).

Table 20.5. Power Doppler sonography (PD US) and contrast-enhanced power Doppler sonography (CEPD US) correlation in 50 patients with suspected appendicitis (%) (From INCESU et al. 2004)

| Parameter | PD US | CEPD US | Significance (p) |
|---|---|---|---|
| Sensitivity | 74 | 100 | <0.01 |
| Specificity | 93 | 93 | >0.05 |
| Accuracy | 80 | 98 | <0.05 |
| Positive predictive value | 96 | 97 | >0.05 |
| Negative predictive value | 61 | 100 | <0.05 |

## 20.6.5
## Other Indications

Acute graft-vs-host disease (aGvHD) of the gastrointestinal tract is one of the major complications after allogeneic haematopoietic cell transplantation. Symptoms include watery diarrhoea, intestinal bleeding, abdominal cramps and ileus. Bowel wall thickening in the ileocaecal region with poor wall stratification or colonic dilatation in bone marrow-transplanted patients, together with the clinical symptoms (nausea, vomiting, aversion to food, weight loss, discomfort in the upper abdomen), might differentiate between infectious bowel disease and aGvHD. High-resolution sonography and colour Doppler imaging proved to be useful tools for detecting acute bowel GvHD, even before clinical symptoms (KLEIN et al. 2001; GORG et al. 2005). No studies exist that evaluate the possible benefit of contrast-enhanced sonography in this context, but we show an example in Figure 20.2.

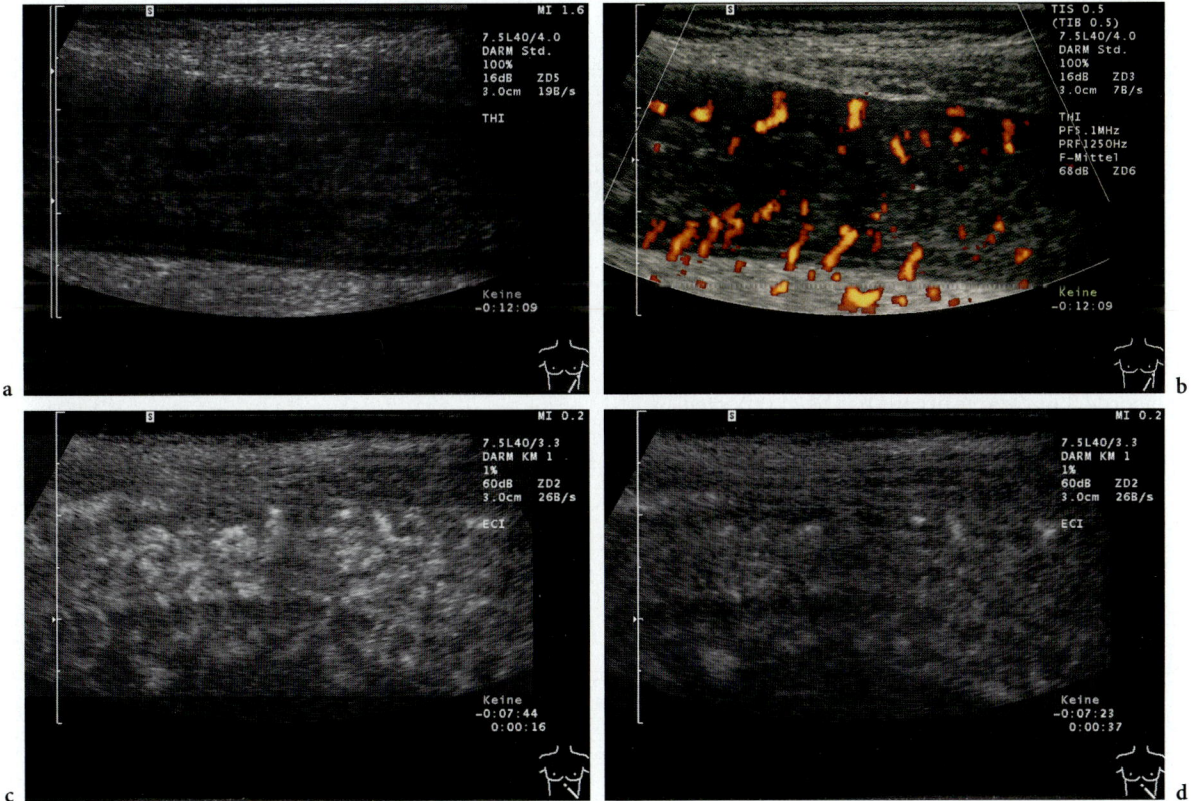

Fig. 20.2. Descending colon of a patient with acute graft-vs-host disease. a B-mode sonography shows increased motility and loss of bowel wall stratification. b Power Doppler sonography shows increased bowel wall perfusion. c Sixteen seconds and d 37 sec after injection of SonoVue: contrast enhancement with microbubbles mainly in the submucosal layer, which was formerly not detectable

## 20.7
## Future Prospects

In recent years, ultrasound has evolved into an easy-to-use imaging method in medicine and in the context of gastrointestinal disorders. Its record of success has grown over the years and the method became the most commonly used imaging modality at the end of the twentieth century. Bowel sonography is currently recommended as the primary imaging procedure in patients with acute and chronic bowel symptoms.

At present, contrast media is used in many applications of modern diagnostic imaging, regardless of which modality is used. Both CT and MRI have gone through the very same process, and contrast agents were first needed to improve the poor quality of morphological images. The same evolution can also be expected for US, given the premises and the high technological quality of present-day equipment. Finally, ultrasound contrast media may become as important for ultrasound in clinical practice as contrast media have been for CT and MRI. Due to recent advantages in sonographic equipment and the application of intravenous contrast agents, contrast-enhanced ultrasonography has been established as a new diagnostic imaging method. Its usefulness for evaluating haemodynamics in the diagnosis of gastrointestinal disorders in various organs has been reported.

It might be expected that improved ultrasound technology and less expensive ultrasound devices will help to spread the use of this technology and to reduce expensive and unnecessary CT and MRI examinations. The use of contrast agents opens totally new prospects within the foreseeable future, on the one hand, and represents a challenge for every sonographer, on the other.

At present, no data are available in the literature concerning contrast-enhanced sonography and infectious colitis, diverticulitis or bowel malignancies.

## References

Blomley M, Cosgrove D (1997) Microbubble echo-enhancers: a new direction for ultrasound? Lancet 349:1855–1856
Blomley MJ, Albrecht T, Cosgrove DO et al (1999) Improved imaging of liver metastases with stimulated acoustic emission in the late phase of enhancement with the US contrast agent SHU 508A: early experience. Radiology 210:409–416
Blomley MJ, Cooke JC, Unger EC et al (2001) Microbubble contrast agents: a new era in ultrasound. Br Med J 322:1222–1225
Bouakaz A, De Jong N, Cachard C (1998) Standard properties of ultrasound contrast agents. Ultrasound Med Biol 24:469–472
Campani R, Calliada F, Bottinelli O (1998) Contrast enhancing agents in ultrasonography: clinical applications. Eur J Radiol 27 (Suppl 2):161–170
Darge K, Troeger J, Duetting T et al (1999) Reflux in young patients: comparison of voiding US of the bladder and retrovesical space with echo enhancement versus voiding cystourethrography for diagnosis. Radiology 210:201–207
Di Sabatino A, Fulle I, Ciccocioppo R et al (2002) Doppler enhancement after intravenous Levovist injection in Crohn's disease. Inflamm Bowel Dis 8:251–257
Duda VF, Rode G, Schlief R (1993) Echocontrast agent enhanced color flow imaging of the breast. Ultrasound Obstet Gynecol 3:191–194
Esteban JM, Aleixandre A, Hurtado MJ et al (2003) Contrast-enhanced power Doppler ultrasound in the diagnosis and follow-up of inflammatory abdominal masses in Crohn's disease. Eur J Gastroenterol Hepatol 15:253–259
Forsberg F, Goldberg BB (1997) New imaging techniques with ultrasound contrast agents. In: Goldberg BB (ed) Ultrasound contrast agents. Martin Dunitz, London, pp 177–192
Goldberg BB, Merton DA, Forsberg F et al (1996) Color amplitude imaging: preliminary results using vascular sonographic contrast agents. J Ultrasound Med 15:127–134
Gorg C, Wollenberg B, Beyer J et al (2005) High-resolution ultrasonography in gastrointestinal graft-versus-host disease. Ann Hematol 84:33–39
Gramiak R, Holen J (1984) CW and pulsed Doppler echocardiography utilizing a stand-alone system. Ultrasound Med Biol 10:215–224
Gramiak R, Shah PM (1968) Echocardiography of the aortic root. Invest Radiol 3:356–366
Harvey CJ, Blomley MJ, Eckersley RJ et al (2000) Pulse-inversion mode imaging of liver specific microbubbles: improved detection of subcentimetre metastases. Lancet 355:807–808
Hata J, Kamada T, Haruma K et al (2005) Evaluation of bowel ischemia with contrast-enhanced US: initial experience. Radiology 236:712–715
Holt S, Samuel E (1979) Grey scale ultrasound in Crohn's disease. Gut 20:590–595
Incesu L, Yazicioglu AK, Selcuk MB et al (2004) Contrast-enhanced power Doppler US in the diagnosis of acute appendicitis. Eur J Radiol 50:201–209
Jeffrey RB Jr, Laing FC, Lewis FR (1987) Acute appendicitis: high-resolution real-time US findings. Radiology 163:11–14
Keyzer C, Zalcman M, De Maertelaer V et al (2005) Comparison of US and unenhanced multi-detector row CT in patients suspected of having acute appendicitis. Radiology 236:527–534
Klein SA, Martin H, Schreiber-Dietrich D et al (2001) A new approach to evaluating intestinal acute graft-versus-host

disease by transabdominal sonography and colour Doppler imaging. Br J Haematol 115:929–934

Kolkman JJ, Falke TH, Roos JC et al (1996) Computed tomography and granulocyte scintigraphy in active inflammatory bowel disease. Comparison with endoscopy and operative findings. Dig Dis Sci 41:641–650

Kratzer W, Tirpitz C von, Mason R et al (2002) Contrast-enhanced power Doppler sonography of the intestinal wall in the differentiation of hypervascularized and hypovascularized intestinal obstructions in patients with Crohn's disease. J Ultrasound Med 21:158–159

Ludwig D, Wiener S, Brüning A et al (1999) Mesenteric blood flow is related to disease activity and risk of relapse in Crohn's disease: a prospective follow-up study. Am J Gastroenterol 94:2942–2950

Meairs S, Daffertshofer M, Neff W et al (2000) Pulse-inversion contrast harmonic imaging: ultrasonographic assessment of cerebral perfusion. Lancet 355:550–551

Mulvagh SL, DeMaria AN, Feinstein SB et al (2000) Contrast echocardiography: current and future applications. J Am Soc Echocardiogr 13:331–342

Nanda NC, Carstensen C (1997) Echo-enhancing agents: safety. In: Nanda NC, Schlief R, Goldberg BB (eds) Advances in echo imaging using contrast enhancers. Kluwer, Dordrecht, pp 115–131

Ophir J, Parker KJ (1989) Contrast agents in diagnostic ultrasound. Ultrasound Med Biol 15:319–333

Parente F, Maconi G, Bollani S et al (2002) Bowel ultrasound in assessment of Crohn's disease and detection of related small bowel strictures: a prospective comparative study versus X-ray and intraoperative findings. Gut 50:490–495

Parente F, Greco S, Molteni M et al (2003) Role of early ultrasound in detecting inflammatory intestinal disorders and identifying their anatomical location within the bowel. Aliment Pharmacol Ther 18:1009–1016

Plikat K, Klebl F, Buchner C et al (2004) Evaluation of intestinal hyperaemia in inflamed bowel by high resolution contrast harmonic imaging (CHI). Ultraschall Med 25:257–262

Rapaccini GL, Pompili M, Orefice R et al (2004) Contrast-enhanced power Doppler of the intestinal wall in the evaluation of patients with Crohn's disease. Scand J Gastroenterol 39:188–194

Ries F, Honisch C, Lambertz M et al (1993) A transpulmonary contrast medium enhances the transcranial Doppler signal in humans. Stroke 24:1903–1909

Robotti D, Cammarota T, Debani P et al (2004) Activity of Crohn disease: value of Color-Power-Doppler and contrast-enhanced ultrasonography. Abdom Imaging 29:648–652

Sallomi DF (2003) The use of contrast-enhanced power Doppler ultrasound in the diagnosis and follow-up of inflammatory abdominal masses associated with Crohn's disease. Eur J Gastroenterol Hepatol 15:249–251

Schacherer D, Schlottmann K (2005) Darmwandsonographie: Indikation, Durchführung, Stellenwert im diagnostischen Konzept bei Darmerkrankungen. Gastroenterol Up2date 1:77–93

Schlottmann K, Klebl F, Zorger N et al (2004) Contrast-enhanced ultrasound allows for interventions of hepatic lesions which are invisible on conventional B-mode. Z Gastroenterol 42: 303–310

Schlottmann K, Fuchs-Koewel B, Demmler-Hackenberg M et al (2005a) High-frequency contrast-harmonic imaging of ophthalmic tumor perfusion. Am J Roentgenol 184:574–578

Schlottmann K, Kratzer W, Schoelmerich J (2005b) Doppler ultrasound and intravenous contrast agents in gastrointestinal tract disorders: current role and future implications. Eur J Gastroenterol Hepatol 17:263–275

Schneider M (1999) Characteristics of SonoVue (trademark). Echocardiography 16:743–746

Schulte-Altedorneburg G, Demharter J, Linné R et al (2003) Does ultrasound contrast agent improve the diagnostic value of colour and power Doppler sonography in superficial lymph node enlargement? Eur J Radiol 48:252–257

Smith MD, Elion JL, McClure RR et al (1984) Left heart opacification with peripheral venous injection of a new saccharide echo contrast agent in dogs. J Am Coll Cardiol 13:1622–1628

Smith MD, Kwan OL, Reiser HJ et al (1989) Superior intensity and reproducibility of SHU-454, a new right heart contrast agent. J Am Coll Cardiol 3:992–998

Tarjan Z, Toth G, Gyorke T et al (2000) Ultrasound in Crohn's disease of the small bowel. Eur J Radiol 35:176–182

von Herbay A, Vogt C, Willers R et al (2004) Real-time imaging with the sonographic contrast agent SonoVue: differentiation between benign and malignant hepatic lesions. J Ultrasound Med 23:1557–1568

# Oral Contrast-Enhanced Bowel Ultrasound

Giovanni Maconi, Salvatore Greco, and Gabriele Bianchi Porro

## CONTENTS

21.1 Introduction  181
21.2 Hydrosonography of the Stomach  181
21.3 Small Intestine Contrast Ultrasonography  182
21.4 Hydrocolonic Sonography  186
References  186

## 21.1
## Introduction

The major limitation of conventional trans-abdominal ultrasound (US) in evaluating the gastrointestinal tract is that it is difficult to achieve a detailed evaluation of the bowel wall structure and its changes due to the presence of air. In fact, luminal gas, in many instances, causes inadequate ultrasonographic imaging of the stomach, small intestine and, particularly, colon.

In the 1990s, it was suggested that it was possible to overcome this limitation and considerably improve ultrasonographic visualisation of the bowel wall of the stomach, small bowel and colon, by filling these organs with water or another echo-poor liquid. Therefore, hydrosonography of the stomach, small bowel or colon, in other words, ultrasonographic examination of the wall of these fluid-filled intestinal tracts, by oral administration or direct instillation of water or non-absorbable solution [i.e., polyethylene glycol (PEG) solution] into the intestinal lumen by a naso-jejunal or rectal probe, have been proposed.

## 21.2
## Hydrosonography of the Stomach

Since US examination of the stomach wall and duodenum may be compromised by artefacts due to the presence of gas, resulting in sub-optimal images, attempts at filling the stomach with water or liquids to reduce acoustic artefacts caused by intra-luminal gas, have been suggested.

Water, orange juice or methylcellulose and simethicone have been used (Lund et al. 1992; Worlicek et al. 1986, 1989). A clear advantage with the use of a specific contrast agent in the detection of bowel wall abnormalities has not been demonstrated. However, compared with water, the orally administered ultrasonographic contrast agents may improve visualisation of the bowel with a decrease in the gas artefact. In particular, cellulose and simethicone have been used to achieve a uniform low level intraluminal echogenicity and reduction of gas artefacts by displacement and absorption of intra-luminal gas since, while drinking water, more air may be ingested resulting in increased artefacts (Harisinghani et al. 1997; Lund et al 1992).

To achieve adequate visualisation of the gastric walls, a variable amount ranging from 500 to 1000 ml of the above-mentioned fluids, should be given to the fasting patient. Immediately prior to the examination, 20 mg of Hyoscine-N-butylscopolamine (Buscopan, Boehringer, Germany) could be injected intravenously to ensure appropriate relaxation of the gastric wall, reducing peristalsis and delaying gastric emptying.

---

G. Maconi, MD
S. Greco, MD
G. Bianchi Porro, MD, PhD
Chair of Gastroenterology, Department of Clinical Sciences, "L. Sacco" University Hospital, Via G.B. Grassi 74, 20157 Milan, Italy

In head-down (angle of inclination 20°) and left lateral position, the fundus and body of the stomach can be better examined. In head-up (angle of inclination 30–40°) left-lateral and supine position, the body and proximal antrum can be displayed, while in head-up right-lateral and standing position a better visualisation of the distal antrum and duodenum can be obtained.

The different parts of the stomach can be examined using a transducer operating at a frequency of 5–12 MHz, but for more distant areas of the fundus and cardia 3.5–5 MHz transducers can guarantee a greater depth of penetration and better visualisation.

While sonography and hydrosonography of the stomach may detect gastric cancer (Ch. 16), gastric submucosal tumours (Ch. 19) and gastroduodenal ulcers, it can not be used for routine assessment of the stomach in dyspeptic patients, endoscopy and endoscopic ultrasound being much more accurate diagnostic tools (Fig. 21.1).

However, when these investigations, for various reasons, can not be performed, or in the case of surveillance of submucosal lesions previously assessed by endoscopic ultrasound, it should not be forgotten that hydrosonography of the stomach can be an effective, cheap, non-invasive and simple alternative. In particular, hydrosonography of the stomach can be considered a valid alternative to endoscopic ultrasound for: (1) diagnosis (and follow-up) of extraluminal gastric compression, and (2) detection and surveillance of gastric submucosal tumours. In this regard, it has been shown that in endosonographically diagnosed gastric submucosal tumours, the lesion can also be visualised (and measured) using trans-abdominal ultrasound of the water-filled stomach in 69% of patients in a study by POLKOWSKI et al. (2002), and in 82.5% of cases, in another study by FUTAGAMI et al. (2001). In the latter study, approximately 95% of gastric submucosal tumours, >20 mm in diameter, were at least detected, and 97% of the lesions, >30 mm in diameter, were correctly diagnosed (FUTAGAMI et al. 2001).

## 21.3
## Small Intestine Contrast Ultrasonography

Like the stomach and duodenum, the small bowel can be easily visualised by trans-abdominal US when filled with water or echo-poor liquids. Water or contrast agents can be directly infused into the small bowel using a naso-jejunal tube by means of a peristaltic pump (FOLVIK et al. 1999) or administered orally (PALLOTTA et al. 1999a).

In both cases, the liquid contrast medium should be non-absorbable and non-fermentable. Isotonic anechoic electrolyte solution containing PEG, which is used for bowel cleansing prior to colonoscopy, is now considered the contrast medium of choice. The ingestion of a variable amount of PEG (up to 1000 ml; range 250–820 ml) provides an adequate distension of the intestinal loops, removes gas making sequential visualisation of the entire small bowel from the duodenum to terminal ileum easier and also allowing measurement of wall thickness and luminal diameter (PALLOTTA et al. 1999a,b, 2000) (Table 21.1).

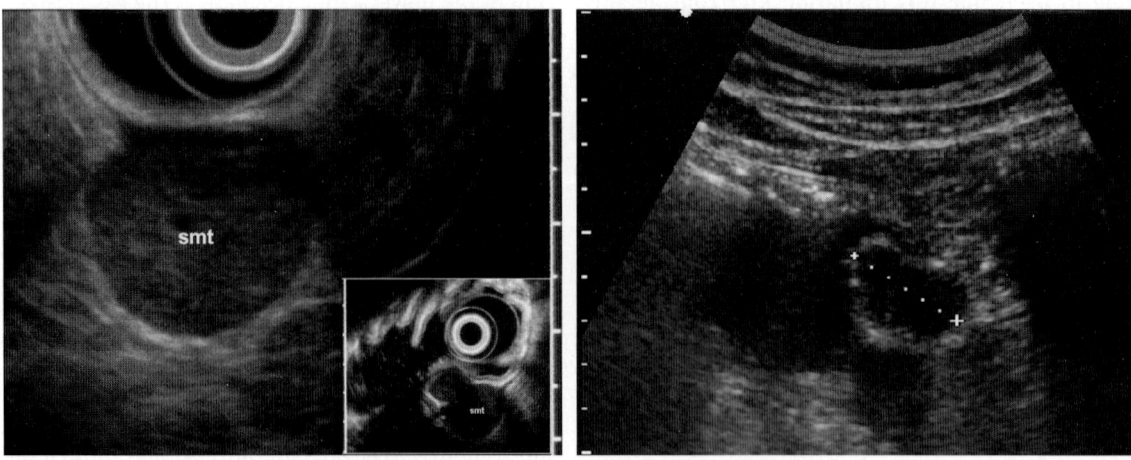

**Fig. 21.1a,b.** Large gastric submucosal tumour (*smt*) at endosonography (**a**) and gastric hydrosonography (**b**). Transabdominal US visualisation of the gastric lesion was possible only after filling the stomach with water

Table 21.1. Type and amount of ultrasonographic contrast media used in small bowel evaluation and duration of examination defined as time to image terminal ileum

| Author | Contrast medium | Amount (ml) Range (mean) | Time (min) to image terminal ileum Range (mean) |
|---|---|---|---|
| PALLOTTA et al. 1999a | PEG 4000 | 200–820 (558) | 17–65 (44) |
| CITTADINI et al. 2001 | PEG 4000 | 500 | 10–90 (31) |
| PALLOTTA et al. 2001 | PEG 4000 | 200–670 (388) | 12–90 (37) |
| PARENTE et al. 2004 | PEG 3350 | 500–800 (624) | 20–60 (31) |
| CALABRESE et al. 2005 | PEG 4000 | 250–500 (375) | 35–90 (40) |
| DELL'AQUILA et al. 2005 | PEG 4000 | 500–800 | 30–60 |
| PALLOTTA et al. 2005 | PEG 4000 | 200–500 (370) | 12–90 (39) |

PEG solutions used in the studies carried out, so far, comprise varying amounts of products such as MACRO-P (Promefarm, Milan, Italy) [containing per litre: PEG 4000 (Macrogol) 58.28 g as the active ingredient; $MgSO_4$ 7.5 g, $NaSO_4$ anhydrous 2.85 g, $NaHCO_3$ 1.69 g, NaCl 0.8 g and KCl 0.74 g and electrolytes] or Klean-Prep (Norgine, Milan, Italy) [containing per litre PEG 3350 59.0 g, anhydrous sodium sulphate 5.68 g, sodium bicarbonate 1.68 g, sodium chloride 1.46 g, and potassium chloride 0.74 g] or Isocolan (Bracco, Milan, Italy) which has a similar composition. Osmolarity of solutions is 280–290 mOsm/kg.

Sonographic assessment of the small bowel should be performed after overnight fasting using increasing amounts of contrast solution from 200 to 500 ml. After ingestion, the contrast solution passes from the stomach to the duodenum, jejunum and ileum, distending the intestinal loops. During the ultrasonographic examination, the morphological aspects of the bowel wall, such as thickening, echo pattern, *valvulae conniventes* and modality of contraction and relaxation, can be analysed (Fig. 21.2).

If distension and visualisation of the entire bowel up to the terminal ileum is not sufficient, further aliquots of contrast solution can be used. The amount of ingested US contrast agent does not seem to affect the luminal diameter or the wall thickness at any level of the small bowel in normal controls (PALLOTTA et al. 1999b).

Bowel examination can be performed immediately after ingestion of the US contrast solution since it is continuously delivered from the stomach into the duodenum and then progressively displaced aborally by peristalsis into the jejunal and ileal loops. Alternatively, it can be performed 10 min after PEG ingestion and then repeated at 10-min intervals until the con-

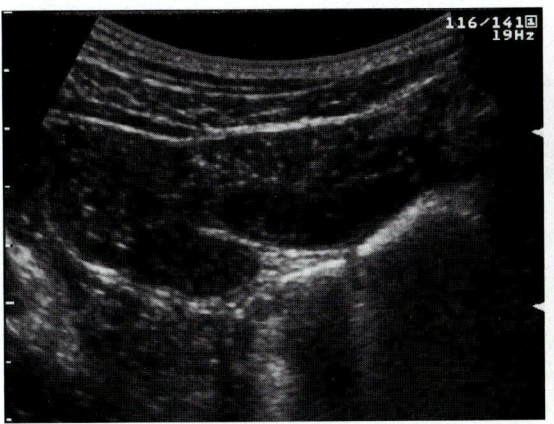 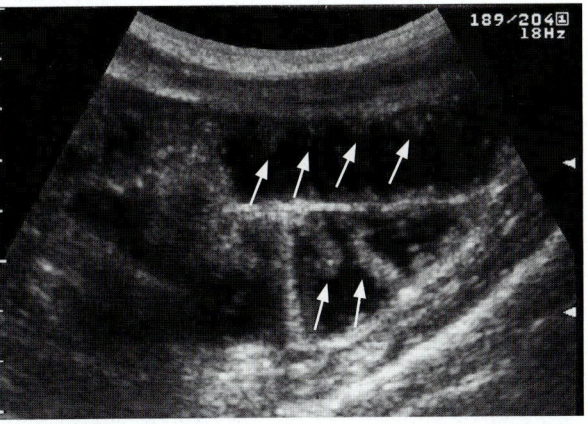

Fig. 21.2a,b. Real-time ultrasonography of small bowel in basal fasting condition (**a**) and following administration of 500 ml of oral contrast agent (**b**). After contrast ingestion, entire small bowel is distended and visualised, and bowel wall and Kerckring's folds may be well delineated (*arrows*)

trast can be seen to flow through the terminal ileum into the caecum.

The mean duration of the entire examination is just over 30 min. On account of the small amount of ingested contrast and palatability, the procedure is well-accepted, safe and tolerable in almost all patients. Indeed, in none of the studies have significant side-effects or major complaints been reported during or immediately after PEG ingestion, apart from one in which mild to moderate nausea was reported in 6.9% and slight abdominal distension in 3.9% of Crohn's disease patients (PARENTE et al. 2004). In this regard, particular caution should be taken in using PEG as contrast ultrasound agent in patients already presenting clear features of small bowel, partial or complete, occlusion at conventional trans-abdominal US. In these cases, as a safer oral contrast agent, variable amounts of tap water can also be used.

The use of oral contrast agents in ultrasonography for the evaluation of small intestine abnormalities has provided accurate results in most studies, showing a specificity ranging between 95.6% and 100%, and sensitivity ranging between 72% and 100%, depending on the underlying disease. In fact, accuracy seems to be greater when patients with Crohn's disease are well represented in the case series (Table 21.2).

In fact, the best results reported in the literature in the detection of small bowel abnormalities are for Crohn's disease patients (PALLOTTA et al. 2001, 2005; PARENTE et al. 2004). In these patients, small intestine contrast US has been shown to be comparable to small bowel X-ray in assessing the number, site and extension of small bowel lesions (Fig. 21.3).

The use of an oral contrast agent seems to offer a clear advantage compared to conventional transabdominal US in detecting proximal small bowel lesions (sensitivity: 80% vs 100%, respectively) and in assessing the number and site of small bowel stenoses in Crohn's disease patients (PARENTE et al. 2004; CALABRESE et al. 2005). As far as the detection of stenosis is concerned, two studies published to date have shown that small intestine contrast US may increase the sensitivity by 15%–18% vs trans-abdominal US in detecting patients with at least one stricture. These studies also showed that US with oral contrast agents has a greater mean sensitivity of 22.2% in detecting patients with at least two or more stenoses (sensitivity: 55.5%–77.7%) (PARENTE et al. 2004; CALABRESE et al. 2005). This advantage is presumably due to the fact that the contrast agent, by favouring the assessment of dilatation of prestenotic jejunal/ileal loops, permits better visualisation of the narrowed segment (Fig. 21.4).

It is worthwhile pointing out that two studies showed that oral contrast US may increase the accuracy in detecting small bowel lesions by inexpert sonologists, both in a consecutive, undiagnosed series of patients (CITTADINI et al. 2001) and, in particular, in Crohn's disease patients where accuracy may become comparable or better than that of an expert sonologist who uses trans-abdominal US (CALABRESE et al. 2005).

Oral contrast US may also be used as a reliable and non-invasive technique in the detection and follow-up of coeliac disease patients. Indeed, with these techniques, a clearer visualisation of ultrasono-

Table 21.2. Sensitivity and specificity of small bowel contrast ultrasonography compared with conventional transabdominal ultrasonography in detecting at least one small bowel lesion assessed by contrast radiology

| Author | Patients | | | Sensitivity | | Specificity | |
| --- | --- | --- | --- | --- | --- | --- | --- |
| | Total | With lesions | With CD | TUS | SICUS | TUS | SICUS |
| PALLOTTA et al. 1999a | 37 | 8 | 5 | n.e. | 100% | n.e. | 95.6% |
| CALABRESE et al. 2005 | 28 | 25 | 25 | 96% | 100% | n.e. | n.e. |
| CITTADINI et al. 2001 | 53 | 25 | 16 | n.e. | 72% | n.e. | 100% |
| PALLOTTA et al. 2001 | 53 | 17 | 8 | n.e. | 100% | n.e. | 97% |
| PARENTE et al. 2004 | 102 | 102 | 102 | 91.4% | 96.1% | n.e. | |
| PALLOTTA et al. 2005 | 91 | 35 | 16 | 57% | 94.3% | 100% | 98% |
| PALLOTTA et al. 2005 | 57 | 55 | 55 | 87.3% | 98.2% | n.e. | |

n.e., Not evaluated; TUS, transabdominal ultrasound; CD, Crohn's disease; SICUS, small intestine contrast ultrasound

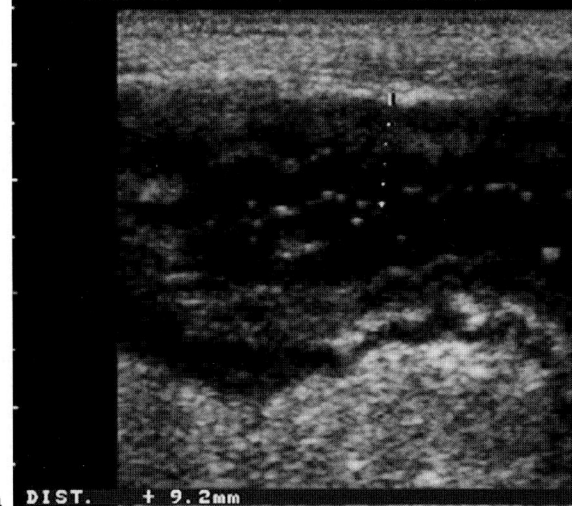

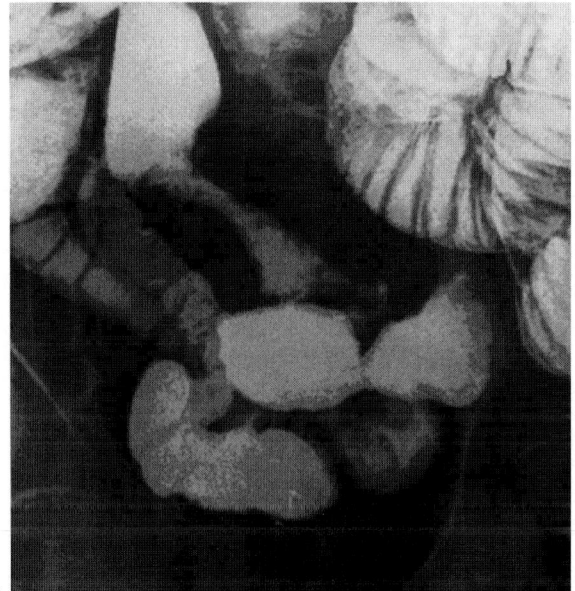

**Fig. 21.3a,b.** Crohn's disease lesions of small intestine well delineated by means of oral contrast ultrasound. The US oral contrast agent allows a more accurate evaluation of mucosal surface showing nodular and ulcerated appearance (**a**) comparable to that at contrast barium radiology (**b**), and providing information regarding thickening and transmural changes of ileal wall

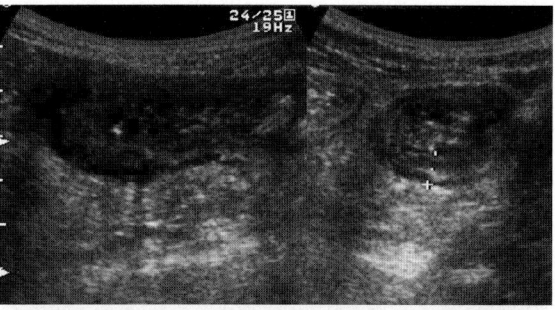

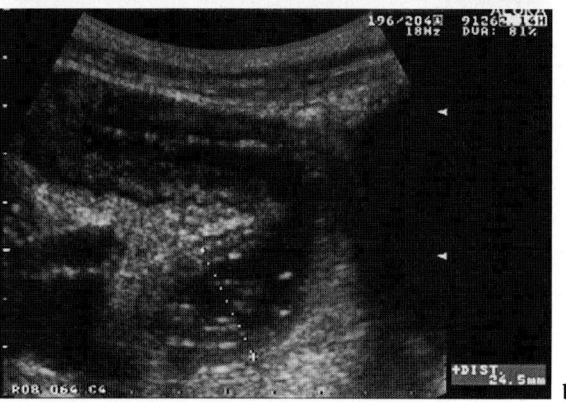

**Fig. 21.4a,b.** Crohn's disease stricture of terminal ileum assessed by (**a**) conventional US (longitudinal and transverse sections) and (**b**) US with oral contrast agent

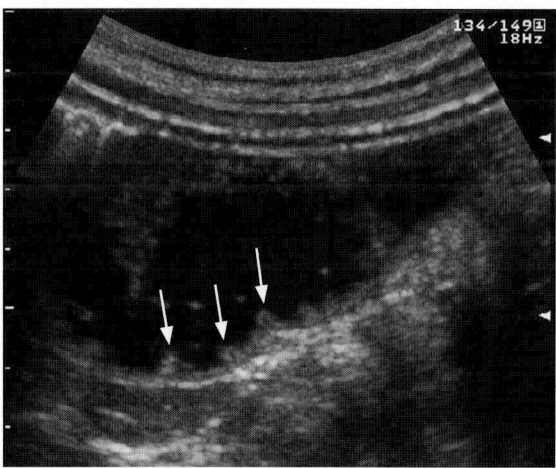

**Fig. 21.5.** Small intestinal contrast ultrasound of coeliac disease patient. Diameter of jejunal loop is significantly greater and number of Kerckring's folds (*arrows*) reduced

graphic signs of coeliac disease can be obtained (see Chap. 9), such as increased loop diameter and jejunal wall thickness, reduced number of Kerckring's folds (including ileal jejunalisation) and increased peristaltic waves (DELL'AQUILA et al. 2005) (Fig. 21.5).

Despite the above-mentioned advantages of small intestine contrast US, some limitations should be taken into account. In most of the studies comparing conventional trans-abdominal US and small intestine contrast US, the same investigator performed first trans-abdominal US and then small intestinal contrast US, thus making less sensitivity of small intestinal contrast US unlikely. Furthermore, compared to trans-abdominal US, small intestine contrast US is a time-consuming procedure, with a mean duration of 40 min. This limitation is not in keeping with the peculiar features of abdominal US, which is a simple, practical and rapidly performed examination. Therefore, for most sonographers, it cannot be considered a routine procedure in clinical practice.

## 21.4
## Hydrocolonic Sonography

In the late 1980s, hydrocolonic sonography has been proposed as a sensitive and less invasive method to image the colon and colonic walls, to be used as an alternative to barium enema and colonoscopy.

Like barium enema and colonoscopy, hydrocolonic sonography requires bowel preparation consisting of a laxative, following which 1500 ml of water should be instilled into the colon, after an intravenous injection of 20 mg of Hyoscine N-butylscopolamine (Buscopan, Boehringer, Germany) for relaxation of the colon. The amount of instilled water depends on distension of the colon, and a relaxant may be necessary to achieve optimal distension and to suppress the sense of urgency of elimination, of the patient.

During and after instilling the water, the sonographic examination can be carried out, preferably using a 3.5–7 MHz transducer and, for detailed evaluation, 5–12 MHz transducers.

The accuracy of hydrocolonic sonography appears to depend on the indication and, therefore, on the study population.

In the detection of colonic polyps and carcinoma and in the prediction of stage of colorectal cancer, hydrocolonic sonography showed a high sensitivity and specificity, in most studies (Bru et al. 2001; Chung et al. 2004; Dixit et al. 1999; Hernandez-Socorro et al. 1995; Limberg 1987, 1990, 1992) but negative results have also been reported (sensitivity <7%, with a false positive rate of 19.2%) (Chui et al. 1994). However, these controversial results depend on the variable presence of overweight patients in the case series, skill of the operators, and the nature, size, stage and site of the neoplastic lesions since a poor accuracy in detecting rectal cancer by hydrocolonic sonography has been reported in most studies.

Early stage neoplasms and polyps, particularly if small in size, are usually detected with lower accuracy. Detection and staging of rectal cancer are frequently underestimated and lesions located in the transverse colon and in both colonic flexures may be difficult to image properly with US (Chung et al. 2004; Dux et al. 1999).

For these and other reasons (i.e., obviously hydrocolonic sonography does not offer the possibility/ opportunity to collect biopsies or remove polyps), although less invasive and expensive than colonoscopy, the use of hydrocolonic sonography, as a screening tool for colorectal cancer, should be evaluated with due care.

However, hydrocolonic sonography may be usefully employed in other circumstances such as the follow-up of inflammatory lesions and the evaluation of colonic lesions that have already been diagnosed at endoscopy or barium enema. Provided the sonographer can image the colonic lesion by hydrocolonic sonography, it is possible to exactly define the extent and colonic wall in which a high grade stenosis is present. In this case, the examination may help to ascertain the T stage of the tumour.

In inflammatory lesions, hydrocolonic sonography may play a useful role in the assessment of disease extension and activity (Limberg and Osswald 1994; Bru et al. 2001). Considering its accuracy, low risk, and cost, hydrocolonic sonography can be useful in the study of disease extension in patients with incomplete colonoscopy, after confirmation of the diagnosis by histology. In patients in whom the diagnosis of inflammatory bowel disease has been established, hydrocolonic sonography may also provide an estimate of disease severity.

## References

Bru C, Sans M, Defelitto MM et al (2001) Hydrocolonic sonography for evaluating inflammatory bowel disease. AJR Am J Roentgenol 177:99–105

Calabrese E, La Seta F, Buccellato A et al (2005) Crohn's disease: a comparative prospective study of transabdominal ultrasonography, small intestine contrast ultrasonography, and small bowel enema. Inflamm Bowel Dis 11:139–145

Chui DW, Gooding GA, McQuaid KR et al (1994) Hydrocolonic ultrasonography in the detection of colonic polyps and tumors. N Engl J Med 331:1685–1688

Chung HW, Chung JB, Park SW, Song SY, Kang JK, Park CI (2004) Comparison of hydrocolonic sonography accuracy in preoperative staging between colon and rectal cancer. World J Gastroenterol 10:1157–1161

Cittadini G, Giasotto V, Garlaschi G, de Cicco E, Gallo A, Cittadini G (2001) Transabdominal ultrasonography of the small bowel after oral administration of a non-absorbable anechoic solution: comparison with barium enteroclysis. Clin Radiol 56:225–230

Dell'Aquila P, Pietrini L, Barone M et al (2005) Small intestinal contrast ultrasonography-based scoring system: a promising approach for the diagnosis and follow-up of celiac disease. J Clin Gastroenterol 39:591–595

Dixit R, Chowdhury V, Kumar N (1999) Hydrocolonic sonography in the evaluation of colonic lesions. Abdom Imaging 24:497–505

Dux M (1999) Hydrocolonic sonography. Abdom Imaging 24:506–507

Folvik G, Bjerke-Larssen T, Odegaard S, Hausken T, Gilja OH, Berstad A (1999) Hydrosonography of the small intestine: comparison with radiologic barium study. Scand J Gastroenterol 34:1247–1252

Futagami K, Hata J, Haruma K et al (2001) Extracorporeal ultrasound is an effective diagnostic alternative to endoscopic ultrasound for gastric submucosal tumours. Scand J Gastroenterol 36:1222–1226

Hernandez-Socorro CR, Guerra C, Hernandez-Romero J, Rey A, Lopez-Facal P, Alvares-Santullano V (1995) Colorectal carcinomas: diagnosis and preoperative staging by hydrocolonic sonography. Surgery 117:609–615

Harisinghani MG, Saini S, Schima W, McNicholas M, Mueller PR (1997) Simethicone coated cellulose as an oral contrast agent for ultrasound of the upper abdomen. Clin Radiol 52:224–226

Limberg B (1987) Diagnosis of inflammatory and neoplastic colonic disease by sonography. J Clin Gastroenterol 9:607–611

Limberg B (1990) Diagnosis of large bowel tumours by colonic sonography. Lancet 335:144–146

Limberg B (1992) Diagnosis and staging of colonic tumors by conventional abdominal sonography as compared with hydrocolonic sonography. N Engl J Med 327:65–69

Limberg B, Osswald B (1994) Diagnosis and differential diagnosis of ulcerative colitis and Crohn's disease by hydrocolonic sonography. Am J Gastroenterol 89:1051–1057

Lund PJ, Fritz TA, Unger EC, Hunt RK, Fuller E (1992) Cellulose as a gastrointestinal US contrast agent. Radiology 185:783–788

Pallotta N, Baccini F, Corazziari E (1999a) Ultrasonography of the small bowel after oral administration of anechoic contrast solution. Lancet 353:985–986

Pallotta N, Baccini F, Corazziari E (1999b) Contrast ultrasonography of the normal small bowel. Ultrasound Med Biol 25:1335–1340

Pallotta N, Baccini F, Corazziari E (2000) Small intestine contrast ultrasonography. J Ultrasound Med 19:21–26

Pallotta N, Baccini F, Corazziari E (2001) Small intestine contrast ultrasonography (SICUS) in the diagnosis of small intestine lesions. Ultrasound Med Biol 27:335–341

Pallotta N, Tomei E, Viscido A et al (2005) Small intestine contrast ultrasonography: an alternative to radiology in the assessment of small bowel disease. Inflamm Bowel Dis 11:146–153

Parente F, Greco S, Molteni M et al (2004) Oral contrast enhanced bowel ultrasonography in the assessment of small intestine Crohn's disease. A prospective comparison with conventional ultrasound, X-ray studies, and ileocolonoscopy. Gut 53:1652–1657

Polkowski M, Palucki J, Butruk E (2002) Transabdominal ultrasound for visualizing gastric submucosal tumors diagnosed by endosonography: can surveillance be simplified? Endoscopy 34:979–983

Worlicek H, Lederer P, Lux G (1986) Ultrasonographic evaluation of the wall of the fluid-filled stomach – case report of a leiomyoblastoma. Hepatogastroenterology 33:184–186

Worlicek H (1986) Sonographic diagnosis of the fluid-filled stomach. Ultraschall Med 7:259–263

Worlicek H, Dunz D, Engelhard K (1989) Ultrasonic examination of the wall of the fluid-filled stomach. J Clin Ultrasound 17:5–14

# Functional Ultrasound of the Gastrointestinal Tract

TRYGVE HAUSKEN and ODD HELGE GILJA

CONTENTS

22.1 Introduction 189
22.2 Distal Stomach 190
22.3 Gastric Emptying 190
22.4 Proximal Stomach and Gastric Accommodation 191
22.5 Antral Peristalsis 192
22.6 Flow of Luminal Contents 193
22.7 Gastroesophageal Reflux Disease 194
22.8 Gallbladder 195
22.9 Ultrasound as a Clinical Tool to Evaluate Patients with Functional Gastrointestinal Disorders 195
References 196

## 22.1 Introduction

Functional ultrasound of the gastrointestinal (GI) tract includes studies of the distal and proximal stomach, gastric and gallbladder emptying, gastric distribution, GI wall motility, and flow of luminal contents in healthy subjects as well as in patients. Furthermore, it includes the effect of different meals and pharmacological intervention.

It is possible to perform ultrasound of the motility in the small and large bowel. However, it is difficult to standardize and cover the entire intestine in one examination. In inflammatory bowel disease, however, is it possible to study stiffness and lack of peristalsis in bowel segments.

T. HAUSKEN, MD, PhD
O. H. GILJA, MD, PhD
Section of Gastroenterology, National Centre for Ultrasound in Gastroenterology, Haukeland University Hospital, Institute of Medicine, University of Bergen, Jonas Liesvei 65, 5021 Bergen, Norway

In the present review, we will focus on the upper part of GI motility.

Imaging methods have much to offer in the understanding of gastric mechanics, as they can be used to assess gastric wall motion and luminal diameter at the same time and the movement of luminal contents (EHRLEIN 1980; CODE 1979; HAUSKEN et al. 1992; KING et al. 1984; HOLT et al. 1980; BOLONDI et al. 1985; HVEEM et al. 1996; BATEMAN and WHITTINGHAM 1982). Fluoroscopic imaging has been used since the turn of the last century for this purpose, but its application in humans is severely constrained by radiation exposure. Scintigraphy is, at present, the "gold standard" for clinical measurement of gastric emptying. Recently, single photon emission computed tomography (SPECT) has been reported as a possible noninvasive alternative (BOURAS et al. 2002). Radiolabelled 99mTc pertechnetate is injected intravenously and accumulates in the gastric mucosa allowing visualization of the stomach. This technique was shown to record changes in postprandial volume to a similar extent to the gastric barostat. Measurement of intraluminal impedance changes is now used to study transport of fluids in the gut (SAVOYE et al. 2003; SIFRIM et al. 2001). This technique involves application of a low-voltage potential difference to closely spaced electrodes on a catheter in the gut lumen and measurement of the resulting current.

Other techniques such as magnetic resonance imaging (MRI) and ultrasound imaging are attractive options since they permit prolonged observation of the human stomach without exposure to radiation. Real time gastric MRI has special appeal but, as yet, its full potential has not been realized due to costs and technical difficulties (MARCIANI et al. 2001).

Ultrasound imaging of gastroduodenal motility has mainly been performed with a transabdominal approach and until recently primarily as 2D ultrasonography (GILJA et al 1995a; HAUSKEN et al. 1992; RICCI et al. 1993; UNDELAND et al. 1997). Three-dimensional ultrasound has, so far, only been applied as an investigational tool in scientific studies due to the complex and time-consuming procedure of image recording and processing (GILJA et al. 1997; BERSTAD et al. 1994). Due to its high availability, modest costs and lack of radiation hazard, 2D real time ultrasonography has found its place in clinical diagnostic practice and not only as an experimental tool.

A number of motility studies have now established ultrasound as a valuable method of studying both the proximal (GILJA et al. 1995) and the distal stomach (HVEEM et al. 1994; HAUSKEN et al. 1992).

juice and between the increased in the of antral area and amounts of ingested water (HVEEM et al. 1994).

Recent studies have shown that fasting and postprandial antral areas increase in patients with functional dyspepsia and diabetes mellitus compared with normal subjects (UNDELAND et al. 1997; HVEEM et al. 1996). The antral area, and hence antral distention, is a significant determinant of postprandial fullness (HAUSKEN et al. 1992).

## 22.2
## Distal Stomach

The width of the antral area is measured in a vertical section in which the antrum, the superior mesenteric vein and the aorta are visualized simultaneously. The outer profile of the muscularis propria is outlined and the area calculated automatically (Fig. 22.1). The values obtained of all measurements are given as the average of two successive measurements.

The relationship between the antral area as measured by ultrasound and the amount of fasting gastric content quantitated by aspiration through the gastroscope and the increment of the antral area after ingestion of graded volumes of water were highly reproducible, with small variations within 1 h and from day to day, and there was a highly significant correlation between the ultrasonographically measured antral area and the amount of fasting gastric

## 22.3
## Gastric Emptying

Scintigraphy is at present the "gold standard" for clinical measurement of gastric emptying. Scintigraphy provides quantitative information about total stomach emptying and intragastric meal distribution of both solid and liquid meals (COLLINS et al. 1988). With the use of a gamma, camera the rate of gastric emptying of a standardized test meal marked with a radioisotope can be calculated. Scintigraphy requires expensive equipment that is often not readily available, is associated with a radiation burden, and cannot detect individual episodes of transpyloric flow.

Using ultrasound, gastric emptying has typically been assessed by changes in either the antral cross-sectional area or diameter (BOLONDI et al. 1985; HOLT et al. 1986). In order to establish ultrasound as an acceptable or even preferred method in assessing gastric emptying, studies have been conducted to compare ultrasound with scintigraphy.

In order to do so, the subjects are usually seated with their back against the gamma camera and the ultrasound transducer is positioned in the region of the umbilicus. The first measurement is performed within 1 min of meal ingestion, followed by subsequent images at intervals depending on which meal is used. Ultrasound $T_{50}$ is defined as the time when the antral area is decreased to half its maximum (HOROWITZ et al. 1993).

With a high- and low-nutrient liquid meal, scintigraphic and ultrasonographic 50% emptying times ($T_{50}$'s) were comparable and longer for dextrose (300 kcal) than for meat soup (20 kcal) (dextrose 107±16 min vs 108±18 min, soup 24±4 min vs 23±5 min). A close correlation was found between scintigraphic and ultrasound $T_{50}$ and the $T_{50}$, and the limits of agreement were good (HVEEM et al. 1996).

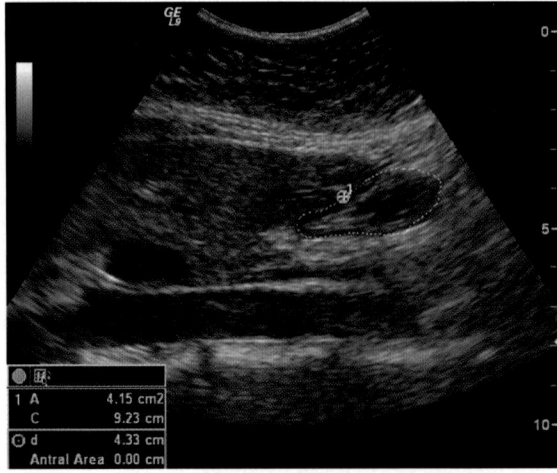

Fig. 22.1. Standardized section of the antrum. Antral area is outlined

Other comparative studies between ultrasound and scintigraphic measurements of gastric emptying have shown a very close relationship between the two methods (Bolondi et al. 1985; Holt et al. 1986). The intraindividual variation in gastric emptying of liquids in normal subjects, however, is relatively large.

## 22.4 Proximal Stomach and Gastric Accommodation

We have developed a sonographic method to monitor postprandial size of the proximal stomach. A proximal gastric area in a sagittal section (Fig. 22.2) is outlined by tracing from the top margin of the fundus and 7 cm downwards along the axis of the stomach as described by Gilja et al. (1995). Diameter on the fundus (Fig. 22.3), defined as the maximal diameter in an oblique frontal section kept within 7 cm along the axis of the proximal stomach, is chosen as the second measure. The subjects are scanned in a sitting position with a 3.25-MHz transducer after ingestion of 500 ml meat soup and the measurements are performed 10 and 20 min postprandially.

The soup emptied from the proximal stomach in a linear manner with a moderate day-to-day variation, low intra- and interobserver error, and the method allows estimation of initial emptying fractions of the proximal stomach (Gilja et al. 1995).

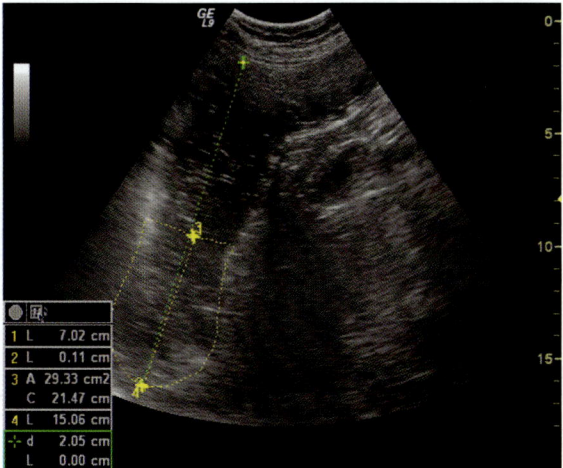

Fig. 22.2. A proximal gastric area in a sagittal section is outlined by tracing from the top margin of the fundus and 7 cm downwards along the axis of the stomach

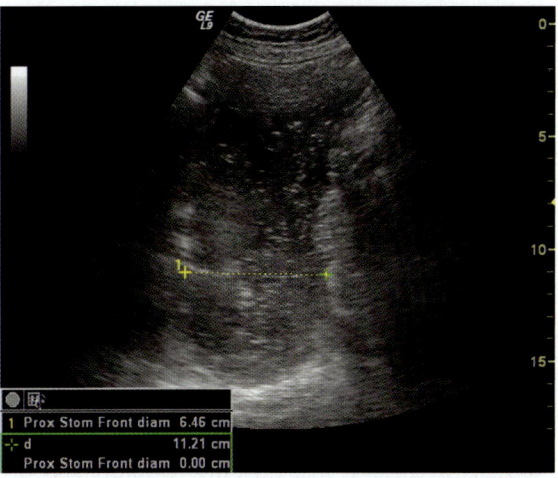

Fig. 22.3. Diameter on the fundus defined as the maximal diameter in an oblique frontal section kept within 7 cm along the axis of the proximal stomach

Ultrasound of the proximal stomach has shown that patients with functional dyspepsia and diabetes have a smaller proximal stomach than healthy subjects (Gilja et al. 1996; Undeland et al. 1998). Sublingual glyceryl trinitrate improves accommodation of the proximal stomach to a meal as measured by ultrasound and reduces postprandial symptoms in a group of patients with functional dyspepsia (Gilja et al. 1997).

In reflux esophagitis patients, the sagittal area of the proximal stomach was significantly larger after a meal, and the patients experienced more epigastric fullness (Tefera et al. 2001, 2002). The findings with both 2D and 3D ultrasound methods in gastroesophageal reflux disease (GERD) patients is consistent with the results of other recently published studies. Zerbib et al. (1999) found a more pronounced relaxation of the proximal stomach in GERD patients using a barostat, and observed an inverse correlation between maximal postprandial relaxation and severity of disease. Penagini et al. (1998) found delayed recovery of proximal gastric tone after intake of a combined solid and liquid meal in GERD patients.

The "gold standard" to study gastric accommodation after a meal has been the barostat. The barostat measures gastric wall relaxation and from that one can infer gastric tone. However, introducing the barostat balloon into the gastric lumen may influence the gastric motility patterns (Moragas et al. 1993; Ropert et al. 1993), and furthermore the examination is invasive and unpleasant. Neither the barostat nor scintigraphy allows estimation of the size of the proximal stomach. On the contrary, ultrasound and SPECT scanning can detect changes in gastric volume in a non-invasive manner. Like ultrasound, SPECT scanning is a non-invasive alternative to the barostat in evaluating gastric relaxation. However, in comparison with meal-induced volume increase, SPECT scanning failed to detect the profound gastric relaxation following glucagon infusion. These findings suggest that SPECT scanning is less suitable than the gastric barostat in detecting gastric relaxation and rather detects the volume of the intragastric contents after meal intake.

An important question is whether imaging methods, such as MRI, SPECT or ultrasonography, can actually be compared to the measurements made by the barostat. We believe that imaging methods and the invasive barostat method do not measure the same aspects of the gastric accommodation process. Thanks to its close contact with the gastric wall, the barostat bag adjusts to changes in proximal gastric pressure by changing the intrabag volume. Thus, changes in volume are believed to reflect changes in muscle tone of the wall. However, the quantitative change in volume seen during barostat examinations is only valid during barostat studies using exactly the same equipment and positioning technique. Imaging methods, however, visualize directly the size of the gastric compartments, thus giving an indirect measure of relaxation and contraction. The volume change seen using imaging can thus be explained by additional secretion, air retention or most probably changes in gastric emptying.

The gastric meal accommodation process has two components: Passive meal distension of the gastric compartments and active muscle relaxation of the gastric wall. The first component is best measured with imaging methods whereas the barostat is best suited for studying the second component. Imaging methods, at this stage, do not distinguish between enlargement of the stomach due to reflex relaxation or due to meal-induced distension; it just measures the totally accommodated volume. Accordingly, it may not be adequate to compare imaging methods to the barostat for validation of gastric accommodation. Gastric accommodation depends on neuromuscular factors and hence it is also a matter of evaluation of the mechanical properties of the stomach. In this sense, the barostat merely detects the existence of change in wall tone, but cannot, like imaging methods, provide data on the distribution of the volume and the normal behavior of the gastric wall. In biomechanics, it is essential to understand the geometry of the organ and the forces and deformation in different directions in order to better understand the active-passive muscle function and mechano-sensation in health and in diseases such as the functional disorders. This warrants 2D and 3D image analysis of the gastric compartments.

The different imaging methods exhibit different spatial and temporal image resolution, and these factors strongly influence accuracy in volume calculation. MRI, and in particular SPECT, imaging have poor spatial and temporal resolution compared to ultrasonography. Ultrasonography can provide temporal resolution above 100 fps, if necessary, and a spatial resolution at submillimeter level. Also, the "stress-factor" of the imaging methods should be considered in this context because dyspeptic patients in general, and vagal reflexes in particular, are very sensitive to psychological stress. Anyone who has been inside a narrow, noisy MR scanner knows how frightening this can be. Naturally, the stress-factor is also substantially involved in studies using the barostat. Simply because functional disorders are so strongly associated with psychological factors, the examination should be performed in a quiet and relaxing atmosphere with a minimum of distress. Ultrasonography satisfies these criteria as it is non-invasive and does not in itself distort the physiological response in stress-responsive individuals. Moreover, due to gravity playing a central role in the propulsion of gastric content, the study of meal accommodation should preferably be performed in a "natural position" such as sitting in a chair. Therefore, methods that enable patients to be seated have an advantage over methods requiring patients to be in a supine position during the examination.

## 22.5
## Antral Peristalsis

Antral contractions (3 per min) are responsible for mixing and grinding of a solid meal into smaller particles (<5 mm) that can pass onto the duodenum. These antral contractions can easily be seen at ultrasonography. The contractions can be occlusive or non lumen-occlusive. An antral contraction is defined as an indentation of the gastric wall greater than one antral wall thickness, which is not due to respiration, pulsation transmitted from the aorta or heart, or to movements of adjacent intestine.

A lumen-occlusive contraction is defined as a contraction in which the ultrasound image shows the gastric walls to come into apposition at some point along the imaged antrum.

Amplitude of antral contractions is measured as a fraction of relaxed area and the motility index is calculated as the amplitude multiplied by frequency.

The motility index as measured by ultrasound was reduced in patients with functional dyspepsia (FD). The effects of acute mental stress on gastric antral motility were reduced by mental stress in the healthy individuals, but not in FD patients (Hausken et al. 1993).

Manometry is the most widely used method for measuring gastric motility (Malagelada and Stanghellini 1985; Husebye 1999). Manometric studies have demonstrated that the patterns of luminal pressure waves are complex both in the fasting and fed states. So far, only two studies assessing concurrent ultrasound and high-resolution manometry have been published.

In the study by Hausken et al. (2002), in the pre- and postprandial period, a total of 44% of antral contractions were not detected by manometry, and only 1/5 of non-occluding contractions.

Hveem et al. (2001) found that only 53% of antral contractions seen ultrasonographically had a temporally associated pressure event in the manometric reference channel. The lumen-occlusive contractions had, in 69%, an associated pressure event. Of the non-lumen-occlusive contractions, only 20% were associated with a pressure event.

The median amplitude of the pressure events in the manometric reference channel was 16 mmHg (range 4–98 mmHg) for lumen-occlusive, and 7 mmHg (range 4–23 mmHg) for non-lumen-occlusive contractions. However, a substantial overlap exists between the two categories of contraction.

In about 50% of antral contractions observed by ultrasound, the corresponding pressure events are not identified in the manometric reference channel. This more than indicates that the knowledge of gastric mechanics, based solely on manometry, is at the least inadequate, missing almost half of the information given by ultrasound with regard to antral contractions.

## 22.6
## Flow of Luminal Contents

Information concerning movement of luminal contents in humans can be obtained by fluoroscopy, scintigraphy, MRI, impedance and duplex sonography. Studies based on scintigraphy and standard ultrasound of the stomach and duodenum will indirectly measure overall rates of gastric emptying, but these methods do not have the temporal resolution to assess on a second-to-second basis. However, promising new MRI methods are being developed. Echo planar imaging, an ultrafast variant of MRI, can provide excellent images both of gastric wall movements and movements of solid and liquid meals.

Ultrasonographic studies by King et al. (1984) using test meals containing bran particles showed that gastric emptying occurred in episodes lasting a few seconds in healthy subjects. The emptying period usually started immediately after relaxation of the antro-pyloro-duodenal segment and was finished before the next peristaltic contraction approached the distal antrum. A brief episode of duodenogastric reflux occurred in about 60% of the peristaltic cycles shortly before the terminal antral contraction. A similar type of reflux was shown in dogs by Malbert and Ruckebusch (1991), who used operatively implanted electromagnetic flowmeter probes. Hausken et al. (1992) showed that using pulsed Doppler combined with real-time ultrasonography (Duplex sonography), it is possible to visualize antro-duodenal motility and transpyloric flow simultaneously. Antegrade and retrograde transpyloric flow is visualized using bidirectional velocity curves. Most contractions of the proximal duodenal bulb precede closure of the pylorus (and the terminal antrum), and duodenal bulb contraction is often accompanied by a short burst of duodenogastric reflux occurring immediately before closure of the pylorus.

Studies of the antro-pyloro-duodenal region are performed with the ultrasound probe positioned at the level of the transpyloric plane, and the antrum, the pylorus and the proximal duodenum are visualized simultaneously. The subjects are studied in a seated position, with a 3.5- to 5-MHz transducer.

In order to study the relation between motility and flow in detail, techniques with a high temporal and spatial resolution are required for the assessment of antro-pyloro-duodenal pressure waves and transpyloric flow. Subjects have to be intubated with a manometric assembly, which is introduced transnasally and positioned in the antro-pyloro-duodenal region using fluoroscopy. The Doppler/ultrasound and manometric recordings have to be synchronized (Hausken et al. 2002).

- First gastric emptying is defined as the first occurrence of gastric emptying after drinking of the soup is initiated. An episode of gastric emptying is defined

as flow across the pylorus with a mean velocity of more than 10 cm/s lasting more than 1 s.
- Occluding peristaltic-related transpyloric emptying is defined as gastric emptying associated with contractile activity in which the ultrasound image shows an occlusion of the stomach wall. Non-occluding peristaltic-related emptying is defined as transpyloric emptying of gastric contents associated with contractile activity of the gastric wall which does not occlude the lumen. During maximal contractions transpyloric flow can still be seen passing back and forth through the open pylorus.
- Non-peristaltic-related transpyloric emptying is defined as transpyloric emptying of gastric contents, without contractions detected on ultrasound or manometry.

Gastric emptying of a low caloric liquid meal follows sequences of emptying-reflux-emptying pulses. About half of the sequences are peristaltic related, but both non-occluding, peristaltic related and non-peristaltic-related emptying sequences occur. Non-peristaltic-related flow sequences often have more alternating emptying-reflux episodes than those associated with peristalsis, and the duration of non-peristaltic-related emptying and reflux pulses are longer. The pressure gradients for all types of emptying are low and the pressure gradients during non-peristaltic-related emptying are significantly lower than during peristaltic related emptying.

Flow can only occur in the presence of an open pylorus. Transpyloric flow can be classified into flow associated with a local increase in the pressure gradient between antrum and duodenum (Pa–Pd) due to antral propagating pressure waves. The second type of flow is independent of peristalsis and is likely to be caused by changes in gastric tone, or by pressure changes outside the stomach such as aortic pulsation and inspiration (HAUSKEN et al. 2002).

The method can be used to study normal physiology and pathophysiology of the gastro-pyloro-duodenal segment and to monitor the effect of medications on transpyloric flow.

Patients with functional dyspepsia often experience early satiety and discomfort after a meal. Using duplex sonography it is possible to relate timing of symptoms and early postprandial emptying in patients with functional dyspepsia (HAUSKEN et al. 1998). Meal-related discomfort was experienced after commencement of transpyloric emptying. An inverse relationship was found between the duration of the tasting period and symptom intensity, suggesting that the time allowed for duodenal tasting might be too short in patients with functional dyspepsia.

Currently available methods for studying gastric emptying do not provide quantitative information about the movement of gastric contents. A new non-invasive method for evaluating stroke volumes using three-dimensional (3D) guided digital color Doppler imaging might help the investigator to quantify net gastric emptying and to estimate the amount of duodenogastric reflux (HAUSKEN et al. 2001). The technique involved color Doppler digital images of transpyloric flow in which the 3D position and orientation of the images were known by using a magnetic location system. In vitro, the system was found to slightly underestimate the reference flow (by average 8.8%). In vivo (five volunteers), stroke volume of gastric emptying episodes lasted on average only 0.69 s with a volume on average of 4.3 ml (range 1.1–7.4 ml), and duodenogastric reflux episodes on average 1.4 s with a volume of 8.3 ml (range 1.3–14.1 ml). It was concluded that with the appropriate instrument settings, orientation determined color Doppler can be used for stroke volume quantification of gastric emptying and duodenogastric reflux episodes.

## 22.7
## Gastroesophageal Reflux Disease

HIRSCH et al. (1996, 1997) performed a comparative study of ultrasonography (abnormal reflux or physiological reflux) with and without the use of color Doppler versus 24-h esophageal pH measurements in 84 high-risk children for suspected gastroesophageal reflux (GER). They found abnormal reflux in 60.7% by pH-metry, in 51.2% by B-mode ultrasonography and in 59.5% by color Doppler ultrasonography. There was agreement between pH-metry and B-mode ultrasonography in 87% of patients as compared to 94% between pH-metry and color Doppler ultrasonography, and increased sensitivity of reflux detection from 84.4% to 98% when color Doppler was added to B-mode ultrasonography. Similarly, JANG et al. (2001) showed that color Doppler sonography was highly sensitive and was thought to be easier to use and more acceptable to the child than pH monitoring. In this study, the two tests showed 81.5% agreement in the detection of GERD. This modality may be clinically useful in screening children for GERD (JANG et al. 2001).

## 22.8
## Gallbladder

As real-time ultrasonography is a cheap, noninvasive, relatively easy, validated and reproducible technique, it can be repeated over time to document time-related changes of gallbladder motor function. Ultimately, functional ultrasonography estimates gallbladder shape and volume in the fasting state and in response to a test meal (liquid or mixed solid-liquid, provided there is sufficient fat content) or exogenous stimulus (e.g., i.v. cholecystokinin). Patients are scanned in the supine, right anterior oblique position. Longitudinal and axial cross-sectional images of the gallbladder in its largest dimensions are obtained in triplicate. Average measurements are used for calculation of the gallbladder volume. The volume of the gallbladder (V) is subsequently calculated using the ellipsoid method as described by DODDS et al. (1985), $V = 0.52 \cdot L \times W \times H$, where L is the length, W is the width, and H is the height or depth of the gallbladder. All subjects are studied in the morning after an overnight fast. Fasting volume of the gallbladder (ml) represents the mean of three volume measurements taken 5 min apart. After taking the fasting volume, gallbladder contraction is stimulated by a fatty meal. Gallbladder contraction and refilling are monitored with ultrasonography and images are taken over time to document time-related changes of gallbladder volume. The difference between the basal volume and the corresponding residual volume represents the gallbladder ejected volume (ml). The gallbladder ejection fraction [GBEF(%)] is calculated according to the formula, GBEF(%) = 1 − (residual volume/fasting volume) × 100.

Although functional ultrasonography of the gallbladder has been mainly used for research purposes in specific referral centers, its simplicity makes such a technique appealing in the clinical setting to assess gallbladder motor function both in healthy and diseased subjects (PALASCIANO et al. 1992). Indications include the study of healthy subjects and of patients during pathophysiologically relevant conditions; in particular when subjects are at risk for gallbladder stasis and gallstone disease or during gallstone disease when a decision concerning medical dissolution therapy is required. A decreased emptying rate of the gallbladder has been demonstrated in patients with gallstones (FISCHER et al. 1982), dyspepsia (MARZIO et al. 1992), diabetes mellitus (STONE et al. 1988), obesity (MARZIO et al. 1988a), and in patients operated on with Billroth type II for duodenal ulcer (MARZIO et al. 1988).

## 22.9
## Ultrasound as a Clinical Tool to Evaluate Patients with Functional GI Disorders

Another advantage of 2D ultrasonography is its clinical applicability; it can easily be performed at the bedside and repeated numerous times in the same subject. At Haukeland University Hospital, we have used the ultrasound meal accommodation test (U-MAT) for the work-up of patients with dyspepsia (Table 22.1) for the past 20 years. Our mainstream clinical proto-

**Table 22.1.** The ultrasound meal accommodation test (UMAT) was developed at Haukeland University Hospital on the basis of close interaction between scientific and clinical work in patients with dyspepsia. Before entering the protocol, the patients have been carefully studied with history, physical examination, blood tests, testing for *H. pylori* and upper endoscopy. In some cases, additional examinations are performed to rule out organic causes of their symptoms. The protocol presented here is the mainstream clinical protocol. In scientific studies, other elements are often added. A 500-ml liquid meal of commercial meat soup (Toro clear meat soup, Rieber & Søn A/S, Bergen, Norway) containing 1.8 g protein, 0.9 g bovine fat, and 1.1 g carbohydrate (20 kcal) is ingested over a period of 4 min. The soup is preheated and then cooled to 37°C to improve imaging quality by reducing the amount of air bubbles. Psychometric evaluation is also performed

| Time | Protocol |
|---|---|
| Fasting | Ordinary ultrasound examination of the liver, gallbladder, biliary tract, spleen, pancreas, kidneys, and large vessels |
| Fasting | Evaluation of symptoms by VAS |
| Fasting | Assessment of motility pattern (phase 1–3) by observing the pattern of contractility in the antrum |
| Fasting | Measurement of area of the distal stomach (AA) |
| Fasting | Visualisation of the proximal stomach to explore whether it has content |
| Meal ingestion | 500 ml of preheated meat soup is ingested in 4 min at a constant speed |
| 2 min pp | Measurement of the sagittal area (SA), the oblique frontal diameter (OFD), and the antral area (AA) |
| 5 min pp | Postprandial symptom evaluation |
| 10 min pp | SA, OFD, and AA measurement |
| 20 min pp | SA, OFD, and AA measurement |
| 30 min pp | SA, OFD, and AA measurement |

col consists of a standard soup meal (500 ml), ultrasound scanning of the proximal and distal stomach using predefined scan sections, calculation of size and volume of the gastric compartments, evaluation of symptoms and psychological assessment. In our experience, ultrasonography used in this context adds valuable clinical information to the management of these patients.

## References

Bateman DN, Whittingham TA (1982) Measurement of gastric emptying by real-time ultrasound. Gut 23:524–527

Berstad A, Hausken T, Gilja OH, Thune N, Matre K, Odegaard S (1994) Volume measurements of gastric antrum by 3-D ultrasonography and flow measurements through the pylorus by duplex technique. Dig Dis Sci 39[12 Suppl]:97S–100S

Bolondi L, Bortolotti M, Santi V, Calletti T, Gaiani S, Labo G (1985) Measurement of gastric emptying time by real-time ultrasonography. Gastroenterology 89:752–759

Bouras EP, Delgado-Aros S, Camilleri M et al (2002) SPECT imaging of the stomach: comparison with barostat, and effects of sex, age, body mass index, and fundoplication. Single photon emission computed tomography. Gut 51:781–786

Code CF (1979) The interdigestive housekeeper of the gastrointestinal tract. Perspect Biol Med 22(2 Pt 2):S49–S55

Collins PJ, Horowitz M, Chatterton BE (1988) Proximal, distal and total stomach emptying of a digestible solid meal in normal subjects. Br J Radiol 61:12–18

Dodds WJ, Groh WJ, Darweesh RMA (1985) Sonographic measurement of gallbladder volume. Am J Radiology 145:1009–1011

Ehrlein HJ (1980) A new technique for simultaneous radiography and recording of gastrointestinal motility in unanesthetized dogs. Lab Anim Sci 30:879–884

Fischer RS, Seltzer F, Rock E, Malmud LS (1982) Abnormal gallbladder emptying in patients with gallstones. Dig Dis Sci 27:1019–1024

Gilja OH, Hausken T, Odegaard S, Berstad A (1995) Monitoring postprandial size of the proximal stomach by ultrasonography. J Ultrasound Med 14:81–89

Gilja OH, Hausken T, Ødegaard S, Berstad A (1996) Ultrasonography of the proximal stomach in patients with functional dyspepsia. Hepato-Gastroenterol 42:86–87

Gilja OH, Detmer PR, Jong JM, Leotta DF, Li XN, Beach KW (1997) Intragastric distribution and gastric emptying assessed by three-dimensional ultrasonography. Gastroenterology 113:38–49

Gilja OH, Hausken T, Bang CJ, Berstad A (1997) Effect of glyceryl trinitrate on gastric accommodation and symptoms in functional dyspepsia. Dig Dis Sci 42:2124–2131

Hausken T, Berstad A (1992) Wide gastric antrum in patients with non-ulcer dyspepsia. Effect of cisapride. Scand J Gastroenterol 27:427–432

Hausken T, Ødegaard S, Matre K, Berstad A (1992) Antroduodenal motility and movements of luminal contents studied by duplex sonography. Gastroenterology 102:1583–1590

Hausken T, Svebak S, Wilhelmsen I et al (1993) Low vagal tone and antral dysmotility in patients with functional dyspepsia. Psychosom Med 55:12–22

Hausken T, Gilja OH, Undeland KA, Berstad A (1998) Timing of postprandial dyspeptic symptoms and transpyloric passage of gastric contents. Scand J Gastroenterol 33:822–827

Hausken T, Li XN, Goldman B, Leotta D, Odegaard S, Martin RW (2001) Quantification of gastric emptying and duodenogastric reflux stroke volumes using three-dimensional guided digital color Doppler imaging. Eur J Ultrasound 13:205–213

Hausken T, Mundt M, Samsom M (2002) Low antroduodenal pressure gradients are responsible for gastric emptying of a low-caloric liquid meal in humans. Neurogastroenterol Motility 14:97–105

Hirsch W, Kedar R, Preiss U (1996) Color Doppler in the diagnosis of the gastroesophageal reflux in children: comparison with pH measurements and B-mode ultrasound. Pediatr Radiol 26:232–235

Hirsch W, Preiss U, Kedar R (1997) Color coded Doppler ultrasound in diagnosis of gastroesophageal reflux. Klin Padiatr 209:6–10

Holt S, McDicken WN, Anderson T, Stewart IC, Heading RC (1980) Dynamic imaging of the stomach by real-time ultrasound – a method for the study of gastric motility. Gut 21:597–601

Holt S, Cervantes J, Wilkinson AA, Wallace JH (1986) Measurement of gastric emptying rate in humans by real-time ultrasound. Gastroenterology 90:918–923

Horowitz M, Edelbroek MA, Wishart JM, Straathof JW (1993) Relationship between oral glucose tolerance and gastric emptying in normal healthy subjects. Diabetologia 36:857–862

Husebye E (1999) The patterns of small bowel motility: physiology and implications in organic disease and functional disorders. Neurogastroenterol Motility 11:141–161

Hveem K, Hausken T, Berstad A (1994) Ultrasonographic assessment of fasting liquid content in the human stomach. Scand J Gastroenterol 29:786–789

Hveem K, Jones KL, Chatterton BE, Horowitz M (1996) Scintigraphic measurement of gastric emptying and ultrasonographic assessment of antral area: relation to appetite. Gut 38:816–821

Hveem K, Sun WM, Hebbard G, Horowitz M, Doran S, Dent J (2001) Relationship between ultrasonically detected phasic antral contractions and antral pressure. Am J Physiol Gastrointest Liver Physiol 281:G95–G101

Jang HS, Lee JS, Lim GY (2001) Correlation of color Doppler sonographic findings with pH measurements in gastroesophageal reflux in children. J Clin Ultrasound 29:212–217

King PM, Adam RD, Pryde A, McDicken WN, Heading RC (1984) Relationships of human antroduodenal motility and transpyloric fluid movement: non-invasive observations with real-time ultrasound. Gut 25:1384–1391

Malagelada JR, Stanghellini V (1985) Manometric evaluation of functional upper gut symptoms. Gastroenterology 88(5 Pt 1):1223–1231

Malbert CH, Ruckebusch Y (1991) Relationships between pressure and flow across the gastroduodenal junction in dogs. Am J Physiol 260:G653–G657

Marciani L, Gowland P, Fillery-Travis A et al (2001) Assessment of antral grinding of a model solid meal with echo-planar imaging. Am J Physiol Gastrointestinal Liver Physiol 280: G844–849

Marzio L, Capone F, Neri M, Mezzetti A, DeAngelis C, Cuccurullo F (1988) Gallbladder kinetics in obese patients. Effect of a regular meal and a low caloric meal. Dig Dis Sci 33:4–9

Marzio L, Di Felice F, Celiberti V, DiGioacchino M, Mezzetti A, Cuccurullo F (1988) Gallbladder emptying in duodenal ulcer patients having undergone Billroth II gastrectomy. Digestion 41:223–228

Marzio L, Di Felice F, Laico MG, Imbimbo B, Lapenna B, Cuccurullo F (1992) Gallbladder hypokinesia and normal gastric emptying of liquids in patients with dyspeptic symptoms. A double-blind placebo-controlled clinical trial with cisapride. Dig Dis Sci 37:262–267

Moragas GM, Azpiroz F, Pavia J (1993) Relation among intragastric pressure postcibal perception, and gastric emptying. Am J Physiol 264:G1112–G1117

Palasciano G, Serio G, Portincasa P et al (1992) Gallbladder volume in adults, and relationship to age, sex, body mass index, and gallstones: a sonographic population study. Am J Gastroenterol 87:493–497

Penagini R, Hebbard G, Horowitz M (1998) Motor function of the proximal stomach and visceral perception in gastro-oesophageal reflux disease. Gut 42:251–257

Ricci R, Bontempo I, Corazziari E, La Bella A, Torsoli A (1993) Real time ultrasonography of the gastric antrum. Gut 34:173–176

Ropert A, des Varannes SB, Bizais Y (1993) Simultaneous assessment of liquid emptying and proximal gastric tone in humans. Gastroenterology 105:667–674

Savoye G, Savoye-Collet C, Oors J, Smout A (2003) Interdigestive transpyloric fluid transport assessed by intraluminal impedance recording. Am J Physiol Gastrointest Liver Physiol 284:G663–G669

Sifrim D, Holloway R, Silny J, Xin Z, Lerut A, Janssens J (2001) Acid and gas reflux in patients with gastroesophageal reflux disease during ambulatory recordings. Gastroenterology 120:1588–1598

Stone BG, Gavaler JS, Belle SH et al (1988) Impairment of gallbladder emptying in diabetes mellitus. Gastroenterology 95:170–176

Tefera S, Gilja OH, Hatlebakk JG, Berstad A (2001) Gastric accommodation studied by ultrasonography in patients with reflux esophagitis. Dig Dis Sci 46:618–625

Tefera S, Gilja OH, Olafsdottir E, Hausken T, Hatlebakk JG, Berstad A (2002) Intragastric maldistribution of a liquid meal in patients with reflux esophagitis assessed by three-dimensional ultrasonography. Gut 2:153–158

Undeland KA, Hausken T, Aanderud S, Berstad A (1997) Lower postprandial gastric volume response in diabetic patients with vagal neuropathy. Neurogastroenterol Motil 9:19–24

Undeland KA, Hausken T, Gilja OH, Aanderud S, Berstad A (1998) Gastric meal accommodation and symptoms in diabetes. A placebo-controlled study of glyceryl trinitrate. Eur J Gastroenterol Hepatol 10:677–681

Zerbib F, des Varannes SB, Ropert A (1999) Proximal gastric tone in gastro-oesophageal reflux disease. Eur J Gastroenterol Hepatol 11:511–515

# Three-Dimensional Ultrasound of the Gastrointestinal Tract

ODD HELGE GILJA

## CONTENTS

23.1 Introduction  199
23.2 Formation of 3D Ultrasonographic Images  199
23.2.1 Data Acquisition  199
23.2.2 Data Digitization  200
23.2.3 Data Storage  200
23.2.4 Data Processing  200
23.2.5 Data Display  201
23.3 Three-Dimensional Ultrasonography of the Stomach  202
23.4 Three-Dimensional Endoscopic Ultrasonography  205
23.5 Three-Dimensional Ultrasonography of the Rectum  207
23.6 Conclusion  208
References  208

## 23.1 Introduction

The digital revolution has made 3D ultrasonography a natural extension of 2D ultrasound scanning. Most frequently this is made by stacking serial 2D ultrasonograms together and utilizing computerized algorithms and equipment to process and display the data; however, in recent years, 2D array matrix probes have been developed to enable real-time 3D scanning.

O. H. GILJA, MD, PhD
Department of Medicine, National Center for Ultrasound in Gastroenterology, Haukeland University Hospital, N-5021 Bergen, Norway

## 23.2 Formation of 3D Ultrasonographic Images

If the relative position in space of a series of 2D sonograms is recorded along with the image data, three-dimensional (3D) ultrasonographic images can be constructed. For most applications, the process of making 3D images based on ultrasonography is divided into five major steps: data acquisition, digitization, storage, processing and display.

### 23.2.1 Data Acquisition

Principally, data acquisition by 3D ultrasonography can be performed in three different ways (SALUSTRI and ROELANDT 1995). Sampling of data may be carried out either by using a 2D probe attached to a motor which moves the probe in a computer-defined way, or by a spatial localizing system connected to a 2D probe, or by electronic 3D probes with the possibility of direct volume acquisition in real time.

Firstly, and most frequently used, are ordinary 2D probes which are inserted into motorized holders and either rotated (GHOSH et al. 1982; ROELANDT et al. 1994), translated (PICOT et al. 1993; ROSS et al. 1993; SACKMANN et al. 1994; SEHGAL et al. 1994; SOHN and GROTEPASS 1990), or tilted (BELOHLAVEK et al. 1993a; HAMPER et al. 1994; MARTIN et al. 1986; MARTIN and BASHEIN 1989; PRETORIUS and NELSON 1995; WAGNER et al. 1994; ZOLLER and LIESS 1994) to acquire a data volume. The rotation scanning is often applied to cardiac imaging, whereas acquisition by tilting or translating is frequently used for transcutaneous abdominal and obstetric scanning. Pullback devices have also been constructed to aid intravascular and intraductal scanning where the transducer is positioned at a distant site in relation to the mechanical holder (CHANDRASEKARAN et al. 1994; MINTZ et al. 1993; ROSENFIELD et al. 1991).

Secondly, acquisition of ultrasonographic data can be assisted by devices that record the exact position and movements of the transducer in space. This has been obtained by utilizing mechanical arms (WHITTINGHAM and BATEMAN 1983; DEKKER et al. 1974; GEISER et al. 1982; NIKRAVESH et al. 1984; RAICHLEN et al. 1986; SAWADA et al. 1985), acoustic sensors (HANDSCHUMACHER et al. 1993; KING et al. 1990, 1991; LEVINE et al. 1989; MORITZ et al. 1976), or magnetic sensors (DETMER et al. 1994; HODGES et al. 1994; KELLY et al. 1994; LEOTTA et al. 1995; PRETORIUS and NELSON 1994). A magnetic sensor, a transducer and a magnetic field generator are depicted in Figure 23.1. Furthermore, gyroscopic and optical devices can be applied to follow the position of the scanhead.

Thirdly, true volumetric 2D array transducers have been developed (GREEN and CAMPBELL 1994). These complex transducers generate a pyramidal volume of ultrasound data, enabling dynamic real-time 3D ultrasonography. The matrix probes have been validated in volume estimation and seem to perform well (BU et al. 2005; QIN et al. 2000; BINDER et al. 2000), also compared with magnetic resonance imaging (MRI) (JENKINS et al. 2004). Clinical applications of real-time 3D ultrasound include measurement of left ventricular volume (ARAI et al. 2004), quantitative assessment of perfusion defects with myocardial contrast agents (CAMARANO et al. 2002), and detection of ischemia during dobutamine-induced stress (AHMAD et al. 2001). In pathological fetal hearts, 3D Echocardiography (3DE) was helpful for localizing multiple cardiac tumors, estimating size and function of the right and left ventricles, and evaluating mechanism of valvular regurgitation and pulmonary obstruction (ACAR et al. 2005).

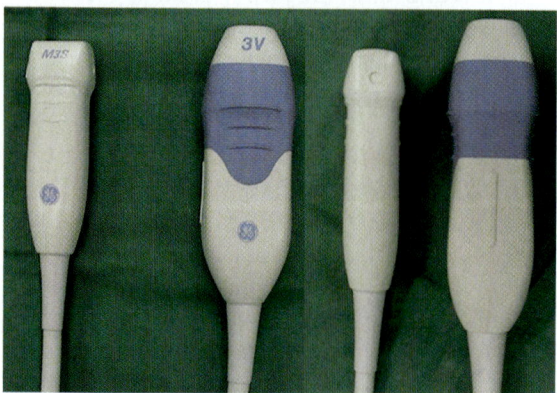

**Fig. 23.1.** Two ultrasound probes viewed from a frontal and lateral perspective. To the left of both panels an ordinary 2D phased array is shown and to the right in both panels a matrix probe, which enables real-time 3D ultrasound scanning, is depicted

## 23.2.2
## Data Digitization

Ultrasound raw data are available in a digital format in most scanners; however, some of the commercially available ultrasound scanners generate analogue output signals. Therefore, in order to be processed by a computer, conversion of ultrasonographic data into a digital format is necessary. Frequently, this is done by video frame grabbing using designated hardware cards in the computer or in the scanner; however, frame grabbing of video signals impairs image resolution; therefore, preferably, raw ultrasound data is digitized directly maintaining the original resolution.

## 23.2.3
## Data Storage

Following data capture and digitization, image data is normally stored temporarily until computer processing can take place. High-resolution 3D ultrasound data give rise to large image files requiring high-capacity storage media such as magneto-optical disks, CD/DVD, or hard disks. The ultimate goal in 3D ultrasonography is to obviate the data storage operation and perform direct data processing and volume estimation in real time, and subsequently store only the clinically relevant images and measurements.

## 23.2.4
## Data Processing

Depending on the mode of acquisition, the image data can be prepared in different ways (BELOHLAVEK et al. 1993b). Only the mainstream flowchart of processing is outlined here.

Firstly, the image data must be converted to a rectangular (Cartesian) coordinate system. Image points are assigned to new positions within a cuberille (regular data volume) on the basis of their pyramidal (if tilting acquisition) coordinates. This scan conversion is usually relatively time-consuming and is performed by computer algorithms.

Secondly, mathematical interpolation is performed to generate values that "fill in the gaps" between 2D slices that are stacked together in the cuberille. After scan conversion and interpolation, the pixels can be treated as spatially correct 3D image elements, known as voxels.

Thirdly, methods for image enhancement are usually applied to improve image contrast and remove artifacts. These techniques include filtering, histogram stretching and sliding, and morphological operations. This step may be important to the overall quality of the final 3D ultrasound image but may not be of great importance for volume measurement. Image enhancement represents an uncertainty because significant clinical information can be lost in the operation.

Fourthly, the cube of image data is now ready for segmentation, i.e., the procedure where the object of interest is separated from the surrounding structures (GREENLEAF et al. 1993). Three fundamental approaches to segmentation have been utilized in 3D ultrasonography:

1. Extraction by visual inspection and manual outlining of contours
2. Semi-automatic separation using visualization algorithms (NIELSON and SHRIVER 1989) aided by operator interaction
3. Fully automatic computer segmentation

The latter method is capable of detecting edges with high contrast but is subject to inaccuracies and artifacts; therefore, automatic segmentation must be used with great care if applied to patient data. Manual segmentation of structures in the 3D data set makes accurate volume estimation and reconstruction of organs or pathology achievable. This method, which primarily supplies quantitative information, is applicable to all areas of sonographic imaging where volume calculation is indicated.

## 23.2.5
## Data Display

The final step in formation of 3D ultrasound images is to display the data so that the inherent voxel information is communicated accurately. Commonly, simple rotation of the object on the computer monitor provides some 3D effects. To further enhance the 3D outcome of the images, stereoglasses have been applied (MARTIN et al. 1995; NELSON and PRETORIUS 1995). Projection of images by optical holography enables the observer to move around the object and examine the spatial relationships from different viewpoints (BAUM and STROKE 1975; KOIVUKANGAS et al. 1986; REDMAN et al. 1969). A typical setup of a 3D ultrasound system is shown in Figure 23.2.

Data processing and display requires specialized computer software to handle the ultrasound images.

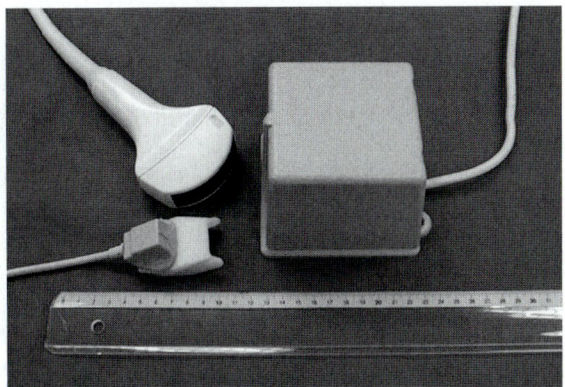

Fig. 23.2. A 3D ultrasound system based on magnetic position and orientation measurement (POM). The Bird System (Ascension Technology Corp., Burlington, Vermont, USA) consists of a sensor that can be attached to the scanhead, a magnetic field generator, and a system control unit (usually hidden in the scanner)

We have developed, in collaboration with Christian Michelsen Research (Bergen, Norway) and Vingmed Sound (Horten, Norway), a software package called EchoPac3D (MARTENS et al. 1997; MARTENS and GILJA 2004). EchoPac3D enables import of image data that are acquired both with mechanical devices and magnetic position sensors, as well as endosonographic acquisitions. Manual segmentation or semi-automatic rendering of structures in the 3D data set makes accurate volume estimation and reconstruction of organs or pathological tissue achievable. The accuracy of volume estimation in this software package has been evaluated in several studies (GILJA et al. 1994; GILJA et al. 1995; THUNE et al. 1996). A display of the EchoPac3D software is shown in Figure 23.3. The 3D ultrasound system used in our lab is outlined more in depth in a previous review (GILJA et al. 1999).

Ultrasound data contains a significant amount of noise and speckle and may exhibit boundary regions several pixels wide. It is important to keep in mind that the quality of the final 3D data display strongly depends on the resolution of the raw data. Transducer frequency and lateral resolution, frame rate of the scanner, accuracy of 3D probe, speed of scanning, and methods of filtering and segmentation, are all factors that influence the final image and subsequently volume measurements. Furthermore, there is no advantage in sampling over a spatial scale that is much smaller than the resolution cell of the display system. The ultrasound sampling conditions using a specific transducer is closely related to the display parameters.

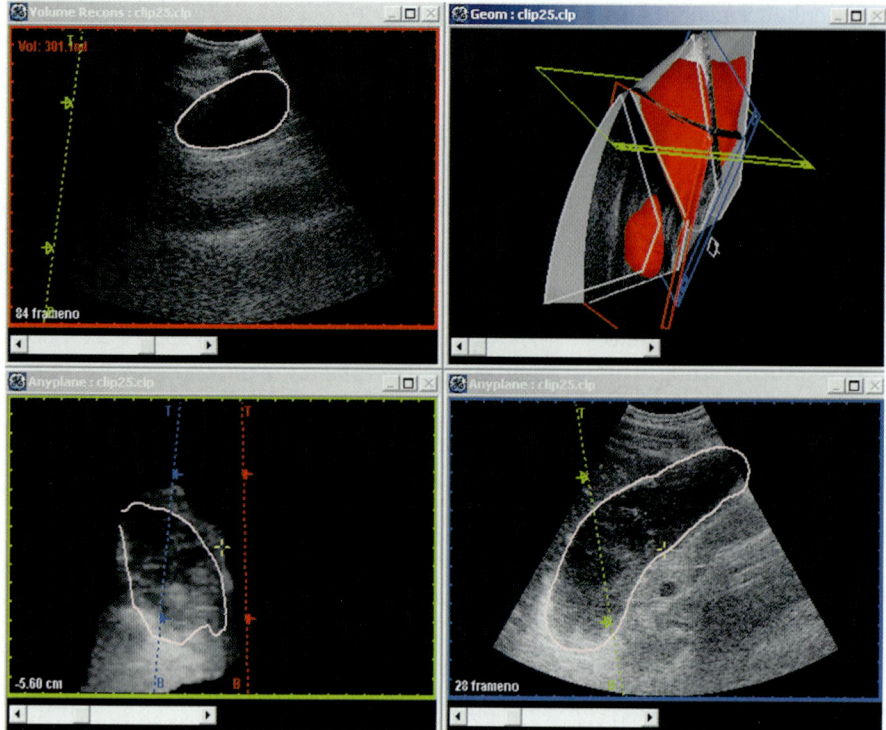

**Fig. 23.3.** A display of EchoPac3D software manufactured by GE-Vingmed Sound (Horten, Norway). In the *upper right panel*, the *red volume* is a reconstructed stomach shown in the geometry window. In the antrum an ultrasound section is displayed and this sagittal section is also depicted in the reconstruction window in the *upper left panel*. The visualization window, enabling application of numerous algorithms, is shown in the *lower right* and *lower left panels*. The software EchoPac3D enables accurate post-processing of 3D ultrasonographic images

## 23.3 Three-Dimensional Ultrasonography of the Stomach

Two-dimensional (2D) ultrasonography has been utilized to assess gastric emptying in patients with functional dyspepsia (BOLONDI et al. 1985; DUAN et al. 1993; HOU et al. 1992; BERSTAD and GILJA 2004), diabetes mellitus (DORLARS et al. 1994), and in infants with gastroesophageal reflux (LI VOTI et al. 1992). In several studies, repeated single 2D ultrasonic sections of the antrum have been applied to measure gastric emptying rates (DESAGA and HIXT 1987; DORLARS et al. 1994; DUAN et al. 1993; HOU et al. 1992; NEWELL et al. 1993). To estimate volumes of the gastric antrum by means of 2D ultrasound, a sum-of-cylinders method (RADBERG et al. 1989) and simple formulas (BOLONDI et al. 1985) have been used. Volume estimation based on 2D sonograms is subject to significant error because assumptions regarding geometrical shape of the antrum need to be made before reliable volume measurements can be performed.

To overcome these limitations, a method for volume estimation of organs and tissue based on three-dimensional (3D) ultrasonography was developed (GILJA et al. 1994). Using a motor device, the transducer was tilted through an angle of 90°, capturing sequential 2D frames before the data set was transferred to a graphic workstation for final 3D processing. This 3D ultrasound system demonstrated excellent accuracy in vitro both on phantoms (THUNE et al. 1996) and on animal organs (GILJA et al. 1994), and intra- and interobserver variation was low. When validated in vivo against MRI, this 3D ultrasound system was in good agreement and presented high precision (GILJA et al. 1995). This system has also been used to study diseases of the liver (HOKLAND and HAUSKEN 1994), and to evaluate patients with functional dyspepsia (BERSTAD et al. 1994; GILJA et al. 1996a; HAUSKEN et al. 1994). Despite the significant achievements with respect to accuracy in volume estimation and 3D reconstruction of tissue and organs, this 3D system could only acquire a 90° fan-like data set from a pre-determined, fixed orientation of the transducer. Accordingly, although highly accurate, a mechanical acquisition system like this poses great limitations to acquisition, because only small volumes can be captured.

Random acquisition of 3D ultrasound data has been achieved by utilizing different devices to locate the exact position and orientation of the transducer in space. To enable scanning of a large organ such as the fluid-filled stomach, a commercially available magnetometer-based position and orientation measurement (POM) device was interfaced to the scanner. This system for magnetic scanhead tracking (Bird, Ascencion Technology, Burlington, Vermont, USA) was validated both with respect to its precision in locating specific points in space (DETMER et al. 1994) and to its accuracy in volume estimation (HODGES et al. 1994; MATRE et al. 1999). In these studies, the sensor system worked satisfactorily in scanning human organs, and high precision and accuracy were revealed in volume estimation.

For the first time, total gastric volumes and intragastric distribution of meals could be studied by ultrasonography (GILJA et al. 1997). In this study, the depth of scanning was adjusted to fit each individual's habitus, averaging 17.6 cm. Sagittal sections of the stomach were recorded throughout its entire length, starting in the proximal part where the transducer was positioned by the left subcostal margin and tilted cranially to image the most superior part of the stomach. After stepwise scanning of the proximal stomach angling from left to right, the transducer was moved and held to insonicate normally to the skin surface. Then the distal stomach was scanned stepwise moving distally to the gastroduodenal junction. The image data and the position and orientation data were transferred to a workstation for final processing. A 3D reconstruction of the total stomach volume based on magnetic scanhead tracking from this first study is depicted in Figure 23.4.

The stomach is a large and geometrically complex organ for study by ultrasonography; therefore, we have validated this 3D ultrasonographic method in vivo in healthy controls. A barostat bag was positioned in the proximal stomach of six healthy subjects who underwent scanning with the Bird magnetic system. In steps of 100 ml, up to 700 ml of meat soup was instilled into and subsequently aspirated from the barostat bag while simultaneous 3D scanning was performed. This 3D ultrasound system correlated very well with infused volumes (Fig. 23.5)

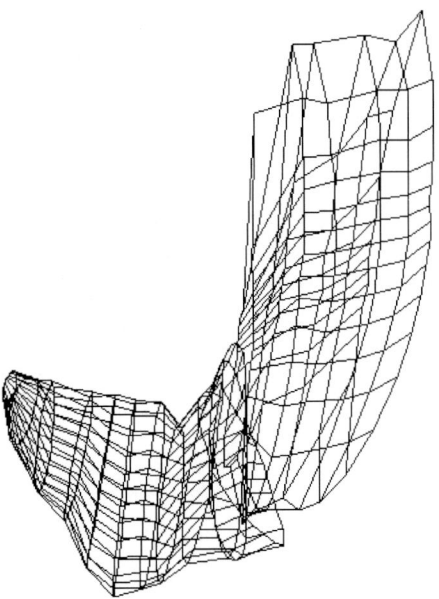

**Fig. 23.4.** A wire-frame outline of the total stomach volume after ingestion of a soup meal serving as contrast medium. The images used for 3D reconstruction are acquired by ordinary 2D ultrasonography and magnetic scanhead tracking enables precise acquisition and reconstruction of the organ

and showed very good agreement with true volumes, as well as low interobserver variation (TEFERA et al. 2002). Patients with reflux esophagitis exhibited an abnormally large volume of the proximal stomach soon after a liquid meal, concomitant with the perception of fullness. The abnormal distention of the proximal stomach may represent an important pathogenetic mechanism in reflux esophagitis.

In functional dyspepsia, poor accommodation of the proximal stomach to a meal has been found in many studies (AHLUWALIA et al. 1994; BERSTAD et al. 1997; GILJA et al. 1996b; TACK et al. 1998). Drinking capacity is often reduced in these patients and drink tests may therefore have a diagnostic potential. A simple drink test in combination with 3D ultrasonography was applied in a test using Toro meat soup, Nutridrink, and water (HJELLAND et al. 2004). The meals were ingested at a rate of 100 ml/min until maximal drinking capacity was reached. Intragastric volume at maximal drinking capacity was determined using 3D ultrasonography (Fig. 23.6). Optimal discrimination between patients and controls was obtained by the combination of symptoms and intragastric volume (S/V) using meat soup as the test meal.

Impaired gastric accommodation may induce dyspeptic symptoms also in postfundoplication patients. Using 3D ultrasonography, postfundoplication patients with and without dyspeptic symptoms were scanned and symptoms were scored postprandially (SCHEFFER et al. 2004). Dyspeptic and nondyspeptic fundoplication patients exhibited similar total gastric volumes at 5 min postprandially compared with controls, whereas smaller total gastric volumes were observed from 15 to 60 min postprandially. Distal stomach volume was more pronounced in dyspeptic fundoplication patients and related with the increase in postprandial fullness sensations. In healthy volunteers, the sensation of fullness was also related to antral volume and area rather than proximal volume (MUNDT et al. 2005).

In another study, we developed an analytical method to describe the 3D geometry of the gastric antrum: gastric fundus and the whole stomach based on 3D ultrasound acquisitions. The Fourier series method was used to simulate the organ surface geometry. The principal curvatures spatial distributions were non-homogeneous in the gastric antrum, gastric fundus, and the stomach due to their complex geometry (Fig. 23.7). An analytical tool for characterizing the complex 3D geometry of an organ such as the human stomach reconstructed by 3D ultrasound was provided (LIAO et al. 2004).

HAUSKEN and co-workers (2001) developed a noninvasive method for evaluating transpyloric flow and duodenogastric reflux stroke volumes using a 3D-guided digital color Doppler imaging model. They studied healthy subjects during ingestion of a soup meal and 10 min postprandially. Cross-sectional color Doppler digital images of duodenogastric reflux episodes were acquired with a 5- to 3-MHz phased-array transducer. The 3D position and orientation data were acquired using a magnetic sensing system. They found high intra- and interindividual variations of the stroke volumes of transpyloric flow episodes during the initial gastric emptying. The duodenogastric reflux episodes lasted on average 2.4 s with a volume of on average of 8.3 ml. This novel method minimized geometric assumptions and angular ambiguity.

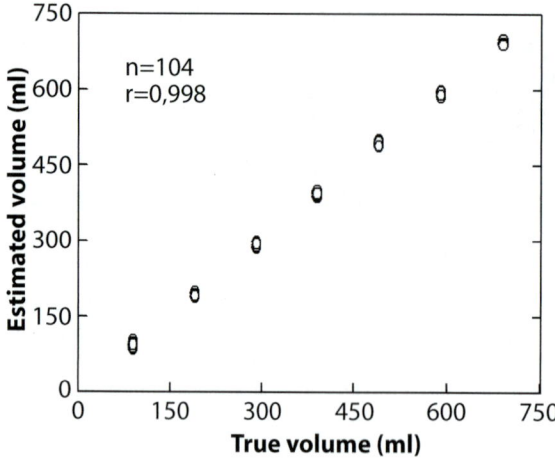

Fig. 23.5. Scatter plot shows the correlation between estimated and true volumes of a barostat bag positioned in the human stomach after scanning by a 3D ultrasound system. Scanning was performed with a 3.5-MHz transducer attached to a Bird system after stepwise instillation and aspiration of the test meal. The magnetic transmitter was positioned just behind the back of the examined subject and within the performance range of the sensor (60 cm)

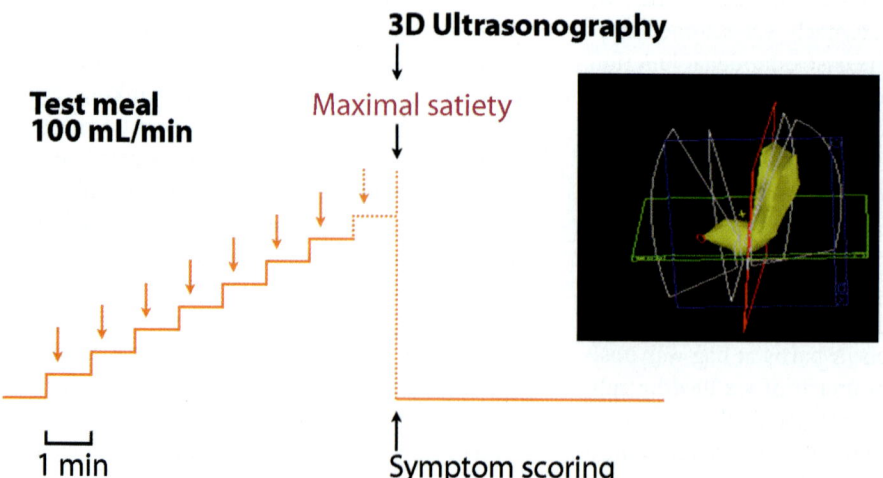

Fig. 23.6. The scanning protocol is shown using 3D ultrasound to determine maximal gastric volume after a meal in patients with functional dyspepsia. Interestingly, the fraction of symptoms per volume (S/V) distinguished best between patients and controls after a soup meal

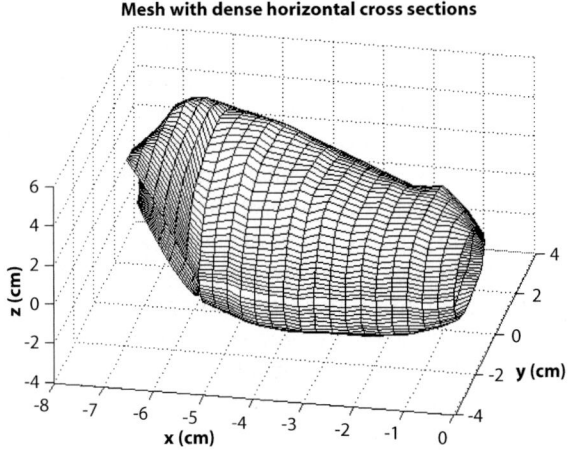

**Fig. 23.7.** A 3D gastric antrum generated by the EchoPac3D program and reconstructed in a new coordinate system. In this geometry, 3D strain can be calculated and visualized following ultrasound scanning

## 23.4
## Three-Dimensional Endoscopic Ultrasonography

Endoscopic ultrasonography (EUS) has gained acceptance as a valuable tool in obtaining diagnostic information in patients with digestive diseases, as it enables detailed visualization of small structures along the gastrointestinal tract; however, its use has been limited to a few centers, partly due to the high demands for skills in both endoscopy and ultrasound scanning. Interpretation of 2D endosonographic images can be challenging, even for experienced operators; therefore, the applicability of new acquisition units allowing endosonographic recordings to be imported into the general 3D reconstruction systems was investigated (MOLIN et al. 1996a; MOLIN et al. 1996b; MOLIN et al. 1997; MOLIN et al. 1999). So far, 3D endosonography has been based on sequential sampling of 2D images, mainly during pull-back of radial scanning probes. The 3D data are usually displayed in an orthogonal window or by any-plane slicing. In one study, endoluminal ultrasound examinations were performed with 360° radial scanning 7.5- and 12-MHz echoendoscope and miniature probes, 8 F as well as 12 and 20 MHz (Olympus, Tokyo, Japan). Acquisition of 2D ultrasound images was achieved by connecting the probes to a computer-controlled linear stepping motor device (Prototype, MKAB, Gothenburg, Sweden) with an acquisition length of 0.5–15 cm and an operating speed at 10 mm/s, resulting in a distance between serial images of 0.1–0.2 mm. Further post-processing was performed using EchoPac3D. These studies demonstrated that 3D endosonography enabled accurate volume estimation of a wide range of tumors (Fig. 23.8), and improved global display of tumor extensions and topographic relations, thus enabling better preoperative planning (ODEGAARD et al. 1999; ODEGAARD et al. 1998). We also explored other methods of 3D acquisition by testing the performance in vitro of a miniature magnetic sensor (MiniBird, Ascension Technology, Burlington, Vermont, USA) for endoluminal US and 3D EUS (MOLIN et al. 2000). The magnetic 6D position and orientation measurement system (POM) was used to track different types of radial scanning endoluminal US probes. The performance of the POM system was similar if ferric or non-ferric US endoscopes were used for EUS. SUMIYAMA et al. (2003) later developed a linear-array 3D EUS with a miniature position sensor attached to the tip of the echoendoscope used in freehand scanning and confirmed its applicability.

In order to improve image quality of the 3D data set by avoiding artifacts from pulsatile organs, ECG-triggered 3D EUS reconstructions were attempted (MOLIN et al. 1998). The authors found that ECG-triggered 3D EUS images could easily be obtained using a stepping motor device during routine examinations, resulting in a clear demonstration of the different wall layers in the longitudinal image axis. The lateral dislocation was 2.40 mm (SD 0.56 mm) in non-ECG triggered examinations resulting in a "fuzzy" image in the axial display, compared with 0.19 mm

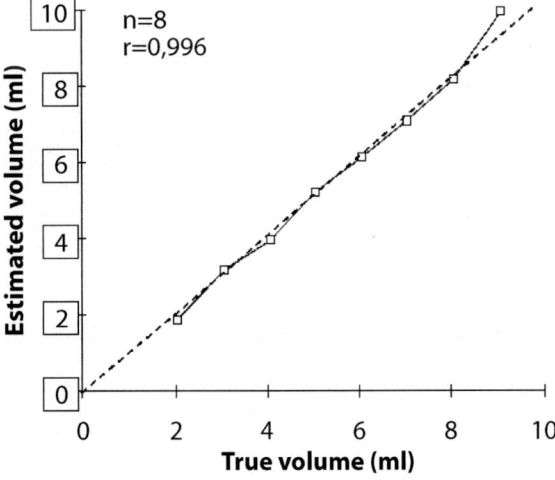

**Fig. 23.8.** The plot shows the association between estimated and true volumes after EUS scanning of a phantom in vitro. The acquisition was performed using Olympus miniprobe 12 MHz (UM-2R)

(SD 0.23 mm) in the ECG triggered scans ($p<0.0027$; Fig. 23.9). This resulted in higher accuracy in the evaluation of small and superficial lesions of the esophageal wall and fundic region of the stomach.

Other researchers have also assessed the clinical usefulness and problems of 3D images obtained by endosonography (NISHIMURA et al. 1997). NISHIMURA and coworkers (1997) studied 18 resected specimens of gastrointestinal lesions and 21 patients. In the resected specimens, the surface images were quite consistent with the macroscopic findings in 17 cases. In two esophageal cancers, 7 out of 10 gastric cancers, and two colonic cancers, the depth of tumor invasion was assessed accurately from the reconstructed images. In the in vivo study, although 3D displays had some limitations, it was particularly useful for esophageal and rectal lesions. They concluded that this new diagnostic method enabled visualization of the total extent of gastrointestinal lesions and appeared to have useful clinical applications.

Another Japanese group used a system of 3D endoscopic ultrasonography to analyze the surface, the echo density, and the echo patterns of cross-sectional images of submucosal lesions. They evaluated the quality of the 3D image and cross-sectional images of lipomas, leiomyomas, and cysts. They stated that analysis of 3D EUS images was useful in making a diagnosis of submucosal lesions (MIYAMOTO et al. 1998). TSUTSUII and coworkers (1998) evaluated the usefulness of 3D sonography using Olympus ultrasound 3D imaging system to spatially clarify digestive lesions. They converted the sequential 2D data into volume data by an image processing software (Medical Design Composer 1.0) developed by the authors. They found that determination of the depth and the extent of tumor invasion was more correctly viewed when arbitrary slicing was applied; however, it was difficult to obtain precise 3D images in lesions greatly influenced by heartbeats.

In another study, volume measurement using tissue characterization of 3D endoscopic ultrasonographic images was performed (YOSHINO et al. 2000), showing good correlation between the volume measured with 3D EUS and the volume obtained using tissue characterization. The tissue characterization volumes were only relatively slightly larger than the volumes measured using 3D EUS, and the authors suggested that there is some promise for tissue characterization in 3D EUS.

HUNERBEIN et al. (1997) aimed at developing a technique for 3D endoscopic ultrasound of the esophagus based on standard endosonographic images. They attached a high-resolution miniprobe (360°, 12.5 MHz) to a stepping motor that enabled ECG-

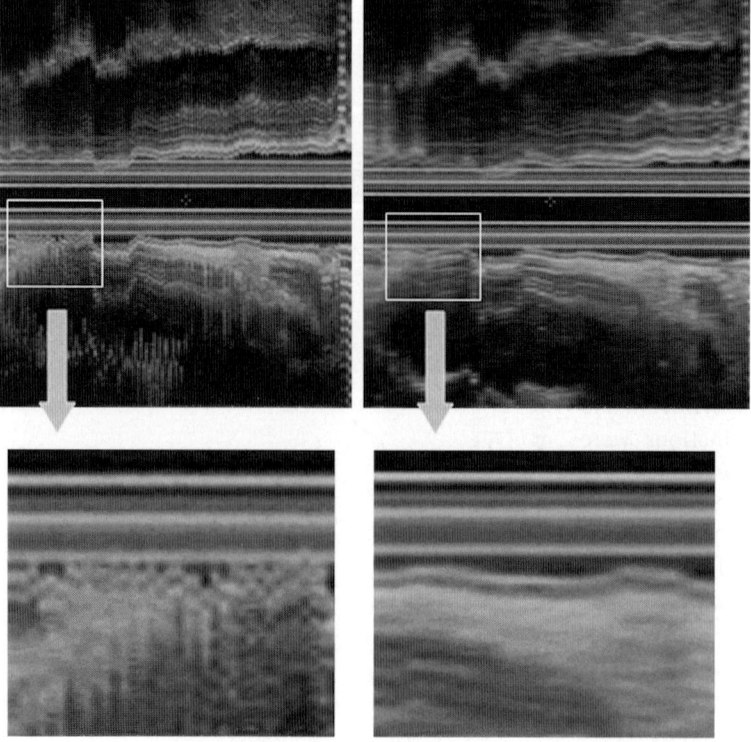

Fig. 23.9. The ECG-triggered 3D EUS reconstructions could be obtained during routine examinations, resulting in a clear demonstration of the different wall layers in the longitudinal image axis. In the *left panel*, a non-ECG triggered EUS acquisition is depicted. Eight-French miniature ultrasound catheters 12–20 MHz (Olympus Optical, Japan) were used. Image distortion was measured as lateral dislocation of the organ wall layers, perpendicular to the probe, in the longitudinal axis of the reconstructed ultrasound image. The lateral dislocation was 2.40 mm (SD 0.56 mm) in non-ECG trigged examinations, resulting in a "fuzzy" image in the axial display, compared with 0.19 mm (SD 0.23 mm) in the ECG-triggered examinations ($p<0.0027$)

triggered withdrawal of the transducer for imaging of esophageal cancer patients. The system enabled the acquisition of accurate 3D ultrasound data within 30–50 s (Fig. 23.10). Computed image processing allowed display of the data in transverse, longitudinal, and oblique sections, or as a 3D reconstruction. Three-dimensional imaging provided accurate visualization of the tumor and surrounding structures in all cases. Longitudinal scan planes and 3D views improved the assessment of longitudinal tumor infiltration and the spatial relation of the tumor to relevant mediastinal structures. They concluded that 3D endoscopic ultrasound of the esophagus was technically feasible and it allowed the assessment of local tumor spread in previously unattainable scan planes.

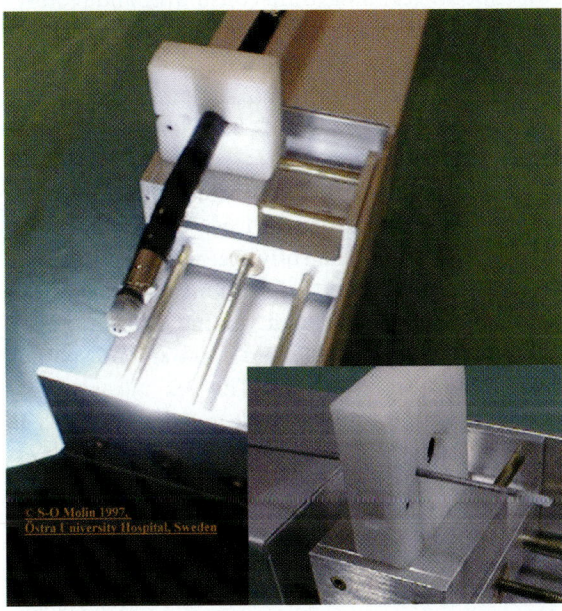

**Fig. 23.10.** A prototype acquisition unit for 3D EUS imaging that can be used both for echoendoscopes and miniprobes. The pullback system allows for a constant speed of transducer movement

## 23.5
## Three-Dimensional Ultrasonography of the Rectum

Transrectal ultrasound is the most sensitive technique for per-operative staging and follow-up of rectal cancer. Major limitations of this technique include the complexity of image interpretation and the inability to examine stenotic tumors or to identify recurrent rectal cancer; therefore, HUNERBEIN and SCHLAG (1997) conducted a prospective study to investigate the value of 3D endosonography for staging of rectal cancer. Three-dimensional endosonography was performed in 100 patients with rectal tumors. Transrectal volume scans were obtained using a 3D multiplane transducer (7.5/10.0 MHz). Stenotic tumors were examined with a 3D front-fire transducer (5.0/7.5 MHz). The volume scans were processed and analyzed on a Combison 530 workstation (Kretztechnik, Zipf, Austria). Display of volume data in three perpendicular planes or as 3D view facilitated the interpretation of ultrasound images and enhanced the diagnostic information of the data. The accuracy of 3D endosonography in the assessment of infiltration depth was 88% compared with 82% with the conventional technique. In the determination of lymph node involvement, 3D and 2D endosonography provided accuracy rates of 79% and 74%, respectively. The 3D scanning allowed the visualization of obstructing tumors using reconstructed planes in front of the transducer. Correct assessment of the infiltration depth was possible in 15 out of 21 patients with obstructing tumors (accuracy 76%). Three-dimensional endosonography displayed suspicious pararectal lesions in 30 patients. Transrectal ultrasound-guided biopsy was extremely precise (accuracy 98%) and showed malignancy in 10 of 30 patients. They concluded that the 3D imaging and ultrasound-guided biopsy seemed capable to improve staging of rectal cancer. The same authors also investigated the value of 3D endorectal ultrasonography for staging of obstructing rectal cancer (HUNERBEIN et al. 1996). In that study, they concluded that this technique may improve therapy planning in advanced rectal cancer by selecting patients who require pre-operative adjuvant therapy. KIM et al. (2002) performed a prospective study to verify whether 3D endorectal ultrasonography (EUS) enhances the accuracy of rectal cancer staging, as compared with conventional EUS. They scanned 33 consecutive patients and the accuracy of 3D EUS was 90.9% for pT2 and 84.8% for pT3, whereas that of conventional EUS was 84.8% and 75.8%, respectively. The lymph node metastasis was accurately predicted by 3D EUS in 28 patients (84.8%), whereas conventional EUS predicted the disorder in 22 patients (66.7%). These differences were not statistically significant, probably due to a low number of patients. The average infiltration grade of the circumference on transverse 3D EUS scans was associated closely with advancement of the TNM stage and lymph node metastasis (KIM et al. 2002).

WILLIAMS et al. (2001) used 3D endoanal sonography to determine the incidence and functional consequences of external sphincter trauma. They examined 55 women after delivery and found ultrasound evidence of postpartum trauma in 13 of 45 women who had a vaginal delivery, involving the external sphincter in five, the puboanalis in nine, and the transverse perineii in three. They concluded that coronal imaging offered by 3D ultrasonography of the external anal sphincter was a useful adjunct to the assessment of trauma. The positive influence of 3D scanning was confirmed by CHRISTENSEN and coworkers (2005) who found that 3D anal endosonography improves diagnostic confidence in detecting damage to the anal sphincter complex. The agreement between two observers was acceptable using 2D but better when using 3D. They concluded that the 3D method may improve the selection of patients for surgical repair of the anal sphincter complex. CHRISTENSEN et al. (2004) also used 3D endosonography in patients with anal carcinoma and found that detection of perirectal lymph nodes and tumor invasion were improved, compared with 2D endosonography. This may affect local tumor staging and thus planning of treatment.

WEST et al. (2004) determined the agreement between hydrogen peroxide-enhanced 3D endoanal ultrasonography (3D HPUS) and endoanal magnetic resonance imaging (MRI) in preoperative assessment of perianal fistulas, and assessed patient preference with regard to these techniques. The methods agreed in 88% for the primary fistula tract, in 90% for the location of the internal opening, in 78% for secondary tracts, and in 88% for fluid collections. They concluded that 3D HPUS and endoanal MRI are equally adequate for the evaluation of perianal fistulas. Both methods are associated with similar discomfort and patients have no preference for either procedure.

## 23.6
## Conclusion

The introduction of 3D ultrasonographic imaging in the field of gastroenterology seems to improve standardization of data acquisition and analysis, and this is particularly relevant for endosonographic imaging. Moreover, acquisition time during an unpleasant procedure for the patient can be reduced. The 3D imaging also makes ultrasonography less operator dependent and facilitates easier interpretation of ultrasonographic images. For volume estimation, there are several studies that demonstrate high accuracy of 3D ultrasonography. Furthermore, when conventional 2D scanning is compared with 3D ultrasonography, studies concluded that 3D ultrasonography performs better than 2D ultrasonography with respect to accuracy and precision in volume calculation (KYEI MENSAH et al. 1996; RICCABONA et al. 1995; SAPIN et al. 1993).

For mapping of complex anatomy, e.g., to aid surgical planning, 3D ultrasonography appears to be a promising tool (BORGES et al. 1996; TROCINO et al. 1996; VANNIER and MARSH 1996; VOGEL et al. 1995); however, there are limitations of 3D ultrasonography that need to be acknowledged. The whole process from acquisition to display of 3D images is, except for real-time 3D scanning, time-consuming and requires dedicated, well-trained operators. The importance of high-quality raw data enabled by careful acquisition cannot be overestimated, as there is principally no new image data in the 3D file compared with the original 2D image.

There is a future for 3D ultrasonography as development in acquisition devices, transducer technology, and computer software and hardware will permit real-time data acquisition and image rendering. On-line display and volume calculation will enhance diagnostic value and allow smooth patient examination and work-up. The 3D ultrasonography may become an important imaging modality in interventional medicine where accurate 3D display is warranted.

## References

Acar P, Dulac Y, Taktak A, Abadir S (2005) Real-time three-dimensional fetal echocardiography using matrix probe. Prenat Diagn 25:370–375

Ahluwalia NK, Thompson DG, Barlow J, Troncon LEA, Hollis S (1994) Relaxation responses of the human proximal stomach to distension during fasting and after food. Am J Physiol 267:G166–G172

Ahmad M, Xie T, McCulloch M, Abreo G, Runge M (2001) Real-time three-dimensional dobutamine stress echocardiography in assessment stress echocardiography in assessment of ischemia: comparison with two-dimensional dobutamine stress echocardiography. J Am Coll Cardiol 37:1303–1309

Arai K, Hozumi T, Matsumura Y, Sugioka K et al (2004) Accuracy of measurement of left ventricular volume and ejection fraction by new real-time three-dimensional echocardiography in patients with wall motion abnormalities secondary to myocardial infarction. Am J Cardiol 94:552–558

Baum G, Stroke GW (1975) Optical holographic three-dimensional ultrasonography. Science 189:994–995

Belohlavek M, Foley DA, Gerber TC, Greenleaf JF, Seward JB (1993a) Three-dimensional ultrasound imaging of the atrial septum: normal and pathologic anatomy. J Am Coll Cardiol 22:1673–1678

Belohlavek M, Foley DA, Gerber TC, Kinter TM, Greenleaf JF, Seward JB (1993b) Three- and four-dimensional cardiovascular ultrasound imaging: a new era for echocardiography. Mayo Clin Proc 68:221–240

Berstad A, Gilja OH (2004) Ultrasonographic alterations in functional dyspepsia. In: Odegaard S, Gilja OH, Gregersen H (eds) Basic and new aspects of gastrointestinal ultrasonography. World Scientific, Singapore, pp 395–420

Berstad A, Hausken T, Gilja OH, Thune N, Matre K, Odegaard S (1994) Volume measurement of gastric antrum by 3-D ultrasonography and flow measurements through the pylorus by duplex technique. Dig Dis Sci 39:97–100

Berstad A, Hausken T, Gilja OH et al (1997) Gastric accommodation in functional dyspepsia. Scand J Gastroenterol 32:193–197

Binder TM, Rosenhek R, Porenta G, Maurer G, Baumgartner H (2000) Improved assessment of mitral valve stenosis by volumetric real-time three-dimensional echocardiography. J Am Coll Cardiol 36:1355–1361

Bolondi L, Bortolotti M, Santi V, Calletti T, Gaiani S, Labo G (1985) Measurement of gastric emptying time by real-time ultrasonography. Gastroenterology 89:752–759

Borges AC, Witt C, Bartel T, Muller S, Konertz W, Baumann G (1996) Preoperative two- and three-dimensional transesophageal echocardiographic assessment of heart tumors. Ann Thorac Surg 61:1163–1167

Bu L, Munns S, Zhang H et al (2005) Rapid full volume data acquisition by real-time 3-dimensional echocardiography for assessment of left ventricular indexes in children: a validation study compared with magnetic resonance imaging. J Am Soc Echocardiogr 18:299–305

Camarano G, Jones M, Freidlin RZ, Panza JA (2002) Quantitative assessment of left ventricular perfusion defects using real-time three-dimensional myocardial contrast echocardiography. J Am Soc Echocardiogr 15:206–213

Chandrasekaran K, Sehgal CM, Hsu TL et al (1994) Three-dimensional volumetric ultrasound imaging of arterial pathology from two-dimensional intravascular ultrasound: an in vitro study. Angiology 45:253–264

Christensen AF, Nielsen MB, Engelholm SA, Roed H, Svendsen LB, Christensen H (2004) Three-dimensional anal endosonography may improve staging of anal cancer compared with two-dimensional endosonography. Dis Colon Rectum 47:341–345

Christensen AF, Nyhuus B, Nielsen MB, Christensen H (2005) Three-dimensional anal endosonography may improve diagnostic confidence of detecting damage to the anal sphincter complex. Br J Radiol 78:308–311

Dekker DL, Piziali RL, Dong EJr (1974) A system for ultrasonically imaging the human heart in three dimensions. Comput Biomed Res 7:544–553

Desaga JF, Hixt U (1987) Sonographic determination of gastric emptying. Ultraschall Med 8:138–141

Detmer PR, Bashein G, Hodges TC et al (1994) 3D ultrasonic image feature localization based on magnetic scanhead tracking: in vitro calibration and validation. Ultrasound Med Biol 20:923–936

Dorlars D, Schilling D, Riemann JF (1994) The feasibility of ultrasonography for the evaluation of stomach motility disorders. Dtsch Med Wochenschr 119:575–580

Duan LP, Zheng ZT, Li YN (1993) A study of gastric emptying in non-ulcer dyspepsia using a new ultrasonographic method. Scand J Gastroenterol 28:355–360

Geiser EA, Christie LGJ, Conetta DA, Conti CR, Gossman GS (1982) A mechanical arm for spatial registration of two-dimensional echocardiographic sections. Cathet Cardiovasc Diagn 8:89–101

Ghosh A, Nanda NC, and Maurer G (1982) Three-dimensional reconstruction of echo-cardiographic images using the rotation method. Ultrasound Med Biol 8:655–661

Gilja OH, Thune N, Matre K, Hausken T, Odegaard S, Berstad A (1994) In vitro evaluation of three-dimensional ultrasonography in volume estimation of abdominal organs. Ultrasound Med Biol 20:157–165

Gilja OH, Smievoll AI, Thune N et al (1995) In vivo comparison of 3D ultrasonography and magnetic resonance imaging in volume estimation of human kidneys. Ultrasound Med Biol 21:25–32

Gilja OH, Hausken T, Odegaard S, Berstad A (1996a) Three-dimensional ultrasonography of the gastric antrum in patients with functional dyspepsia. Scand J Gastroenterol 31:847–855

Gilja OH, Hausken T, Wilhelmsen I, Berstad A (1996b) Impaired accommodation of proximal stomach to a meal in functional dyspepsia. Dig Dis Sci 41:689–696

Gilja OH, Detmer PR, Jong JM et al (1997) Intragastric distribution and gastric emptying assessed by 3D-ultrasonography. Gastroenterology 113:38–49

Gilja OH, Hausken T, Berstad A, Odegaard S (1999) Measurements of organ volume by ultrasonography. Proc Inst Mech Eng [H] 213:247–259

Green K, Campbell G (1994) Nitric oxide formation is involved in vagal inhibition of the stomach of the trout (Salmo gairdneri). J Auton Nerv Syst 50:221–229

Greenleaf JF, Belohlavek M, Gerber TC, Foley DA, Seward JB (1993) Multidimensional visualization in echocardiography: an introduction. Mayo Clin Proc 68:213–220

Hamper UM, Trapanotto V, Sheth S, DeJong MR, Caskey CI (1994) Three-dimensional US: preliminary clinical experience. Radiology 191:397–401

Handschumacher MD, Lethor JP, Siu SC et al (1993) A new integrated system for three-dimensional echocardiographic reconstruction: development and validation for ventricular volume with application in human subjects. J Am Coll Cardiol 21:743–753

Hausken T, Thune N, Matre K, Gilja OH, Odegaard S, Berstad A (1994) Volume estimation of the gastric antrum and the gallbladder in patients with non-ulcer dyspepsia and erosive prepyloric changes, using three-dimensional ultrasonography. Neurogastroenterol Mot 6:263–270

Hausken T, Li X-N, Goldman B, Leotta DF, Odegaard S, Martin RW (2001) Quantification of gastric emptying and duodenogastric reflux stroke volumes using three-dimensional guided digital color Doppler imaging. Eur J Ultrasound 13:205–213

Hjelland IE, Ofstad AP, Narvestad JK, Berstad A, Hausken T (2004) Drink tests in functional dyspepsia: Which drink is best? Scand J Gastroenterol 39:933–937

Hodges TC, Detmer PR, Burns DH, Beach KW, Strandness DE Jr (1994) Ultrasonic three-dimensional reconstruction: in vitro and in vivo volume and area measurement. Ultrasound Med Biol 20:719–729

Hokland J, Hausken T (1994) An interactive volume rendering method applied to ultrasonography of abdominal structures. IEEE Ultrason Symp Proc 3:1567–1571

Hou XH, Deng YB, Zhang JK (1992) Measurement of gastric emptying in non-ulcer dyspepsia. Chung Hua Nei Ko Tsa Chih 31:623–625, 658

Hunerbein M, Schlag PM (1997) Three-dimensional endosonography for staging of rectal cancer. Ann Surg 225:432–438

Hunerbein M, Below C, Schlag PM (1996) Three-dimensional endorectal ultrasonography for staging of obstructing rectal cancer. Dis Colon Rectum 39:636–642

Hunerbein M, Gretschel S, Ghadimi BM, Schlag PM (1997) Three-dimensional endoscopic ultrasound of the esophagus. Preliminary experience. Surg Endosc 11:991–994

Jenkins C, Bricknell K, Hanekom L, Marwick TH (2004) Reproducibility and accuracy of echocardiographic measurements of left ventricular parameters using real-time three-dimensional echocardiography. J Am Coll Cardiol 44:878–886

Kelly IM, Gardener JE, Brett AD, Richards R, Lees WR (1994) Three-dimensional US of the fetus. Work in progress. Radiology 192:253–259

Kim JC, Cho YK, Kim SY, Park SK, Lee MG (2002) Comparative study of three-dimensional and conventional endorectal ultrasonography used in rectal cancer staging. Surg Endosc 16:1280–1285

King DL, King DL Jr, Shao MY (1990) Three-dimensional spatial registration and interactive display of position and orientation of real-time ultrasound images. J Ultrasound Med 9:525–532

King DL, King DL Jr, Shao MY (1991) Evaluation of in vitro measurement accuracy of a three-dimensional ultrasound scanner. J Ultrasound Med 10:77–82

Koivukangas J, Ylitalo J, Alasaarela E, Tauriainen A (1986) Three-dimensional ultrasound imaging of brain for neurosurgery. Ann Clin Res 18 (Suppl 47):65–72

Kyei Mensah A, Zaidi J, Pittrof R, Shaker A, Campbell S, Tan SL (1996) Transvaginal three-dimensional ultrasound: accuracy of follicular volume measurements. Fertil Steril 65:371–376

Leotta DF, Detmer PR, Gilja OH et al (1995) Three-dimensional ultrasound imaging using multiple magnetic tracking systems and miniature magnetic sensors. Proc IEEE Int Ultrasonics Symp, Seattle Washington, pp 1415–1418

Levine RA, Handschumacher MD, Sanfilippo AJ et al (1989) Three-dimensional echocardiographic reconstruction of the mitral valve, with implications for the diagnosis of mitral valve prolapse. Circulation 80:589–598

Liao D, Gregersen H, Hausken T, Gilja OH, Mundt M, Kassab G (2004) Analysis of surface geometry of the human stomach using real-time 3-D ultrasonography in vivo. Neurogastroenterol Motil 16:315–324

LiVoti G, Tulone V, Bruno R et al (1992) Ultrasonography and gastric emptying: evaluation in infants with gastroesophageal reflux. J Pediatr Gastroenterol Nutr 14:397–399

Martens D, Gilja OH (2004) The EchoPAC-3D software for 3D image analysis. In: Odegaard S, Gilja OH, Gregersen H (eds) Basic and new aspects of gastrointestinal ultrasonography. World Scientific, Singapore

Martens D, Hausken T, Gilja OH, Steen EN, Alker HJ (1997) 3D processing of ultrasound images using a novel echopac-3D software. Ultrasound Med Biol 23 (S1):136

Martin RW, Bashein G (1989) Measurement of stroke volume with three-dimensional transesophageal ultrasonic scanning: comparison with thermodilution measurement. Anesthesiology 70:470–476

Martin RW, Bashein G, Zimmer R, Sutherland J (1986) An endoscopic micromanipulator for multiplanar transesophageal imaging. Ultrasound Med Biol 12:965–975

Martin RW, Legget M, McDonald J et al (1995) Stereographic viewing of 3D ultrasound images: A novelty or a tool? Proc IEEE Int Ultrasonics Symp 2:1431–1434

Matre K, Stokke EM, Martens D, Gilja OH (1999) In vitro volume estimation of kidneys using three-dimensional ultrasonography and a position sensor. Eur J Ultrasound 10:65–73

Mintz GS, Pichard AD, Satler LF, Popma JJ, Kent KM, Leon MB (1993) Three-dimensional intravascular ultrasonography: reconstruction of endovascular stents in vitro and in vivo. J Clin Ultrasound 21:609–615

Miyamoto M, Aoyama N, Sakashita M et al (1998) Three-dimensional endoscopic ultrasonography for SMT. Digestion 59:194

Molin SO, Nesje LB, Gilja OH, Hausken T, Odegaard S (1996a) Modalities for three-dimensional endoscopic and laparoscopic ultrasonography: in vitro and in vivo evaluation. Endoscopy 28:S38

Molin SO, Nesje LB, Gilja OH, Hausken T, Odegaard S (1996b) Adoption of conventional endosonography for 3D visualization of GI tract. Scand J Gastroenterol 31:33

Molin SO, Jirås A, Hall-Angerås M, Falk A, Martens D, Gilja OH, Nesje LB, Odegaard S (1997) Virtual reality in surgical practice. In vitro and in vivo evaluations. In: Sieburg H, Weghorst S, Morgan K (eds) Studies in health technology and informatics. IOS Press and Ohmsha, pp 246–253

Molin SO, Engstrøm A, Nesje LB, Gilja OH, Odegaard S (1998) Improvement of 3D EUS using ECG- and respiratory triggered acquisition. Eur J Ultrasound 7:54

Molin S, Nesje LB, Gilja OH, Hausken T, Martens D, Odegaard S (1999) 3D-endosonography in gastroenterology: methodology and clinical applications. Eur J Ultrasound 10:171–177

Molin SO, Liedman B, Lundell L et al (2000) Performance of a miniature magnetic position sensor for 3D-EUS imaging. Endoscopy 32:50

Moritz WE, Shreve PL, Mace LE (1976) Analysis of an ultrasonic spatial locating system. IEEE Trans Instrum Meas 25:43–50

Mundt MW, Hausken T, Smout AJ, Samsom M (2005) Relationships between gastric accommodation and gastrointestinal sensations in healthy volunteers. A study using the barostat technique and two- and three-dimensional ultrasonography. Dig Dis Sci 50:1654–1660

Nelson TR, Pretorius DH (1995) Visualization of the fetal thoracic skeleton with three-dimensional sonography: a preliminary report. Am J Roentgenol 164:1485–1488

Newell SJ, Chapman S, Booth IW (1993) Ultrasonic assessment of gastric emptying in the preterm infant. Arch Dis Child 69:32–36

Nielson GM, Shriver B (1989) Visualization in scientific computing. IEEE Computer Society Press, Los Alamitos

Nikravesh PE, Skorton DJ, Chandran KB, Attarwala YM, Pandian N, Kerber RE (1984) Computerized three-dimensional finite element reconstruction of the left ventricle from cross-sectional echocardiograms. Ultrason Imaging 6:48–59

Nishimura K, Niwa Y, Goto H, Hase S, Arisawa T, Hayakawa T (1997) Three-dimensional endoscopic ultrasonography of gastrointestinal lesions using an ultrasound probe. Scand J Gastroenterol 32:862–868

Odegaard S, Nesje LB, Gilja OH, Hausken T, Molin SO, Martens D (1998) Diseases of the gastrointestinal tract examined with 3D endoscopic ultrasonography. In: Bismuth H, Galmiche JP, Huguier M, Jaeck D. Eighth World Congress of the Int Gastro-Surgical Club, Monduzzi Editore, 15-4-0098, pp 827–831

Odegaard S, Nesje LB, Molin SO, Gilja OH, Hausken T (1999) Three-dimensional intraluminal sonography in the evaluation of gastrointestinal diseases. Abdom Imaging 24:449–451

Picot PA, Rickey DW, Mitchell R, Rankin RN, Fenster A (1993) Three-dimensional colour Doppler imaging. Ultrasound Med Biol 19:95–104

Pretorius DH, Nelson TR (1994) Prenatal visualization of cranial sutures and fontanelles with three-dimensional ultrasonography. J Ultrasound Med 13:871–876

Pretorius DH, Nelson TR (1995) Fetal face visualization using three-dimensional ultrasonography. J Ultrasound Med 14:349–356

Qin JX, Jones M, Shiota T, Greenberg NL et al (2000) Validation of real-time three-dimensional echocardiography for quantifying left ventricular volumes in the presence of a left ventricular aneurysm: in vitro and in vivo studies. J Am Coll Cardiol 36:900–907

Radberg G, Asztely M, Cantor P et al (1989) Gastric and gallbladder emptying in relation to the secretion of cholecystokinin after a meal in late pregnancy. Digestion 42:174–180

Raichlen JS, Trivedi SS, Herman GT, St. John Sutton MG, Reichek N (1986) Dynamic three-dimensional reconstruction of the left ventricle from two-dimensional echocardiograms. J Am Coll Cardiol 8:364–370

Redman JD, Walton WP, Fleming JE, Hall AM (1969) Holographic display of data from ultrasonic scanning. Ultrasonics 7:26–29

Riccabona M, Nelson TR, Pretorius DH, Davidson TE (1995) Distance and volume measurement using three-dimensional ultrasonography. J Ultrasound Med 14:881–886

Roelandt JR, ten Cate FJ, Vletter WB, Taams MA (1994) Ultrasonic dynamic three-dimensional visualization of the heart with a multiplane transesophageal imaging transducer. J Am Soc Echocardiogr 7:217–229

Rosenfield K, Losordo DW, Ramaswamy K et al (1991) Three-dimensional reconstruction of human coronary and peripheral arteries from images recorded during two-dimensional intravascular ultrasound examination. Circulation 84:1938–1956

Ross JJ Jr, D'Adamo AJ, Karalis DG, Chandrasekaran K (1993) Three-dimensional transesophageal echo imaging of the descending thoracic aorta. Am J Cardiol 71:1000–1002

Sackmann M, Pauletzki J, Zwiebel FM, Holl J (1994) Three-dimensional ultrasonography in hepatobiliary and pancreatic diseases. Bildgebung 61:100–103

Salustri A, Roelandt JR (1995) Ultrasonic three-dimensional reconstruction of the heart. Ultrasound Med Biol 21:281–293

Sapin PM, Schroeder KD, Smith MD, DeMaria AN, King DL (1993) Three-dimensional echocardiographic measurement of left ventricular volume in vitro: comparison with two-dimensional echocardiography and cineventriculography. J Am Coll Cardiol 22:1530–1537

Sawada H, Fujii J, Aizawa T et al. (1985) Three dimensional reconstruction of the human left ventricle from multiple cross-sectional echocardiograms: comparison with biplane cineventriculography using Simpson's rule. J Cardiogr 15:439–447

Scheffer RC, Gooszen HG, Wassenaar EB, Samsom M (2004) Relationship between partial gastric volumes and dyspeptic symptoms in fundoplication patients: a 3D ultrasonographic study. Am J Gastroenterol 99:1902–1909

Sehgal CM, Broderick GA, Whittington R, Gorniak RJ, Arger PH (1994) Three-dimensional US and volumetric assessment of the prostate. Radiology 192:274–278

Sohn C, Grotepass J (1990) 3-dimensional organ image using ultrasound. Ultraschall Med 11:295–301

Sumiyama K, Suzuki N, Tajiri H (2003) A linear-array freehand 3-D endoscopic ultrasound. Ultrasound Med Biol 29:1001–1006

Tack J, Piessevaux H, Coulie B, Caenepeel P, Janssens J (1998) Role of impaired gastric accommodation to a meal in functional dyspepsia. Gastroenterology 115:1346–1352

Tefera S, Gilja OH, Olavsdottir E, Hausken T, Hatlebakk JG, Berstad A (2002) Intragastric maldistribution of a liquid meal in patients with reflux oesophagitis assessed by three dimensional ultrasonography. Gut 50:153–158

Thune N, Hausken T, Gilja OH, Matre K (1996) A practical method for estimating enclosed volumes using 3D ultrasound. Eur J Ultrasound 3:83–92

Trocino G, Salustri A, Roelandt JR, Ansink T, van Herwerden L (1996) Three-dimensional echocardiography of a flail tricuspid valve. J Am Soc Echocardiogr 9:91–93

Tsutsuii A, Okamura S, Okita Y et al. (1998) Usefulness of three-dimensional display of digestive lesions by endoscopic ultrasonography. Digestion 59 (S3):194

Vannier MW, Marsh JL (1996) Three-dimensional imaging, surgical planning, and image-guided therapy. Radiol Clin North Am 34:545–563

Vogel M, Ho SY, Lincoln C, Yacoub MH, Anderson RH (1995) Three-dimensional echocardiography can simulate intraoperative visualization of congenitally malformed hearts. Ann Thorac Surg 60:1282–1288

Wagner S, Gebel M, Bleck JS, Manns MP (1994) Clinical application of three-dimensional sonography in hepatobiliary disease. Bildgebung 61:104–109

West RL, Dwarkasing S, Felt-Bersma RJ, Schouten WR, Hop WC, Hussain SM, Kuipers EJ (2004) Hydrogen peroxide-enhanced three-dimensional endoanal ultrasonography and endoanal magnetic resonance imaging in evaluating perianal fistulas: agreement and patient preference. Eur J Gastroenterol Hepatol 16:1319–1324

Whittingham TA, Bateman DN (1983) Measurement of stomach volume by real-time ultrasound. Ultrasound Med Biol (Suppl 2):459–463

Williams AB, Bartram CI, Halligan S, Spencer JA, Nicholls RJ, Kmiot WA (2001) Anal sphincter damage after vaginal delivery using three-dimensional endosonography. Obstet Gynecol 97:770–775

Yoshino J, Nakazawa S, Inui K, Wakabayashi T et al (2000) Volume measurement using tissue characterization of three-dimensional endoscopic ultrasonographic images. Endoscopy 32:624–629

Zoller WG, Liess H (1994) 3-D ultrasound in gastroenterology. Bildgebung 61:95–99

# Percutaneous Gastrointestinal Biopsy

Ilario de Sio, Loredana Tibullo, and Camillo Del Vecchio-Blanco

CONTENTS

24.1 Introduction  213
24.2 Indications and Contraindications  214
24.3 Technique  214
24.4 Results  216
References  218

## 24.1 Introduction

Fine-needle biopsies (FNBs) accomplished with ultrasound (US) and/or computed tomography (CT) guidance have been a widely accepted procedure in diagnosing abdominal and retroperitoneal space-occupying lesions (Droese et al. 1984; Memel et al. 1996). Compared with CT, US has been shown to be safer, more cost-effective, and faster; moreover it does not require ionizing radiation and therefore is not of any radiation risk to the patient or operator (Dodd et al. 1996; Sheafor et al. 1998). Since 1975 US-guided FNBs have been performed mostly in solid abdominal and retroperitoneal organs such as liver, pancreas, spleen, kidney, and lymph node masses, with a high diagnostic accuracy, low complication rate (ranging from 0.05 to 0.23% in multi-institutional and mono-institutional series, respectively) and a very low mortality rate (0.001–0.038%). (Livraghi et al. 1983; Smith 1984; Fornari et al. 1989; Nolsoe et al. 1990; Smith 1991).

Gastrointestinal tract lesions, both inflammatory and/or neoplastic, may be visualized by US as a "target" or "bull's-eye" lesion, or as a "pseudokidney" mass (Figs. 24.1, 24.2; Bluth et al. 1979; Fakhry and Berk 1981; Goerg et al. 1990; Lim 1996; Lutz and Petzoldt 1976; Morgan et al. 1980; Rapaccini et al. 1986; Schwerk et al. 1979). In particular, although the diagnosis of gastrointestinal tract tumor is conventionally based on biopsy performed during endoscopy, since 1980 many authors have reported the possibility of diagnosing of gastrointestinal neoplasia by means of a US-guided FNB (Abbit 1991; Allen and Irwin 1997; Ballo and Guy 2001; Bhaduri et al. 1999; Bree et al. 1991; Carson et al. 1998, Das and Pant 1994; Dodd et al. 1998; Farmer et al. 2000; Green et al. 1988; Heriot et al. 1998; Ho et al. 2003; Javid et al. 1999; Ledermann et al. 2001; Marco-Domenech et al. 2001; Shidham et al. 1998; Solbiati et al. 1986; Torp-Pedersen et al. 1984; Tudor et al. 1999). Sonographically guided fine-needle aspiration

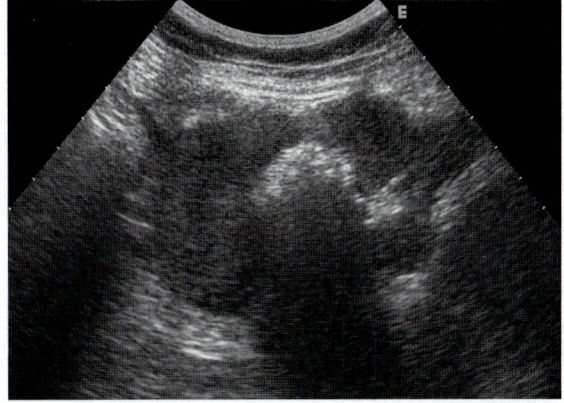

**Fig. 24.1.** The pseudo-kidney sign. The strong echogenic centre (corresponding to the lumen content) is surrounded by an echo-poor rim (thickened bowel wall) in a case of colonic adenocarcinoma

I. de Sio, MD
Gastroenterology Unit, Ultrasonography Section, II University of Naples, Via S. Pansini 5, 80131 Naples, Italy
L. Tibullo, MD, PhD
Department of Internal Medicine and Gastroenterology Ultrasonography Section, II University of Naples. Via S. Pansini 5, 80131 Naples, Italy
C. Del Vecchio-Blanco, MD
Department of Internal Medicine and Gastroenterology, II University of Naples, Via S. Pansini 5, 80131 Naples, Italy

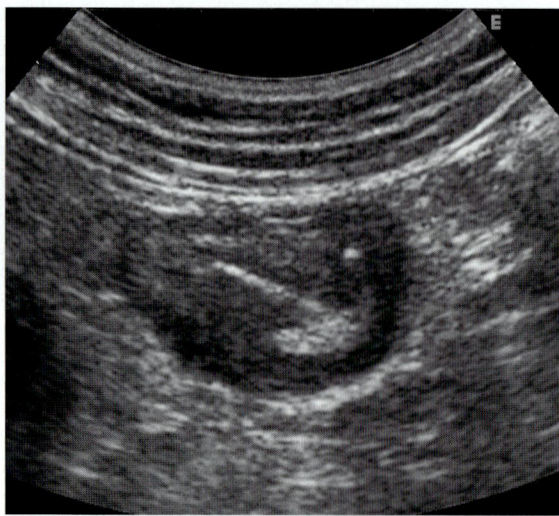

**Fig. 24.2.** The "target-like" pattern in a case of gastric adenocarcinoma

biopsy of a bowel wall lesion was first performed in 1981 by ENNIS and MACERLEAN (1981).

## 24.2
## Indications and Contraindications

Percutaneous US-guided FNB of a gastrointestinal mass is performed mainly when:
1. The lesion is well visualized at US study.
2. The lesion is endoscopically inaccessible (i.e., localized between the ligament of Treitz and the ileocecal valve).
3. The lesion is situated in the submucosa (as frequently seen in gastrointestinal lymphoma), is intramural, or develops in the subserosa (i.e., in gastrointestinal stromal tumors), and is thus not accessible by conventional endoscopic biopsy.
4. A previous biopsy during endoscopy is non-diagnostic or only necrotic material is obtained.
5. Endoscopy cannot be performed for uncooperative patients or for contraindications.
6. It is impossible to obtain an adequate biopsy sample during endoscopy due to presence of severe stenosis.

Contraindications are represented only by a severe coagulative impairment (i.e., platelet count ≤40000/mm$^3$; prothrombin time ≤40%) and by distention of bowel loops.

## 24.3
## Technique

Percutaneous FNBs are frequently performed under US guidance with a real-time convex transducer (3.5–5 MHz) by both a "free-hand" technique and a biopsy-guided attachment. Fine needles (i.e., needles with an outer diameter <1 mm–20 gauge) of both the "cutting" or "non-cutting" type, are frequently used to obtain a cytological and/or histological diagnosis (BALLO and GUY 2001; CARSON et al. 1998; ENNIS and MAC ERLEAN 1981; GREEN et al. 1988; LEDERMANN et al. 2001; MARCO-DOMENECH et al. 2001; SOLBIATI et al. 1986; TORP-PEDERSEN et al. 1984; JAVID et al. 1999). Some authors have also used large (1.2 mm–18 G) cutting needles (BALLO and GUY 2001; CARSON et al. 1998; FARMER et al. 2000; LEDERMANN et al. 2001; MARCO-DOMENECH et al. 2001; TUDOR et al. 1999). The use of large cutting needles has been experimentally demonstrated to be safe (AKAN et al. 1998) and not associated with increased mortality and/or morbidity (MARCO-DOMENECH et al. 2001; TUDOR et al. 1999). Patients must fast from the night prior to the biopsy and usually bowel preparation or antibiotic prophylaxis are not needed (TUDOR et al. 1999). All patients sign a written informed consent. The procedure is usually performed both on an inpatient/outpatient basis (BALLO and GUY 2001) and often without local anesthesia; however, some authors use local anesthesia by infiltration of 5–10 ml of 1% lidocaine hydrochloride into the abdominal wall by means of a 25-G needle (Ho et al. 1998). In many cases, color and power Doppler are useful to evaluate and avoid large vessels along the needle

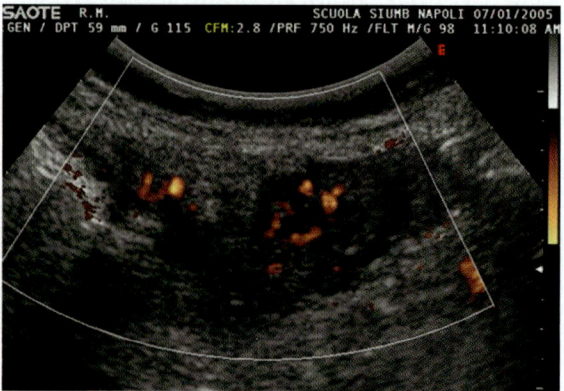

**Fig. 24.3.** Power Doppler of a diffuse thickened gastric wall shows clear vascular signals (to be avoided during fine needle biopsy)

tract (Fig. 24.3) (Marco-Domenech et al. 2001; Ho et al. 2003). Briefly, percutaneous FNB is frequently performed by two operators, one holding the transducer and the second manipulating the needle. In "pseudokidney" lesions, it is important to place the needle in the hypoechoic rim, thus avoiding crossing the echogenic center (Fig. 24.4), which corresponds to the mucosa and the lumen of gastrointestinal loop. When a "non-cutting" needle is used, it is fitted to a 10- to 20-ml syringe attached to an aspiration piston, and is monitored while advancing in the lesion. When the tip of the needle (shown on the scan) is in the tumor wall, the piston is completely retracted and the needle is moved back and forth three or four times in the tumor (Torp-Pedersen et al. 1984).

When aspiration is completed, the negative pressure is equilibrated and the needle is withdrawn. After withdrawal of the needle, the syringe is disconnected, filled with air and reconnected and the material in the needle is expelled onto a glass slide and smeared. The specimen is then air dried and fixed in ethanol; Papanicolau and May–Grunwald–Giemsa are the standard staining techniques used, whereas if a carcinoid tumor is suspected, the Grimelius staining method is used (Solbiati et al. 1986).

When a "cutting-type" needle is used, the needle is advanced until lesion indentation is seen, then the trigger mechanism is fired and the needle is withdrawn, obtaining a histological sample (Fig. 24.5; Tudor et al. 1999).

Core-needle biopsy samples are fixed in formalin and embedded in paraffin wax; 3- to 4 μm-thick sections are cut and then stained with hematoxylin/eosin. Further immunohistochemical analysis of the material is then possible for specific indications requested. In all cases, the presence of a cytopathologist, to assess specimen adequacy during the procedure, would result in a high diagnostic outcome (Ballo and Guy 2001); however, if this is not possible, two needle punctures during the first session should be performed.

After the procedure is completed, the outpatients are observed from 2 to 4 h in order to monitor eventual immediate complications such as persistent pain, fever or bleeding at puncture site. Some authors prefer to perform an ultrasound control before discharging patients. In our Department, we performed FNBs of gastrointestinal masses, with US guidance, by using a 3.5- to 5 MHz convex probe equipped with a biopsy device. All the procedures were performed in outpatients with no general or local anesthesia and we used both fine-cutting and non-cutting needles.

Ultrasound-guided FNBs (Ledermann et al. 2001) have been performed mostly in suspected primary or metastatic neoplastic gastrointestinal lesions, also in those patients with HIV infection (Bhaduri et al. 1999) in which gastrointestinal manifestations (such as opportunistic infections or lymphoproliferative or neoplastic disease) occurs in about 50% of the patients, and endoscopic diagnosis is not possible due to the submucosal nature of the disease (Fig. 24.6).

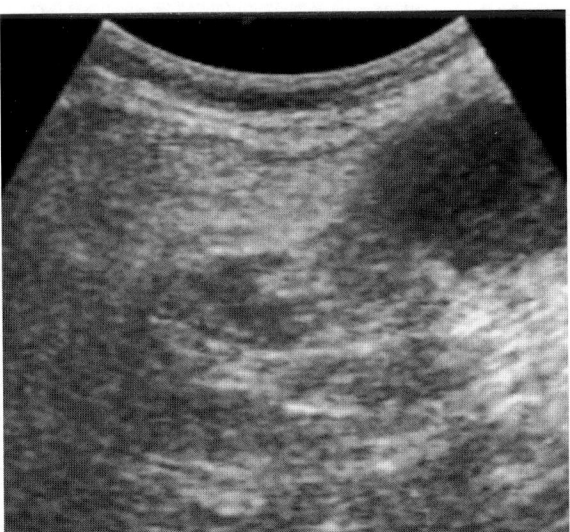 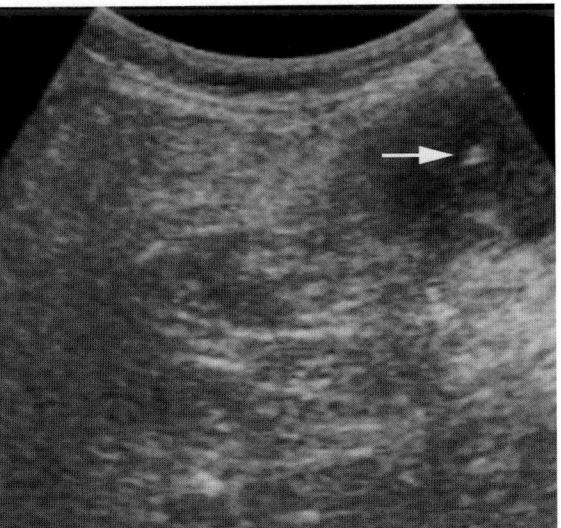

**Fig. 24.4. a** Transverse sonogram of abdomen shows gastric hypoechoic wall thickening. **b** Ultrasound-guided fine-needle aspiration biopsy (non-cutting needle) of the lesion (*arrow* indicates the tip of the needle): cytological diagnosis of gastric adenocarcinoma

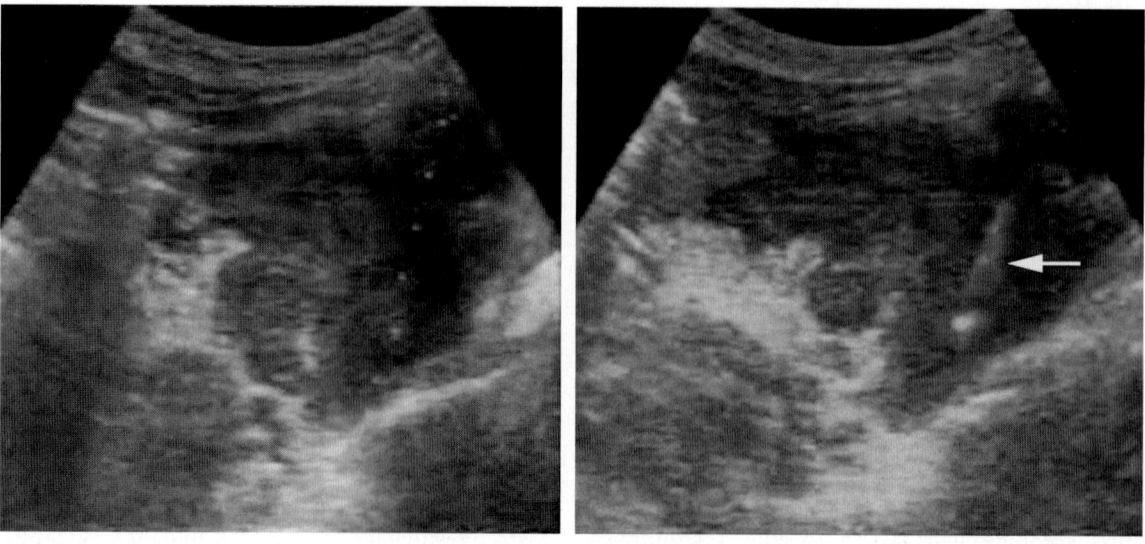

**Fig. 24.5. a** A diffuse thickening of the gastric wall (endoscopic biopsy resulted non diagnostic). **b** Ultrasound-guided fine-needle biopsy with a cutting needle. The needle is well visualized (*arrow*): histological diagnosis of gastric lymphoma

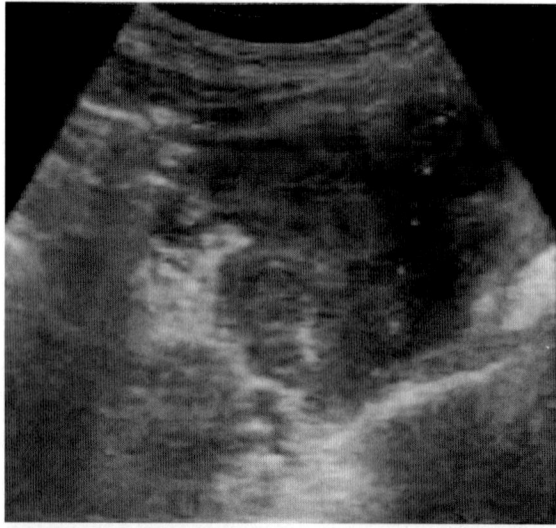

**Fig. 24.6.** Ultrasound-guided fine-needle biopsy of bowel wall involvement: *arrow* indicates the needle tip. Final diagnosis: intestinal lymphoma

## 24.4 Results

Table 24.1 summarizes the most important studies published on the use of FNBs of gastrointestinal wall lesions. Because of the relatively small population, and the absence of a clear gold standard in order to assess the true-negative and false-negative results, few data are available regarding sensitivity, specificity, and overall diagnostic accuracy of the procedure. When the data are reported, sensitivity, specificity, diagnostic accuracy, predictive positive value, and predictive negative value are 90–91%, 100% (no false-positive results), 80–100, 100, and 67%, respectively, thus equal to those obtained in other malignant abdominal diseases (BALLO and GUY 2001; JAVID et al. 1999; TORP-PEDERSEN et al. 1984). The procedure is well tolerated, no mortality has been reported, and only four complications have been described following percutaneous US-guided FNBs of gastrointestinal tract lesions (one case of hemoperitoneum, one of sepsis, one of small parietal hematoma, and one of bile peritonitis; JAVID et al. 1999; MARCO-DOMENECH et al. 2001; TUDOR et al. 1999).

Patients with indications for percutaneous FNBs of gastrointestinal tract lesions are not commonly encountered. In fact, as reported by SOLBIATI et al.

Table 24.1. Published studies on the use of percutaneous fine-needle biopsies of gastrointestinal wall lesions

| Reference | Number | Site | Needle type | Gauge | Complications |
|---|---|---|---|---|---|
| ENNIS MACERLEAN (1981) | 7 | B | NC | | No |
| TORP-PEDERSEN et al. (1984)[a] | 78 | S–SB–C | NC | 23 | No |
| SOLBIATI et al. (1986) | 24 | S–SB–C | NC | 22 | No |
| GREEN et al. (1988) | 3 | S | NC | 22 | No |
| DAS and PANT (1994) | 78 | S–C | NC | | No |
| CARSON et al. (1998) | 44 | S–SB–C | NC–C | 18, 22 | No |
| TUDOR et al. (1999) | 10 | SB | C | 18 | Yes[d] |
| BHADURI et al. (1999) | 3 | S–SB | | | No |
| JAVID et al. (1999)[b] | 50 | C | NC | 22 | Yes[e] |
| FARMER et al. (2000) | 12 | S–SB–C | C | 18 | No |
| MARCO-DOMENECH et al. (2001) | 42 | S–SB–C | C–NC | 18, 21, 22 | Yes[f] |
| BALLO and GUY (2001)[c] | 20 | S–SB–C | NC | 18, 22 | No |
| LEDERMANN et al. (2001) | 7 | SB–C | NC–C | 18, 22 | No |

S stomach, SB small bowel, C colon, C cutting type, NC non-cutting type
[a] Authors report a positive predictive value and a negative predictive value of FNB of 100 and 67%, respectively
[b] Authors report a sensitivity and specificity of 91.8% and 100%, respectively
[c] Authors report a diagnostic accuracy of 100%
[d] One small hematoma
[e] One case of hemoperitoneum, one case of sepsis
[f] One case of bile peritonitis

(1986), they represent only 1.5% of all abdominal biopsies performed in the same period.

Our experience is quite similar (unpublished data). In fact, US-guided FNBs of gastrointestinal masses represent only 1.7% (34 out of 1876) of all abdominal US-guided FNBs over a 15-year period. We performed FNBs of the gastric wall in 13 cases, and of the bowel wall in 21 cases (sigmoid colon 12 cases; small bowel 9 cases).

The indications to the procedure were impossibility to perform endoscopy in 8 cases, non-diagnostic endoscopic biopsies in 20 cases (Fig. 24.7), and endoscopically inaccessible lesion in 6 cases (Fig. 24.8). No complications occurred and the procedure was well tolerated in all patients; however, an alternative approach to diagnosis of gastrointestinal diseases may be needed in some cases. In particular when the lesion is clearly visible at ultrasound, US-guided FNB could be considered a simple, rapid, relatively non-invasive and accurate procedure.

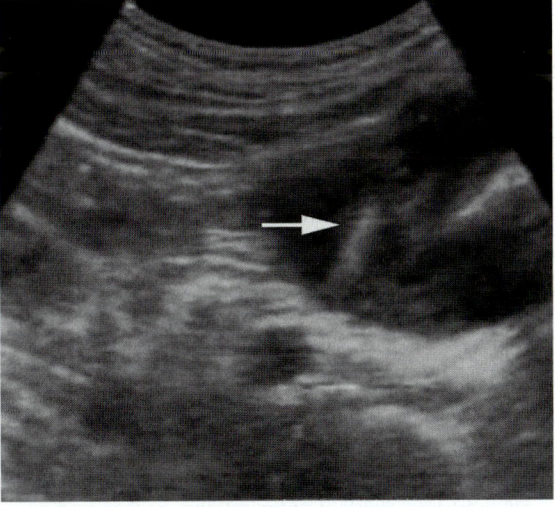

Fig. 24.7. Ultrasound-guided fine-needle biopsy with a cutting needle in a case of endoscopically negative biopsies. The needle tip is clearly visible in hypoechoic gastric wall (*arrow*). Final diagnosis: gastric adenocarcinoma

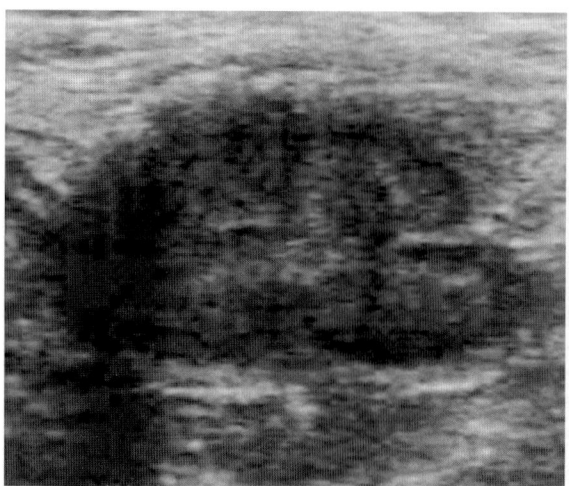 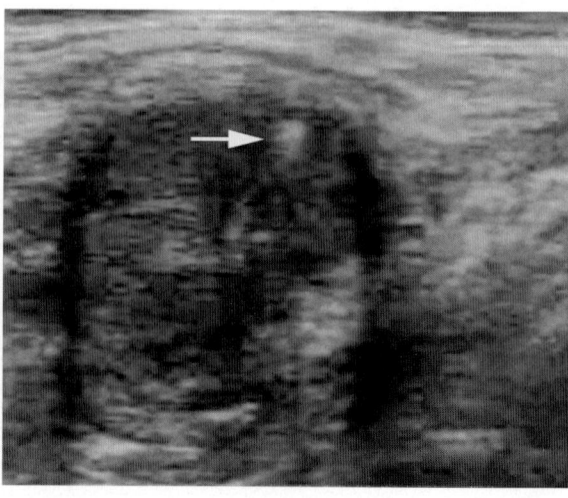

Fig. 24.8. **a** Hypoechoic abdominal mass in left hypochondrium in patient with abdominal pain and fever. **b** Ultrasound-guided fine-needle aspiration (*arrow* indicates needle tip). Final diagnosis: jejuneal metastasis from bronchial cancer

## References

Abbitt PL (1991) Percutaneous fine-needle aspiration of bowel wall abnormalities under ultrasonic guidance. J Clin Ultrasound 19:310–314

Akan H, Ozen N, Incesu L et al (1998) Are percutaneous transgastric biopsies using 14, 16 and 18 G Tru-Cut needles safe? An experimental study in the rabbit. Australas Radiol 42:99–101

Allen DC, Irwin ST (1997) Fine needle aspiration cytology of gastric carcinoma. Ulster Med J 66:111–114

Ballo MS, Guy CD (2001) Percutaneous fine-needle aspiration of gastrointestinal wall lesions with image guidance. Diagn Cytopathol 24:16–20

Bhaduri S, Wiselka MJ, Rogers PM (1999) A review of ultrasound-guided percutaneous biopsy of gastrointestinal tract in HIV-infected patients. HIV Med 1:43–46

Bluth EI, Merrit CRB, Sullivan LA (1979) Ultrasonic evaluation of the stomach, small bowel and colon radiology. 124:791–792

Bree RL, McGough MF, Schwab RE (1991) CT or US-guided fine-needle aspiration biopsy in gastric neoplasms. J Comput Assist Tomogr 15:565–569

Carson BW, Brown JA, Cooperberg PL (1998) Ultrasonographically guided percutaneous biopsy of gastric, small bowel and colonic abnormalities: efficacy and safety. J Ultrasound Med 17:739–742

Das DK, Pant CS (1994) Fine needle aspiration cytologic diagnosis of gastrointestinal tract lesions. A study of 78 cases. Acta Cytol 38:723–729

Dodd LG, Esola CC, Memel DS et al (1996) Sonography: the undiscovered jewel of interventional radiology. Radiographics 16:1271–1288

Dodd LG, Nelson RC, Mooney EE et al (1998) Fine-needle aspiration of gastrointestinal stromal tumors. Am J Clin Pathol 109:439–443

Droese M, Altmannsberger M, Kehl A et al (1984) Ultrasound guided percutaneous fine needle aspiration biopsy of abdominal and retroperitoneal masses: accuracy of cytology in the diagnosis of malignancies, cytologic tumor typing and use of antibodies to intermediate filaments in selected cases. Acta Cytol 28:368–384

Ennis MG, MacErlean DP (1981) Biopsy of bowel wall pathology under ultrasound control. Gastrointest Radiol 15:17–20

Fakhry JR, Berk RN (1981) The "target" pattern: characteristic sonographic feature of stomach and bowel abnormalities. Am J Roentgenol 137:969–972

Farmer KD, Harries SR, Fox BM et al (2000) Core biopsy of the bowel wall: efficacy and safety in the clinical setting. Am J Roentgenol 175:1627–1630

Fornari F, Civardi G, Cavanna L et al (1989) Complications of ultrasonically guided fine-needle abdominal biopsy. Scand J Gastroenterol 24:949–955

Goerg C, Schwerk WB, Goerg K (1990) Gastrointestinal lymphoma: sonographic findings in 54 patients. Am J Roentgenol 155:795–798

Green J, Katz S, Phillips G et al (1988) Percutaneous sonographic needle aspiration biopsy of endoscopically negative gastric carcinoma. Am J Gastroenterol 83:1150–1153

Heriot AG, Kurnar D, Thomas V et al (1998) Ultrasonically guided fine-needle aspiration cytology in the diagnosis of colonic lesions. Br J Surg 85:1713–1715

Ho L, Thomas J, Fine SA et al (2003) Usefulness of sonographic guidance during percutaneous biopsy of mesenteric masses. Am J Roentgenol 180:1563–1566

Javid G, Gulzar GM, Khan B et al (1999) Percutaneous sonography-guided fine needle aspiration biopsy of colonscopic biopsy negative colonic lesions. Indian J Gastroenterol 18:146–148

Ledermann HP, Binkert C, Frohlich E et al (2001) Diagnosis of symptomatic intestinal metastases using transabdominal sonography and sonographically guided puncture. Am J Roentgenol 176:155–158

Lim JH (1996) Colorectal cancer: sonographic findings. Am J Roentgenol 167:45–47

Livraghi T, Damascelli B, Lombardi C et al (1983) Risk in fine needle abdominal biopsy. J Clin Ultrasound 11:77–81

Lutz H, Petzoldt R (1976) Ultrasonic patterns of space occupying lesions of stomach and intestine. Ultrasound Med Biol 133:677–680

Marco-Domenech SF, Gil-Sanchez S, Fernandez-Garcia P et al (2001) Sonographically guided percutaneous biopsy of gastrointestinal tract lesions. Am J Roentgenol 176:147–151

Memel DS, Dodd GD, Esola CC (1996) Efficacy of sonography as a guidance technique for biopsy of abdominal, pelvic and retroperitoneal lymph nodes. Am J Roentgenol 167:957–962

Morgan CL, Trought WS, Oddson TA et al (1980) Ultrasound patterns of disorders affecting the gastrointestinal tract. Radiology 135:129–135

Nolsoe C, Nielsen L, Torp-Pederson S et al (1990) Major complications and deaths due to interventional ultrasonography: a review of 8000 cases. J Clin Ultrasound 18:179–184

Rapaccini GL, Sabelli C, Caturelli E et al (1986) Real-time ultrasound as screening procedure in gastrointestinal tract disease. Ital J Gastroenterol 18:85–87

Schwerck W, Braun B, Dombrowsky H (1979) Real time ultrasound examination in the diagnosis of gastrointestinal tumours. J Clin Ultrasound 7:425–431

Sheafor DH, Paulson EK, Simmons CM et al (1998) Abdominal percutaneous interventional procedures: comparison of CT and US guidance. Radiology 207:705–710

Shidham VB, Weiss JP, Quinn TJ et al (1998) Fine needle aspiration cytology of gastric solitary fibrous tumor. A case report. Acta Cytol 42:1159–1166

Smith EH (1984) The hazards of fine-needle aspiration biopsy. Ultrasound Med Biol 10:629–634

Smith EH (1991) Complications of percutaneous abdominal fine-needle biopsy. Radiology 178:253–258

Solbiati L, Montali G, Croce F et al (1986) Fine-needle aspiration biopsy of bowel lesions under ultrasound guidance: indications and results. Gastrointest Radiol 11:172–176

Torp-Pedersen S, Gronval S, Holm HH (1984) Ultrasonically guided fine-needle aspiration biopsy of gastrointestinal mass lesions. J Ultrasound Med 3:65–68

Tudor GR, Rodgers PM, West KP (1999) Bowel lesions: percutaneous US-guided 18-gauge needle biopsy: preliminary experience. Radiology 212:594–597

# Subject Index

3D-endoanal sonography 207
3D-endosonography 205
– of the rectum 207
3D-ultrasound 199
– of the stomach 202

## A
Abdominal free fluid 87
Abscess(es), intra-abdominal 68
Accordion sign 117
Afferent loop syndrome 31
Amoebiasis 121
Antral area 190
Antral contractions 193
Antral peristalsis 192
Appendagitis 8
Appendices epiploicae, torsion of 24
Appendicitis
– acute 4, 176
– clinical features 4
– computed tomography 6
– magnetic resonance imaging 7
– sonographic signs 5
Ascariasis 122
Ascaris lumbricoides 122
Ascites 113, 152

## B
Bacterial ileocecitis 104, see also Infectious Ileocecitis
Barber pole sign 46
Bezoar, small bowel 29
Bochdaleck hernia 43
Bull's-eye sign 141

## C
Carcinoid tumor 159
Carcinomatosis, peritoneal 151
– sonographic findings 151
Clostridium difficile 116
Clostridium difficile colitis 115, 185
Coeliac disease 16, 85
Colonic carcinoma 186, see also Colorectal cancer
Colonic polyps 186
Colorectal cancer 129
– pathology 129
– transabdominal sonographic findings 130
– transrectal sonographic findings 131, 132
Contrast agent
– intravenous 170
– oral 183
Contrast harmonic imaging 173, 184

Crohn's disease 15, 61
– disease activity 63
– pathological features 61
– sonographic features 62

## D
Dapaong tumour 125
Diaphragmatic hernia 43
Diverticulitis
– acute colonic 21, 22
– right-sided 23
Diverticulosis 19
– diagnostic methods 20
– sonographic features 20
Doughnut sign 49
Duodenogastric reflux 193, 204
Dyspepsia, functional dyspepsia 194, 203

## E
EchoPac3D 201
Echovist 171, see also SHU-454
Ectopic pancreas 161
Ectopic pregnancy 8
Entamoeba hystolitica 121
Enteritis 101
Eosinophilic enteritis 95

## F
Familial Mediterranean fever 17
Femoral hernia 37
Fine-needle aspiration 156
Fine-needle biopsy 213
– accuracy 216
– complications 216, 217
– contraindications 214
– indications 214
– technique 214
Fistula(e)
– in Crohn's disease 66
– perianal 208

## G
Gallbladder emptying 90
Gallbladder function 195
Gallstone ileus 30
Gastric accomodation 191, 203
Gastric anisakiasis 138
Gastric cancer 135
– advanced 138
– early 136
– staging of 140

Gastric emptying 190, 194
Gastric ulcer, benign 138
Gastric volume(s) 203
Gastric wall, normal 135
Gastroenteritis 101
Gastroesophageal reflux 44, 194
Gastrointestinal stromal tumor 161
Graft-vs-host-disease 177

## H
Haemangioma 161
Hernia(s), abdominal 35
- Bochdaleck 43
- complications of 39
- diaphragmatic 43
- femoral 37
- hiatal 43, 44
- para-oesophageal type of 44
- sliding type of 44
- incarcerated 39
- inguinal 35
- internal 41
- irriducible 39
- morgagni 43
- obstructed 39, 42
- peritoneo-pericardial 43
- postoperative follow up 41
- Richter's 39
- Spigelian 39
- strangulated 41
- umbelical 39
- ventral 38
Hydrocolonic sonography 186 see also Hydrosonography, colon
Hydrosonography
- colon 186
- gastric 181
- small bowel 183

## I
Incarcerated hernia 39
Infectious enteritis 101
Infectious ileocecitis 7, 16, 104, see also Bacterial ileocecitis
Inflammatory mass, intraabdominal 68, 176
Inguinal hernia 35
Internal hernia 41
Intussusception 48
- colocolic 50
- double 50
- hydrostatic reduction 50
- ileocecal 32
- ileocolic 50
- jejunogastric 51
- small bowel 50
- transient 50, 88
Irriducible hernia 39
Ischaemia, bowel 176
Ischemic colitis 24, 55
- computed tomography findings 56
- sonographic findings 56

## L
Levovist 171
Lipoma 161
Lymph nodes, mesenteric 11, 65
- cavitation 89
Lymphangectasia, primary intestinal 93
Lymphangioma 161
Lymphoma 13, 143
- gastrointestinal 143, 148
- differential diagnosis 144
- follow up 147
- staging 144, 146
- intestinal 89
- Non-Hodgkin, gastric 143

## M
Malrotation of midgut 44
Meckel's diverticulum 7
Mesenteric cyst 46
Mesenteric hypertrophy 65
Mesenteric lymphadenitis 111, see also Lymph nodes, mesenteric
Metastasis, peritoneal 151, see also Carcinomatosis, Peritoneal
Mesothelioma, peritoneal 156
Morgagni hernia 43
Mucocele of the appendix 9
Mycobacterium avium complex 16, 149

## N
Neutropenic enterocolitis 106

## O
Obstructed hernia 39, 42
Obstruction, intestinal 27, 66
- colonic 32
- small bowel 28
Occlusion, intestinal 66, see also Obstruction, Intestinal
Oesophagostomiasis 124
Oesophagostomum bifurcum 124
Omental cake 113, 154
Omental infarction 8
Ovarian torsion 24

## P
Paralytic ileus 32
Peanut sign 47
Perforation, intestinal 70
Perianal fistulas 208
Peritoneo-pericardial hernia 43
Peritonitis, tubercolous 112, see also Tuberculosis, peritoneal
Phlegmon 68
Pneumatosis cystoides intestinalis 161
Polyethylen glycol (PEG) solution 183
Primary mesenteric lymphadenitis 17
Primary sclerosing cholangitis 16
Proximal stomach 191
Pseudomembranous colitis 115
- clinical manifestations 116
- computed tomography 118
- endoscopy 116
- sonography 116
Pseudomyxoma peritoneii 9, 151
Pseudopolyposis, colonic 77

## R

Rectal cancer 207
Rectal wall, normal 133
Reflux esophagitis 191, 203
Richter's hernia 39

## S

Salmonellosis 102
Schwannoma 161
Shigellosis 104
SHU-454171
SHU-563-A 172
SHU-580171, *see aslo* Levovist
Sinus track 66
Small bowel adenocarcinoma 89
Small bowel contrast ultrasound 183, *see also* Hydrosonography, small bowel
SonoVue 172
Spigelian hernia 39
Stenosis 66, 176184
Strangulated hernia 41
Stricture 111, *see also* Stenosis
Submucosal tumors 159

## T

Toxic megacolon 79, 116
Transpyloric flow 193, 194
Trichuriasis 124
Trichuris trichiura 124
Triple-circle sign 50, 51

Tuberculosis
– intestinal 16, 109
– differential diagnosis 113
– pathology 109
– sonographic findings 110
– peritoneal 112
– ascites 112
– mesenteric thickness 113
– omental cake 113
Typhoid fever 102

## U

Ulcerative colitis 74
– clinical features 74
– differential diagnosis 80
– pathological features 75
– sonographic features 76
– disease activity 78
Umbelical hernia 39
Ureter stones 8

## V

Ventral hernia 38
Volvulus
– caecal 47
– gastric 46, 47
– midgut 45
– small bowel 44

## W

Whipple's disease 94, 149
Whirlpool sign 45
White bowel 149

# List of Contributors

GABRIELE BIANCHI PORRO, MD, PhD
Chair of Gastroenterology
Department of Clinical Sciences
'L.Sacco' University Hospital
Via G.B. Grassi 74
20157 Milan
Italy

ETIENNE DANSE, MD, PhD
Department of Radiology
St-Luc University Hospital
Université Catholique de Louvain
10, Avenue Hippocrate
1200 Brussels
Belgium

SEVERIN DAUM, MD
Medizinische Klinik und Poliklinik I
Gastroenterologie,
Infektiologie und Rheumatololgie
Charité – Universitätsmedizin Berlin
Campus Benjamin Franklin
Hindenburgdamm 30
12200 Berlin
Germany

CAMILLO DEL VECCHIO BLANCO, MD
Department of Internal Medicine
and Gastroenterology, II
University of Naples
Via S. Pansini 5
80131 Naples
Italy

ILARIO DE SIO, MD
Gastroenterology Unit
Ultrasonography Section, II
University of Naples
Via S. Pansini 5
80131 Naples
Italy

MIRELLA FRAQUELLI, MD, PhD
Department of Gastroenterology
and Endocrinology
IRCCS Fondazione Ospedale Maggiore
Mangiagalli e Regina Elena
Pad. Granelli 3 piano
Via F. Sforza 35
20122 Milan
Italy

DAPHNE GEUKENS, MD
Department of Radiology
University Hospital Center
6000 Charleroi
Belgium

ODD HELGE GILJA, MD, PhD
Section of Gastroenterology
National Centre for Ultrasound
in Gastroenterology
Haukeland University Hospital
Institute of Medicine
University of Bergen
Jonas Liesvei 65
5021 Bergen
Norway

SALVATORE GRECO, MD
Chair of Gastroenterology
Department of Clinical Sciences
'L.Sacco' University Hospital
Via G.B. Grassi 74
20157 Milano
Italy

NORBERT GRITZMANN, MD
Prim. Univ. Prof., Department of Radiology
and Nuclear Medicine
KH Barmherzige Brüder Salzburg
Kajetanerplatz 1
5020 Salzburg
Austria

Ken Haruma, MD, PhD
Professor of Internal Medicine
Division of Gastroenterology
Department of Internal Medicine
Kawasaki Medical School
577, Matsushima
Kurashiki-city
Okayama 701-0192
Japan

Jiro Hata, MD
Department of Clinical Pathology
and Laboratory Medicine
Kawasaki Medical School,
577, Matsushima
Kurashiki-city
Okayama, 701-0192
Japan

Trygve Hausken, MD, PhD
Professor, Section of Gastroenterology
National Centre for Ultrasound
in Gastroenterology
Haukeland University Hospital
Institute of Medicine
University of Bergen
Jonas Liesvei 65
5021 Bergen
Norway

Jörg C. Hoffmann, MD
Medizinische Klinik und Poliklinik I
Gastroenterologie
Infektiologie und Rheumatololgie
Charité – Universitätsmedizin Berlin
Campus Benjamin Franklin
Hindenburgdamm 30
12200 Berlin
Germany

Tomoari Kamada, MD
Division of Gastroenterology
Department of Internal Medicine
Kawasaki Medical School
577, Matsushima
Kurashiki-city
Okayama 701-0192
Japan

Hiroaki Kusunoki, MD
Division of Gastroenterology
Department of Internal Medicine
Kawasaki Medical School
577, Matsushima
Kurashiki-city
Okayama 701-0192
Japan

Dong Ho Lee, MD
Professor of Radiology
Department of Radiology
and Center for Imaging Science
Kyung Hee University Hospital
1, Hoeki-dong, Dongdaemun-gu
Seoul
Korea

Jae Hoon Lim, MD
Professor of Radiology
Department of Radiology
Samsung Medical Center
Sungkyunkwan University School of Medicine
50 Ilwon-dong, Kangnam-ku
Seoul 135-710
Korea

Giovanni Maconi, MD
Chair of Gastroenterology
Department of Clinical Sciences
'L.Sacco' University Hospital
Via G.B. Grassi 74
20157 Milan
Italy

Noriaki Manabe, MD
Division of Gastroenterology
Department of Internal Medicine
Kawasaki Medical School
577, Matsushima
Kurashiki-city
Okayama 701-0192
Japan

Elisa Radice, MD
Chair of Gastroenterology
Department of Clinical Sciences
'L.Sacco' University Hospital
Via G.B. Grassi 74
20157 Milan
Italy

MOTONORI SATO, MD
Division of Gastroenterology
Department of Internal Medicine
Kawasaki Medical School
577, Matsushima
Kurashiki-city
Okayama 701-0192
Japan

DORIS SCHACHERER, MD
Department of Internal Medicine I
University of Regensburg
Franz-Josef-Strauss-Allee 11
93042 Regensburg
Germany

JÜRGEN SCHÖLMERICH, MD
Professor, Department of Internal Medicine I
University Regensburg
Franz-Josef-Strauss-Allee 11
93042 Regensburg
Germany

TOSHIAKI TANAKA, MD
Division of Gastroenterology
Department of Internal Medicine
Kawasaki Medical School
577, Matsushima
Kurashiki-city
Okayama 701-0192
Japan

LUCIANO TARANTINO, MD
Interventional Ultrasound Unit
Department of Medicine
S. Givanni di Dio Hospital
Via Mario Vergara Padre, 187
80027 Frattamaggiore, Naples
Italy

LOREDANA TIBULLO, MD, PhD
Department of Internal Medicine and
Gastroenterology Ultrasonography Section, II
University of Naples
Via S. Pansini 5
80131 Naples
Italy

S. BOOPATHY VIJAYARAGHAVAN, MD, DMRD
SONOSCAN, Ultrasonic Scan Center
15B, Venkatachalam Road
Coimbatore-641 002
Tamil Nadu
India

MARTIN ZEITZ, MD
Professor, Medizinische Klinik I
Charité – Universitätsmedizin Berlin
Campus Benjamin Franklin
Hindenburgdamm 30
12200 Berlin
Germany

# Medical Radiology  Diagnostic Imaging and Radiation Oncology
*Titles in the series already published*

## Diagnostic Imaging

**Innovations in Diagnostic Imaging**
Edited by J. H. Anderson

**Radiology of the Upper Urinary Tract**
Edited by E. K. Lang

**The Thymus - Diagnostic Imaging, Functions, and Pathologic Anatomy**
Edited by E. Walter, E. Willich, and W. R. Webb

**Interventional Neuroradiology**
Edited by A. Valavanis

**Radiology of the Pancreas**
Edited by A. L. Baert,
co-edited by G. Delorme

**Radiology of the Lower Urinary Tract**
Edited by E. K. Lang

**Magnetic Resonance Angiography**
Edited by I. P. Arlart, G. M. Bongartz, and G. Marchal

**Contrast-Enhanced MRI of the Breast**
S. Heywang-Köbrunner and R. Beck

**Spiral CT of the Chest**
Edited by M. Rémy-Jardin and J. Rémy

**Radiological Diagnosis of Breast Diseases**
Edited by M. Friedrich and E.A. Sickles

**Radiology of the Trauma**
Edited by M. Heller and A. Fink

**Biliary Tract Radiology**
Edited by P. Rossi,
co-edited by M. Brezi

**Radiological Imaging of Sports Injuries**
Edited by C. Masciocchi

**Modern Imaging of the Alimentary Tube**
Edited by A. R. Margulis

**Diagnosis and Therapy of Spinal Tumors**
Edited by P. R. Algra, J. Valk, and J. J. Heimans

**Interventional Magnetic Resonance Imaging**
Edited by J. F. Debatin and G. Adam

**Abdominal and Pelvic MRI**
Edited by A. Heuck and M. Reiser

**Orthopedic Imaging**
Techniques and Applications
Edited by A. M. Davies
and H. Pettersson

**Radiology of the Female Pelvic Organs**
Edited by E. K.Lang

**Magnetic Resonance of the Heart and Great Vessels**
Clinical Applications
Edited by J. Bogaert, A.J. Duerinckx, and F. E. Rademakers

**Modern Head and Neck Imaging**
Edited by S. K. Mukherji
and J. A. Castelijns

**Radiological Imaging of Endocrine Diseases**
Edited by J. N. Bruneton
in collaboration with B. Padovani
and M.-Y. Mourou

**Trends in Contrast Media**
Edited by H. S. Thomsen,
R. N. Muller, and R. F. Mattrey

**Functional MRI**
Edited by C. T. W. Moonen
and P. A. Bandettini

**Radiology of the Pancreas**
2nd Revised Edition
Edited by A. L. Baert. Co-edited by
G. Delorme and L. Van Hoe

**Emergency Pediatric Radiology**
Edited by H. Carty

**Spiral CT of the Abdomen**
Edited by F. Terrier, M. Grossholz, and C. D. Becker

**Liver Malignancies**
Diagnostic and
Interventional Radiology
Edited by C. Bartolozzi
and R. Lencioni

**Medical Imaging of the Spleen**
Edited by A. M. De Schepper
and F. Vanhoenacker

**Radiology of Peripheral Vascular Diseases**
Edited by E. Zeitler

**Diagnostic Nuclear Medicine**
Edited by C. Schiepers

**Radiology of Blunt Trauma of the Chest**
P. Schnyder and M. Wintermark

**Portal Hypertension**
Diagnostic Imaging-Guided Therapy
Edited by P. Rossi
Co-edited by P. Ricci and L. Broglia

**Recent Advances in Diagnostic Neuroradiology**
Edited by Ph. Demaerel

**Virtual Endoscopy and Related 3D Techniques**
Edited by P. Rogalla, J. Terwisscha
Van Scheltinga, and B. Hamm

**Multislice CT**
Edited by M. F. Reiser, M. Takahashi,
M. Modic, and R. Bruening

**Pediatric Uroradiology**
Edited by R. Fotter

**Transfontanellar Doppler Imaging in Neonates**
A. Couture and C. Veyrac

**Radiology of AIDS**
A Practical Approach
Edited by J.W.A.J. Reeders
and P.C. Goodman

**CT of the Peritoneum**
Armando Rossi and Giorgio Rossi

**Magnetic Resonance Angiography**
2nd Revised Edition
Edited by I. P. Arlart,
G. M. Bongratz, and G. Marchal

**Pediatric Chest Imaging**
Edited by Javier Lucaya
and Janet L. Strife

**Applications of Sonography in Head and Neck Pathology**
Edited by J. N. Bruneton
in collaboration with C. Raffaelli
and O. Dassonville

**Imaging of the Larynx**
Edited by R. Hermans

**3D Image Processing**
Techniques and Clinical Applications
Edited by D. Caramella
and C. Bartolozzi

**Imaging of Orbital and Visual Pathway Pathology**
Edited by W. S. Müller-Forell

**Pediatric ENT Radiology**
Edited by S. J. King and A. E. Boothroyd

**Radiological Imaging of the Small Intestine**
Edited by N. C. Gourtsoyiannis

**Imaging of the Knee**
Techniques and Applications
Edited by A. M. Davies
and V. N. Cassar-Pullicino

**Perinatal Imaging**
From Ultrasound to MR Imaging
Edited by Fred E. Avni

**Radiological Imaging of the Neonatal Chest**
Edited by V. Donoghue

**Diagnostic and Interventional Radiology in Liver Transplantation**
Edited by E. Bücheler, V. Nicolas, C. E. Broelsch, X. Rogiers, and G. Krupski

**Radiology of Osteoporosis**
Edited by S. Grampp

**Imaging Pelvic Floor Disorders**
Edited by C. I. Bartram and J. O. L. DeLancey
Associate Editors: S. Halligan, F. M. Kelvin, and J. Stoker

**Imaging of the Pancreas**
Cystic and Rare Tumors
Edited by C. Procacci and A. J. Megibow

**High Resolution Sonography of the Peripheral Nervous System**
Edited by S. Peer and G. Bodner

**Imaging of the Foot and Ankle**
Techniques and Applications
Edited by A. M. Davies, R. W. Whitehouse, and J. P. R. Jenkins

**Radiology Imaging of the Ureter**
Edited by F. Joffre, Ph. Otal, and M. Soulie

**Imaging of the Shoulder**
Techniques and Applications
Edited by A. M. Davies and J. Hodler

**Radiology of the Petrous Bone**
Edited by M. Lemmerling and S. S. Kollias

**Interventional Radiology in Cancer**
Edited by A. Adam, R. F. Dondelinger, and P. R. Mueller

**Duplex and Color Doppler Imaging of the Venous System**
Edited by G. H. Mostbeck

**Multidetector-Row CT of the Thorax**
Edited by U. J. Schoepf

**Functional Imaging of the Chest**
Edited by H.-U. Kauczor

**Radiology of the Pharynx and the Esophagus**
Edited by O. Ekberg

**Radiological Imaging in Hematological Malignancies**
Edited by A. Guermazi

**Imaging and Intervention in Abdominal Trauma**
Edited by R. F. Dondelinger

**Multislice CT**
2nd Revised Edition
Edited by M. F. Reiser, M. Takahashi, M. Modic, and C. R. Becker

**Intracranial Vascular Malformations and Aneurysms**
From Diagnostic Work-Up to Endovascular Therapy
Edited by M. Forsting

**Radiology and Imaging of the Colon**
Edited by A. H. Chapman

**Coronary Radiology**
Edited by M. Oudkerk

**Dynamic Contrast-Enhanced Magnetic Resonance Imaging in Oncology**
Edited by A. Jackson, D. L. Buckley, and G. J. M. Parker

**Imaging in Treatment Planning for Sinonasal Diseases**
Edited by R. Maroldi and P. Nicolai

**Clinical Cardiac MRI**
With Interactive CD-ROM
Edited by J. Bogaert, S. Dymarkowski, and A. M. Taylor

**Focal Liver Lesions**
Detection, Characterization, Ablation
Edited by R. Lencioni, D. Cioni, and C. Bartolozzi

**Multidetector-Row CT Angiography**
Edited by C. Catalano and R. Passariello

**Paediatric Musculoskeletal Diseases**
With an Emphasis on Ultrasound
Edited by D. Wilson

**Contrast Media in Ultrasonography**
Basic Principles and Clinical Applications
Edited by Emilio Quaia

**MR Imaging in White Matter Diseases of the Brain and Spinal Cord**
Edited by M. Filippi, N. De Stefano, V. Dousset, and J. C. McGowan

**Diagnostic Nuclear Medicine**
2nd Revised Edition
Edited by C. Schiepers

**Imaging of the Kidney Cancer**
Edited by A. Guermazi

**Magnetic Resonance Imaging in Ischemic Stroke**
Edited by R. von Kummer and T. Back

**Imaging of the Hip & Bony Pelvis**
Techniques and Applications
Edited by A. M. Davies, K. J. Johnson, and R. W. Whitehouse

**Imaging of Occupational and Environmental Disorders of the Chest**
Edited by P. A. Gevenois and P. De Vuyst

**Contrast Media**
Safety Issues and ESUR Guidelines
Edited by H. S. Thomsen

**Virtual Colonoscopy**
A Practical Guide
Edited by P. Lefere and S. Gryspeerdt

**Vascular Embolotherapy**
A Comprehensive Approach
Volume 1
Edited by J. Golzarian. Co-edited by S. Sun and M. J. Sharafuddin

**Vascular Embolotherapy**
A Comprehensive Approach
Volume 2
Edited by J. Golzarian. Co-edited by S. Sun and M. J. Sharafuddin

**Head and Neck Cancer Imaging**
Edited by R. Hermans

**Vascular Interventional Radiology**
Current Evidence in Endovascular Surgery
Edited by M. G. Cowling

**Ultrasound of the Gastrointestinal Tract**
Edited by G. Maconi and G. Bianchi Porro

**Imaging of Orthopedic Sports Injuries**
Edited by F. M. Vanhoenacker, M. Maas, J. L. M. A. Gielen

**Parallel Imaging in Clinical MR Applications**
Edited by S. O. Schoenberg, O. Dietrich, and F. M. Reiser

**MR and CT of the Female Pelvis**
Edited by B. Hamm and R. Forstner

**Ultrasound of the Musculoskeletal System**
S. Bianchi and C. Martinoli

**Radiology of the Stomach and Duodenum**
Edited by A. H. Freeman and E. Sala

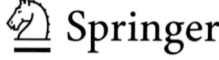

# MEDICAL RADIOLOGY   Diagnostic Imaging and Radiation Oncology
*Titles in the series already published*

## RADIATION ONCOLOGY

**Lung Cancer**
Edited by C.W. Scarantino

**Innovations in Radiation Oncology**
Edited by H. R. Withers
and L. J. Peters

**Radiation Therapy
of Head and Neck Cancer**
Edited by G. E. Laramore

**Gastrointestinal Cancer –
Radiation Therapy**
Edited by R.R. Dobelbower, Jr.

**Radiation Exposure
and Occupational Risks**
Edited by E. Scherer, C. Streffer,
and K.-R. Trott

**Radiation Therapy of Benign Diseases**
A Clinical Guide
S. E. Order and S. S. Donaldson

**Interventional Radiation
Therapy Techniques – Brachytherapy**
Edited by R. Sauer

**Radiopathology of Organs and Tissues**
Edited by E. Scherer, C. Streffer,
and K.-R. Trott

**Concomitant Continuous Infusion
Chemotherapy and Radiation**
Edited by M. Rotman
and C. J. Rosenthal

**Intraoperative Radiotherapy –
Clinical Experiences and Results**
Edited by F. A. Calvo, M. Santos,
and L.W. Brady

**Radiotherapy of Intraocular
and Orbital Tumors**
Edited by W. E. Alberti and
R. H. Sagerman

**Interstitial and Intracavitary
Thermoradiotherapy**
Edited by M. H. Seegenschmiedt
and R. Sauer

**Non-Disseminated Breast Cancer**
Controversial Issues in Management
Edited by G. H. Fletcher and S.H. Levitt

**Current Topics in
Clinical Radiobiology of Tumors**
Edited by H.-P. Beck-Bornholdt

**Practical Approaches to
Cancer Invasion and Metastases**
A Compendium of Radiation
Oncologists' Responses to 40 Histories
Edited by A. R. Kagan with the
Assistance of R. J. Steckel

**Radiation Therapy in Pediatric Oncology**
Edited by J. R. Cassady

**Radiation Therapy Physics**
Edited by A. R. Smith

**Late Sequelae in Oncology**
Edited by J. Dunst and R. Sauer

**Mediastinal Tumors. Update 1995**
Edited by D. E. Wood and C. R. Thomas, Jr.

**Thermoradiotherapy
and Thermochemotherapy**
Volume 1:
Biology, Physiology, and Physics
Volume 2:
Clinical Applications
Edited by M.H. Seegenschmiedt,
P. Fessenden, and C.C. Vernon

**Carcinoma of the Prostate**
Innovations in Management
Edited by Z. Petrovich, L. Baert,
and L.W. Brady

**Radiation Oncology
of Gynecological Cancers**
Edited by H.W. Vahrson

**Carcinoma of the Bladder**
Innovations in Management
Edited by Z. Petrovich, L. Baert,
and L.W. Brady

**Blood Perfusion and
Microenvironment of Human Tumors**
Implications for Clinical Radiooncology
Edited by M. Molls and P. Vaupel

**Radiation Therapy of Benign Diseases**
A Clinical Guide
2nd Revised Edition
S. E. Order and S. S. Donaldson

**Carcinoma of the Kidney and Testis,
and Rare Urologic Malignancies**
Innovations in Management
Edited by Z. Petrovich, L. Baert,
and L.W. Brady

**Progress and Perspectives in the
Treatment of Lung Cancer**
Edited by P. Van Houtte,
J. Klastersky, and P. Rocmans

**Combined Modality Therapy of
Central Nervous System Tumors**
Edited by Z. Petrovich, L. W. Brady,
M. L. Apuzzo, and M. Bamberg

**Age-Related Macular Degeneration**
Current Treatment Concepts
Edited by W. A. Alberti, G. Richard,
and R. H. Sagerman

**Radiotherapy of Intraocular
and Orbital Tumors**
2nd Revised Edition
Edited by R. H. Sagerman,
and W. E. Alberti

**Modification of Radiation Response**
Cytokines, Growth Factors,
and Other Biolgical Targets
Edited by C. Nieder, L. Milas,
and K. K. Ang

**Radiation Oncology for Cure and Palliation**
R. G. Parker, N. A. Janjan,
and M. T. Selch

**Clinical Target Volumes in Conformal and
Intensity Modulated Radiation Therapy**
A Clinical Guide to Cancer Treatment
Edited by V. Grégoire, P. Scalliet,
and K. K. Ang

**Advances in Radiation Oncology
in Lung Cancer**
Edited by Branislav Jeremić

**New Technologies in Radiation Oncology**
Edited by W. Schlegel, T. Bortfeld,
and A.-L. Grosu

**Technical Basis of Radiation Therapy**
4th Revised Edition
Edited by S. H. Levitt, J. A. Purdy, C. A.
Perez, and S. Vijayakumar

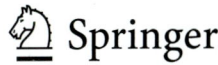

Printing and Binding: Stürtz GmbH, Würzburg

```
RC          Ultrasound of the
804         gastrointestinal
.U4         tract.
U486
2007

                        35010000546695
$139.00
```

| | DATE | | |
|---|---|---|---|
| | | | |
| | | | |
| | | | |
| | | | |
| | | | |
| | | | |
| | | | |
| | | | |
| | | | |
| | | | |
| | | | |
| | | | |
| | | | |

**BAKER & TAYLOR**